SMALLPOX AND THE
LITERARY IMAGINATION
1660–1820

Smallpox was a much feared disease until modern times, responsible for many deaths worldwide and reaching epidemic proportions amongst the British population in the seventeenth and eighteenth centuries. This is the first substantial critical study of the literary representation of the disease and its victims between the Restoration and the development of inoculation against smallpox around 1800. David Shuttleton draws upon a wide range of canonical texts including works by Dryden, Johnson, Steele, Goldsmith and Lady Mary Wortley Montagu, the latter having experimented with vaccination against smallpox. He reads these texts alongside medical treatises and the rare, but moving writings of smallpox survivors, showing how medical and imaginative writers developed a shared tradition of figurative tropes, myths and metaphors. This fascinating study uncovers the cultural impact of smallpox, and the different ways writers found to come to terms with the terror of disease and death.

DAVID E. SHUTTLETON is Lecturer in English at the University of Wales Aberystwyth.

SMALLPOX AND THE LITERARY IMAGINATION
1660–1820

DAVID E. SHUTTLETON

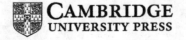

CAMBRIDGE
UNIVERSITY PRESS

University Printing House, Cambridge CB2 8BS, United Kingdom

Cambridge University Press is part of the University of Cambridge.

It furthers the University's mission by disseminating knowledge in the pursuit of
education, learning and research at the highest international levels of excellence.

www.cambridge.org
Information on this title: www.cambridge.org/9780521872096

© David E. Shuttleton 2007

First published 2007
First paperback edition 2012

A catalogue record for this publication is available from the British Library

ISBN 978-0-521-87209-6 Hardback

Contents

Contents

Illustrations

Acknowledgements

The completion of this study was supported by an award from the Arts and Humanities Research Council. My research was also supported by the Senate Fund of the University of Wales Aberystwyth and by a visiting fellowship from the William Andrews Clark Memorial Library, UCLA, and I thank all the institutions concerned. I also thank the library staff of the following institutions for their kind assistance: The British Library, London; the Williams Clark Memorial Library and the UCLA Louise Darling Biomedical Library (Special Collections), Los Angeles; the National Library of Scotland and the Royal College of Physicians Edinburgh, and Edinburgh University Library (Special Collections). Parts of Chapter 1 appeared in a substantially different form as 'Contagion by Conceit: Menstruosity and the Rhetoric of Smallpox into the Age of Inoculation', in Claire L. Carlin, ed. *Imagining Contagion in Early-Modern Europe* (Palgrave Macmillan, 2005), pp. 228–42. I thank the British Academy for their support with illustrations.

Of the many individuals who have kindly lent professional support to my work on smallpox, my particular thanks go to Janet Todd and Karina Williamson; and also to George S. Rousseau, not only for his professional support, but also for his dynamic role in founding and chairing the 'Framing and Imagining Disease Colloquia' in which I was able to develop my ideas when this study was at an early stage. I also extend thanks to all the participants who contributed to the stimulating discussions we had in Leicester, Paris, Oxford and London. My thanks also go to Claire Carlin for inviting me to the valuable colloquium on contagion hosted by the Centre for Religious Studies at the University of Victoria, BC, and to all the participants. Nearer home, I am particularly indebted to Claire Jowitt and Sarah Prescott for kindly reading sections of my manuscript when they had pressing research work of their own: many thanks for your unstinting professional support and friendship. I would also like to thank Bill Zachs for his professional support, for his exceptional generosity in loaning rare books and for a 'literary' friendship which has continued over the years since we were post-graduate students. Many thanks also to Patricia Duncker for her professional support and friendship over all the years we worked together in Wales and since. Thanks also to Andrew Hadfield for his encouragement and for his help with Spenserian allusions. I also thank Linda Bree for having faith in this project, and all the other staff at Cambridge University Press for their highly professional work in seeing this book through the press. I also thank the generous anonymous readers who offered invaluable criticism of the manuscript at various stages in its development (though any errors are, naturally my own). Last, but far from least, I thank my partner Will Datson for his invaluable practical help in running our household/s, with computing, copy-editing and digital imaging, but above all for his love and friendship over the last twenty-five years. If this book is dedicated to anyone, it is to you Will, but the subject is just 'too gruesome . . .'.

Prologue

In 1701, Henry, Second Earl of Clarendon communicated a 'curious' story to the diarist Samuel Pepys. It concerned the events leading up to the sudden death of the Earl's wife Theodosia, Lady Cornbury, back in March 1661. In the middle of that February the Earl of Newborough 'and another Scotch gentleman' had been house-guests:

After dinner, as we were standing and talking together in the room, says my Lord Newborough to the other Scotch gentleman, (who was looking very steadfastly at my wife,) 'What is the matter that thou hast had thine eyes fixed upon my Lady Cornbury ever since she came into the room? Is she not a fine woman? Why doest thou not speak?' – 'She's a handsome Lady indeed,' (said the gentleman,) 'but I see her in blood.' Whereupon my Lord Newborough laughed at him: and all the company going out of the room, we parted: and I believe none of us thought more of the matter; I am sure I did not. My wife was at that time perfectly well in health, and looked as well as ever she did in her life. In the beginning of the next month she fell ill of the smallpox: she was always very apprehensive of that disease, and used to say, if she ever had it she should dye of it. Upon the ninth day after the smallpox appeared, in the morning, she bled at the nose, which quickly stop't; but in the afternoon the blood burst out again with great violence at her nose and mouth, and about eleven of the clock that night she dyed, almost weltering in her blood.[1]

Clarendon's grief had prevented him investigating this 'thing so very extraordinary' and tracing the mysterious 'Scotch gentleman', but his tale of clairvoyance still carries a peculiar resonance, encapsulating some of the horror surrounding a sudden-onset disease which defied all the predictive and curative efforts of known medicine. The anecdote invites us to consider the potentially active powers of the imagination while also drawing together several characteristic elements in traditional understandings of smallpox: the vulnerability of those weakened by fear, the corruption of the blood and an emphasis upon visual horror. Perhaps it even bears traces of a vestigial belief in *fascination*, the malevolent power of a bewitching, contagious gaze working by occult sympathy or, as some Epicurean

commentators had come to describe, by an exchange of minuscule simu-
lacra, 'seeds' or 'exuvias' sloughed off from the surface of objects and
persons and carried through the air.[2] Did the Scotch gentleman merely
predict Lady Cornbury's death, or did the touch of his bloody vision
somehow trigger the eruption of a disease which had long 'infected' Lady
Cornbury's apprehensive imagination?

Reading Clarendon's anecdote in the 1820s, the poet Samuel Taylor
Coleridge made a marginal note suggesting how *he* would have set about
investigating this odd occurrence:

It would have been necessary to cross-examine this Scotch Deuteroptis [i.e. 'second-
seer'], whether he had not seen the duplicate or spectrum of *other* persons in blood.
It might have been the result of an inflammatory condition of his own brains, or a
slight pressure on the region of the optic nerve. I have repeatedly seen the
phantasm of the page I was reading all spotted with blood, or with the letters all
blood.[3]

Lady Cornbury's death and Coleridge's interpretative comments belong
neatly at either end of the historical period covered by my own study of
how smallpox informed the literary imagination; the poet's hermeneutic
gloss usefully exemplifying the process of retrospective re-reading that any
such project inevitably involves. Coleridge approaches Clarendon's story as
a case for forensic examination and retrospective diagnosis. Contrary to
what might be our expectations of a romantic poet, we find him immediately turning to anatomy and the physiology of the nervous system in
support of a purely materialist explanation for this bloody imagining. But
then Coleridge, who was writing a hundred years after the first adoption of
inoculation in England and over twenty years after Edward Jenner's earliest
experiments with vaccination, was a hypochondriac whose own imagination obsessed over disease. The febrile poet took a keen interest in medical
and other natural science.[4]

In seeking to test an historical account of smallpox against more
'advanced' scientific knowledge Coleridge's commentary makes no allow-
ances for a text written when the 'scientific' understanding of the disease
was significantly different. In so doing it resembles the *post-facto* strategy
adopted by many medical historians writing in the nineteenth and early
twentieth centuries. Often retired physicians who delighted in exposing the
now absurd if quaint mistaken beliefs of their ancestors, in these triumphalist narratives the gradual 'conquest' of smallpox stands centre-stage as a
major victory in a progressive process of paradigmatic breakthroughs.[5]
Empiricists may well share Coleridge's desire to reduce Clarendon's

evocative tale down to a matter of faulty organic perception, but what is to be made of the relationship *between* imaginative and scientific responses to disease? Coleridge's marginal note seeks to explain away a mysterious insight into smallpox, but nonetheless the poet's imagination was clearly drawn to the gruesome tale of Lady Cornbury's death. With its theme of tragic foreknowledge – the ancient Gaels' so-called 'second sight' – and its potentially punitive image of a woman almost drowning in her own blood (to welter can mean 'to wallow about in dirt or moral degradation'), Clarendon's account contains all the supernatural, gory elements necessary to inspire just the kind of imaginative, romantic poem for which the young Coleridge had become justly famous. Indeed the elderly poet had good reason to be drawn to a story of smallpox.

In February 1774, as a private volunteer in the 15th Light Dragoons the twenty-one-year-old Coleridge had been ordered to spend two weeks quarantined in Henley Pest House as the lone nurse of a fellow soldier struck down by smallpox. His patient recovered, but the traumatic experience had a lasting impact upon the already distraught writer.[6] But smallpox had not finished with Coleridge. In 1799, while the now married poet was away studying in Germany, his second-born child Berkeley was to die at the age of nine months immediately after contracting smallpox by inoculation, and not before infecting his young mother Sara. It not only left her young face permanently pitted, but as she reported to her husband, her once beautiful hair was left 'utterly spoiled': 'I have had it all cut off close to my head, and I believe I must get some false hair until my own is grown, only I am affriad [sic] you will not like it'. Sara felt obliged to wear a wig – by then unfashionable – for the rest of her life.[7] Coleridge never suffered smallpox himself, but like most people born throughout the era of my study he could not avoid being intimately acquainted with this deadly and disfiguring disease.

Introduction: imagining smallpox

The circumstances surrounding Lady Cornbury's death in 1661 may have been unusual, but it came at a time when smallpox was rapidly emerging as the most dominant pathological killer.[1] In his *History of Epidemics in Britain* (1894), the pioneering late-Victorian medical historian Charles Creighton remarks that 'from the beginning of the Stuart period, smallpox is mentioned in letters, especially from London, in such a way as to give the impression of something which, if not new, was much more formidable than before'.[2] In particular the deaths of Prince Henry and Princess Mary, brother and sister of Charles II, within months of their return from exile in 1660, served to alert the whole nation to the increased danger of what earlier medical texts often describe as a relatively mild disease of childhood. The bills of mortality confirm that by the late seventeenth century smallpox had overtaken the Plague, leprosy and syphilis as the most common cause of premature death throughout Britain and much of Continental Europe. Epidemiologists have since offered various theories for this apparent increase in virulence but all agree that the greater mobility of populations and associated expansion of cities at this time of rapid growth in trade were probably major factors in eroding natural immunity levels and accelerating the spread of this contagious viral infection to epidemic, occasionally pandemic proportions. With the adoption of the middle-eastern folk-practice of variolation (inoculation), first introduced into royal circles by Lady Mary Wortley Montagu in the early 1720s, followed by Edward Jenner's experimental development of effective vaccination using serum derived from cow-pox in the 1790s, smallpox also accrued historical significance as one of the few diseases for which the often theory-bound eighteenth-century medical profession developed effective preventive techniques. With the constant threat of death or disfigurement and the emergence of controversial prophylactic techniques, the long eighteenth century is a crucial era of intensified literary representation.

Writing in the early 1950s the medical historian Genevieve Miller opened her comprehensive account of *The Adoption of Inoculation for*

Smallpox in England and France, by observing that the 'Age of Reason could just as truthfully be labelled the age of Smallpox; the Augustan Age in England may be characterised not solely by its neoclassical literature . . . but in a downright earthy way by its chief disease'.[3] Her period labels are somewhat dated, but note the implied tension between an elevated neo-classical literary aesthetics and the sordid earthiness of smallpox. The suggestion is that in their desire for rational order neoclassical writers turned away from pustules and the loathsome somatic, domestic and communal disorder enacted by smallpox. Part of the aim of my study is to demolish any such false distinction between a purportedly transcendent literary practice and the dirty reality of smallpox. In fact John Dryden's first published poem was an elegy 'Upon the Death of Lord Hastings' con-tributed to the memorial volume *Lachrymae Musarum: The Tears of the Muse: exprest in elegies written by divers persons of nobility and worth, upon the death of the most hopefull, Henry Lord Hastings* (1649), prompted by the death of one of the poet's schoolfellows, who had died of smallpox at the age of nineteen on the eve of the day originally planned for his wedding, in June 1649.[4] Responding to Dryden's comparisons between Hastings's pock-marked corpse and a 'constellation', Samuel Johnson was later to make the glib observation that 'Lord Hastings died of smallpox; and his poet has made of the pustules first rose-buds, and then gems; at last exalts them into stars'.[5] Johnson's strictures (his target was metaphysical intellec-tualism) were to be repeated by later critics who felt obliged to dismiss Dryden's attention to pustules as a uniquely unfortunate, adolescent lapse in literary taste.[6] In the twentieth century Bonamy Dobrée went so far as to suggest that a poem containing some good lines is rendered 'horrific with dire metaphysical conceits on the more loathsome manifestations of the smallpox'.[7] But as Aaron Santesso has recently observed, Dryden was simply addressing a common disease; a 'description of smallpox is exotic enough today for modern critics to seize on it as lurid and sensationalistic, but at the time of the elegy's composition, smallpox was very common, even an everyday sight'.[8] Indeed Dryden and the other contributors to *Lachrymae Musarum*, were working with established tropes, traceable back at least as far as the loyalist poems generated by the recovery of Charles I from the smallpox in 1633 (in a typical example, Jeremy Terrent invites his reader to consider the royal pustules as not the 'Eruption of ill Humours' but 'small Starres to shew him Heavenly').[9]

As Dryden's elegy illustrates, disgust for the pathogenic was allied to fascination. What Barbara Maria Stafford describes as a neo-classical 'aesthetic of immaculateness', epitomised by white skin and smooth marble, was rooted in what Steven Connor summarises as 'a panicky and unstable response to the nauseating phantasmagoria of rotting, eruptive and squamous skins that constituted the actual bodyscape in the eighteenth century'.[10] Smallpox may have evaded understanding and defied control but many writers felt impelled to confront this 'loathsome', high-visibility disease and in so doing gave it a face, a motivational personality, a history and, if not always a politics, then certainly a morality.[11] Moreover, as I detail in my opening chapter, while smallpox haunted the social imaginary like an ever-present spectre, the purported power of the imagination, particularly the fear-struck female imagination, traditionally played a crucial role in professional and popular understandings of the pathogenic origins and contagious action of the disease.

Smallpox and the Literary Imagination is predicated on a claim that existing accounts of smallpox by traditional historians and literary critics alike are impoverished in so far as they have both tended to down-play the role of the literary imagination in the cultural framing of the disease.[12] As already noted, the former have presented a progressive narrative marked by breakthroughs in models of pathology and prophylactic technologies. In such accounts, where historical medical texts are simply tested for accuracy in the light of current knowledge, the use of figurative language is passed-over while more obviously imaginative sources such as poems are only included to provide illustrative 'background colour'. Neither Miller in her still standard history of inoculation, nor Donald R. Hopkins in *The Greatest Killer; Smallpox in History* (2002) – his recently reprinted global history of the disease – wholly ignore such literary material, but they disregard the definitional and potentially therapeutic function of such imaginative con-structs. And while smallpox has not been wholly ignored by recent literary scholars working in a post-structuralist theoretical climate concerned with semiotic analysis, intertextuality, and the emergence of inter- or cross-disciplinary studies, such attention has been somewhat piece-meal.[13]

My study is organised under four thematic headings – disease, death, disfigurement and prevention – but this does not represent a radical rejection of diachronic historicity. While I do not always pursue a strictly chronological narrative, attention has been paid to questions of development in the sequential ordering of the discussion (under 'Death' for example, a chapter devoted to seventeenth-century elegiac poetry is followed by one tracing mortuary representation in the era of the novel). Under 'Disease', an opening chapter considering the role of the imagination in contemporary understandings of the pathology of smallpox concentrates on medical mod-els and case-histories. This is complemented in Chapter 2 by attention to how the disease is represented in the testamentary writings of those who survived smallpox for, despite a relatively recent turn towards illness as narrative and the perspective of patients in our understanding of disease, barely any attention has been paid to the voices of these victims.[14] Under 'Death', Chapters 3 and 4 expand upon the one substantial study of the poetics of smallpox, forming the final chapter in Raymond Anselment's *The Realms of Apollo: Literature and Healing in Seventeenth-Century England* (1995), which was confined almost exclusively to seventeenth-century elegies.[15] In Chapter 4 I trace this mortuary tradition into the age of sensibility. Under 'Disfigurement', Chapter 5 examines the cultural emphasis upon women as the victims of disfigurement, a recent concern of some feminist literary historians engaged with reassessing the literary career of the period's most famous smallpox survivor, Lady Mary Wortley Montagu. Isobel Grundy and Jill Campbell in particular have provided revisionist readings of the relationship between Montagu's transgressive roles as aristocratic woman writer and medical innovator.[16] More generally Campbell and also Felicity Nussbaum have analysed the pervasive figure of the 'scarred woman' in the context of contemporary attitudes towards gender, ageing and embodiment.[17] These studies have tended to overlook the contribution to this cultural formation of contemporary medical models (as discussed in my opening chapter), in which smallpox was over-determined in relation to femininity as a monstrous 'breeding'. My own account of these punitive and consolatory representations of smallpox as 'Beauty's Enemy' is complemented, in Chapter 6, by a comparative analysis of the contrasting figure of the 'scarred man'. Under 'Prevention', the final two chapters address literary responses to inoculation and vaccination: in an important essay Tim Fulford and Debbie Lee have discussed Jenner's propagandist use of pastoral poetry in promoting vaccination, but little consideration has been given to the earlier poetic, novelistic and dramatic efforts to promote inoculation or address the ethical dilemmas it posed.[18] My aim throughout has been to recover the many neglected literary responses to smallpox – in medical treatises, moral essays, poems, novels, plays and, not least, in the neglected auto-pathographical writings of actual survivors – but it will be useful to preface any further discussion of my critical approach to this rewarding material with a very brief account of the extra-textual behaviour of the *Variola* virus.

By 1977, the year of the last recorded case of naturally acquired smallpox, the World Health Organisation recognised ten strains of the virus *Variola Major*.[19] Suffice to note here that the two dominant types identifiable in historical accounts seem to have been the severe strain once known as 'malignant' or 'confluent' (or sometimes 'black') smallpox (Type 2), with a mortality rate of about 75 per cent and the 'distinct', or semi-confluent smallpox (Type 3), with a 25 per cent mortality rate.[20] Although not the most contagious of diseases, smallpox could spread rapidly through households and entire communities, disrupting family and wider social stability. Writing in 1804 the poet Robert Bloomfield, regretfully recalling his own father's hurried, night-time burial, talked of a disease whose 'horrid nature could inspire a dread / That cuts the bonds of custom like a thread'.[21]

Quarantine measures were enacted on the basis of the reasonable belief that pestilential particles could be carried from the sickness chamber on clothes, bedding and other soft textured objects. Though smallpox could be spread through the handling of infected clothes, the primary source of infection was in fact from particles of moisture in a sufferer's breath and from the corpses of victims, but aerial infection could occur over distances of hundreds of yards. The virus usually entered the body through the nose and mouth (rarely through cuts in the skin surface). For a non-immune person, there was an incubation period of usually twelve to fourteen days, in which time the victim was a non-infectious, so-called passive carrier. Thereafter they became highly infectious, remaining so until the removal of all scabs or, in the event of death, until decomposition.

Smallpox displayed a very distinctive symptom pattern, well-recognised by early-modern physicians as a characteristic fever, the first sign being a high temperature accompanied by head and back aches, followed by general debility and sometimes vomiting. After a few days victims developed the characteristic rash, starting with the face, arms and upper torso, but often spreading over the whole body. This erupted into fluid filled pustules that suppurated, giving off an offensive odour, polluting clothing and bedding. If pustules formed on the lips or mouth they could render eating and even drinking very difficult or, in severe cases, impossible.

Smallpox was commonly castigated for being 'doubly cruel' because it did not simply herald likely death, but disfigured its victims. Severe cases were sometimes rendered unrecognisable even by close relations. In an elegy of 1661 to Henry, Duke of Gloucester, the royal physician Martin Lluelyn, who had attended the prince on his deathbed, remarks how 'Most fevers Limbecks though with these they burn, / They leave the featur'd carcasse to the Urne, / But thine was borne of that offensive race, / Arm'd to destroy, she first strove to deface'.[22] Lluelyn's verses conveniently provide a

succinct description of the range of painful symptoms besetting victims at
the height of the illness:

> The sharp disquiets of an aching brain,
> A heart in sunder torne, yet whole to pain.
> Eyes darting forth dimme fires, instead of sight;
> At once made see, and injur'd by the Light;
> Faint pulse; and tongue to thirsty cinders dry'd:
> When the reliefe of thirst must be deny'd.
> The Bowels parcht, limbs in tormenting throwes
> To coole their heat, while heat from cooling growes.
> Slumbers which wandering phansies keep awake,
> And sense not lead by objects, but mistake . . .[23]

As indicated here victims were often blinded by swellings and ulceration
and frequently became delirious. The severity of symptoms and survival
rates depended upon the type of smallpox contracted, but also to some
extent on an individual's age and state of health at the time of exposure.[24]
Death could come rapidly as a result of general toxaemia and it could be
traumatic with haemorrhage to the lungs or stomach, as was evidently the
case with the fearful Lady Clarendon. Even mild cases could easily succumb to secondary bacteriological infections.

Smallpox did leave many survivors disfigured by characteristic 'pitted'
scars, but it often led to other complications. The poet Thomas Blacklock,
discussed in Chapter 6, was one of a significant minority of survivors left
blind either as a result of corneal scarring after ulceration, or more drasti-
cally after having the eyes destroyed by gangrene. Opportunistic secondary
infections could lead to other types of permanent disablement. For example, when Benjamin Hoadly – subsequently Bishop of Winchester and the
leading churchman of his generation – contracted smallpox as a student
'the intervention of an unskilled surgeon, left him crippled'; obliged to
kneel on a stool to preach, he always used crutches at home and sticks in
public.[25] Complications could be very protracted. Josiah Wedgwood, who
survived contracting smallpox in the Burslam epidemic of 1742 when he
was eleven years old, was left with a badly scarred face, but more seriously,
with a secondary infection in his right knee which left him with a painful,
immobilising abscess eventually requiring him to have his leg amputated in
1768 when he was 37.[26] The poet and essayist Jane Bowdler was an invalid
for life after surviving smallpox in 1759 when she was sixteen.[27] Clinical
evidence gathered in the early twentieth century that smallpox left some
male survivors impotent is supported by the fact that the poet Blacklock is
just one of several male victims to be discussed who had childless marriages.

There are moments throughout the literature of smallpox when writers suggest that this particularly offensive, insulting disease outruns the worst fears of the imagination. Discussing Lady Mary Wortley Montagu as smallpox's most famous survivor, art historian Marcia Pointon remarks on how the 'horror of this illness and its symptoms are hard now to imagine'.[28] Even for those for whom the gruesome symptoms were an everyday reality, smallpox seemed to confound the powers of description. In 1799, when trying to convey the emotional drain of witnessing baby Berkeley's tormented, pox-ridden condition – and no doubt feeling inhibited by her husband's obvious literary proficiency – Sara Coleridge wrote in desperation that what 'I felt is impossible to write', yet the letters in which she struggles to record this traumatising experience are one of the most moving records we have of the domestic impact of the disease. 'He was blind', she writes, 'his nose was clogged that he could not suck and his dear gums and tongue were covered and he was so hoarse that he could not cry; but he made *a horrid noise in his throat* which when I dozed for a minute I always heard in my dreams'.[29] Sara's struggle towards adequate representation did not simply leave us with silence.

Examining the many elegies in which such feelings of literary inadequacy are most commonly expressed, Anselment concludes that as a subject smallpox presented poets with a distinct set of problems in which 'the figurative and the literal are indeed ambivalently bound together'; desperate to salvage something of the body's lost integrity and beauty 'the noisomeness of smallpox must be confronted and cannot be forgotten, yet it also has to be denied or transformed'. Less convincingly, in seeking to distinguish the cultural iconography of smallpox from that of leprosy, bubonic plague and syphilis, Anselment also claims that the former was peculiarly resistant to metaphoric appropriation. He suggests that although a diverse range of poets emphasised its peculiar cruelty, fierceness, foulness, and 'envious' nature, unlike the plague, they do not present smallpox as 'divine punishment for some unspecified sin or national transgression'; '[t]heirs is not the metaphoric meaning Susan Sontag finds in dreaded disease; they did not fashion figurative embodiments of evil in which the ills of society are "projected onto a disease" and "the disease (so enriched with meaning) is projected onto the world"'.[30] The grotesque, repulsive face of smallpox undoubtedly posed an aesthetic challenge. It may not have accrued *the same* meanings as the other eruptive diseases but, as will emerge below, writers did adapt established formulas and as a 'foul pox', 'cruel plague' or 'leprous Fury' smallpox was often freighted with moral and sometimes overtly political meanings. Even Anselment's larger claim is somewhat undermined by some of his own examples, especially in the many elegies prompted by the royal deaths in 1660 which readily interpret such increased virulence as providential punishment for collective sin. This specific matter is addressed in Chapter 3 below, but here I want to stay focused on the suggestion that smallpox comes near to fulfilling Sontag's implicit desire for a disease that resists metaphoric appropriation.

In an influential statement at the opening of *Illness as Metaphor* Sontag declares that in undertaking her project of cultural critique she seeks to demythologise and thereby liberate illness – specifically tuberculosis and cancer – from the dark-night of metaphor: 'My point is that illness is not metaphor, and that the most truthful way of regarding illness – and the healthiest way of being ill – is one most purified of, most resistant to, metaphoric thinking'.[31] Writing on sickness narratives, Howard Brody is one of several commentators who have since questioned the value of Sontag's project: 'When Sontag generalizes from destructive uses of metaphor to all attribution of meaning to illness, however, she overreaches her argument' for at 'one point she states "Nothing is more punitive than to give disease a meaning – that meaning being invariably a moralistic one"'.[32] For Brody, the act of imposing a meaning on disease is not something we can choose to do or not to do; we should 'not dismiss the importance of metaphor as a way that real people grapple with the experience of sickness' not least because 'it is precisely by giving meaning to illness that one succeeds in alleviating suffering'.[33] Out of a similar concern with the therapeutic role of illness narratives, Anne Hunsaker Hawkins even suggests that Sontag's 'observations that "the healthiest way of being ill" is the one that "is most purified of, most resistant to, metaphoric thinking" seems itself a coping device – moreover, a coping device based on the questionable assumption that language and perception can be devoid of metaphor'. What Sontag failed to acknowledge, Hawkins insists, 'is that myths about illness may be enabling as well as disabling'.[34]

These objections are also partly those of Roy Porter and G. S. Rousseau at the close of *Gout, the Patrician Malady* (1998) where, in defending their own richly textual approach concerned with figuration and narration in medical writings, literary texts, journals, diaries, verbal testimonies and pictorial evidence, they note how this goes against the philosophical position of Sontag who 'argued, passionately and compassionately, for the desirability of demystifying disease: disease should be a scientific category not a cultural and moral sign or stigma'. However sincere in its aim, they are compelled to conclude that 'the witness of history weighs heavily *against* this position' because '[p]eople and cultures have always given meaning to disease'.[35] Addressing the other side of the same equation Sander L. Gilman makes the important observation that the 'infected individual is never value-neutral, that is, solely a person exhibiting specific pathological signs or symptoms'; like 'any complex text, the signs of illness are read within the conventions of an interpretative community that comprehends them in the light of earlier, powerful readings of what are understood to be similar or parallel texts'.[36] The origin of the label 'smallpox' offers a perfect illustration of how this process might work reciprocally: the term was first adopted in the early sixteenth century as a way of distinguishing the 'lesser' or 'small' pox from the 'Great Pox', the newly emergent syphilis which in its first stage produces similar pocky lesions.[37] But this superficial similarity of cutaneous symptoms meant that smallpox never wholly cast off a taint of association with venereal disease.

Early modern scholars debated the origins of smallpox, but many would have agreed with the leading early-Georgian physician Richard Mead when he declared it 'a modern disease' which must have been unknown to the ancients because making such 'dreadful havoc among mankind' they 'would have minutely described it, had they been acquainted with it'.[38] There was general consensus that it had been carried into Europe in the eleventh century from its assumed origins in the over-heated climate of Northern Africa by Islamic invaders or – in what amounted to the same racial slur – by returning crusaders.[39] Thus, in 1748 when William Wagstaffe turned Mead's scholarly account of history of smallpox into facetious doggerel verse he reflected upon the irony that 'The European Acquisitions, / In these religious Expeditions, / Being only to bear back these Boils; / Trophies accurst! Infernal Spoils'. Taking up hints in Mead, Wagstaffe equates the importation of smallpox with that of syphilis as the filthy products of oriental luxury.[40] To reinforce this xenophobic message Wagstaffe alludes to one Reiske who claimed to have found a 'vellum' in the medical library at Leiden proving that 'ARABIA's pois'nous Earth / Gave to this Pox its motley Birth. / The Year, the Sun's refulgent Ray / Saw MAHOMET shoot into the Day'.[41] Such blatant associations between smallpox and a demonised Eastern 'other' exploited the fact that the first writer to offer a coherent account of the disease was the tenth century Arabian physician Rhazes (Abū Bakr Muhammad ibn Zakariya al Rāzi).[42] In retrospect, the persistent notion that smallpox was a filthy foreign import takes on tragic irony in the light of the disastrous impact of the disease when it was introduced by European colonial adventurers, accidentally or otherwise, into non-immune indigenous populations, particularly in the Americas.[43]

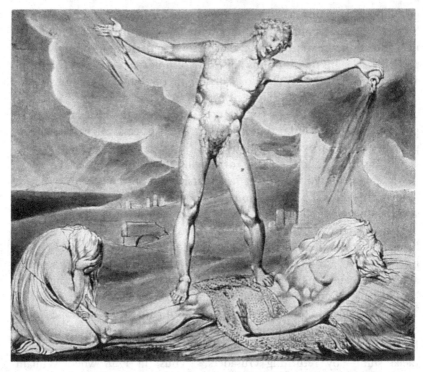

1. William Blake, 'Satan smiting Job with Boils', from *The Book of Job* (1825). Poets and theological writers often identified Job's 'boils' with the symptoms of smallpox.

Smallpox is never named in the Bible, but righteous Christians, equating it with leprosy and the other highly visible, eruptive diseases which are, read it as further evidence of the corrupt legacy of original sin.[44] In his notorious *Sermon against the dangerous and sinful practice of inoculation*, delivered in London in 1722, the high-church preacher Edmund Massey famously identified smallpox with the plague of 'boils' inflicted by Satan upon Job.[45] (Illustration 1) Despite ridicule from physicians and other churchmen, Massey's neat argument that the devil was the first inoculator and therefore the procedure is a blasphemous affront to divine authority could not be ignored. Massey's exegesis later finds support from the theologian Patrick Delany, a Dublin associate of Swift. Delany not only offers a detailed exposition of how Job's distemper must have been smallpox but by drawing upon descriptive passages in the Psalms he also identifies King David's sickness 'which he considered the chastisement of God, upon him for his sins' to have also been smallpox: 'for there is no other distemper, in which all these characters, universal soreness and unsoundness of flesh, corruption, stench, temporary blindness ... and loss of beauty, are at once united'.[46] Delany was particularly struck by the aptness of the verse 'When thou with rebukes dost correct man for iniquity, thou makest his beauty to consume away, like a moth, fretting a garment' (Psalm XXXIX, xi).[47] Contemporary allusions to smallpox as a 'plague' or 'Leprous Fury' were sometimes tied to Job's testing distemper or alternatively to the healing of Lazarus; an elegy of 1709 typically refers to the smallpox victim as 'A *Lazar* scarce to his dear Kindred known'.[48] But far more frequently, as I shall be addressing at length, as a disease which posed such a threat to beauty, small-pox was largely cast as the legacy of female transgression. When Dryden asks 'Was there no milder way but the small-pox, / The very filthiness of Pandora's box?' a mythic association between wayward femininity and disease is ren-dered all the more glaring through the use of sexual innuendo ('box' was a seventeenth-century slang term for the female genitals).[49]

As the influential work of the structural anthropologist Mary Douglas has shown, punitive interpretations of disease and associated taboos con-cerning the sources of contamination, stem from a desire to impose a sense of order on the irrational.[50] Drawing on Freud, Gilman presents a subtle argument for seeing all imaginative representations of disease as attempts at imposing a reality principle, often achieved through such stigmatising acts of distancing projection on to the diseased 'other':

The fixed structures of art provide us with a sort of carnival during which we fantasize about our potential loss of control, perhaps even revel in the fear that it generates within us, but we always believe that this fear exists separate from us. This sense of the carnivalesque provides us with exactly the missing fixity for our understanding of the world which the reality of disease denies. For illness is a real loss of control that results in our becoming the Other whom we have feared, whom we have projected onto the world. These images of disease, whether in art or in literature, are not in flux, even though they represent collapse. They are solid, fixed, images, that remain constantly between the world of art representing disorder, disease, and madness and the source of our anxiety about self-control.[51]

After Foucault it has become a commonplace of cultural and literary studies to address disease as a discursive construct.[52] Compared however with such pathological labels as, for example, nineteenth-century 'hysteria' or 'homosexuality', the evident materiality of smallpox and its obvious corporeal impact might seem to throw the mud of a deeply mistrusted biologism in the face of a post-structuralism which insists on the primacy of language. But as Gilman observes in a related context, it 'is not that syphilis is as phantasmagoric as masturbatory insanity, but that the social reality of each [i.e. the "real" disease and the "imagined" one] is constructed on the basis of specific ideological needs and structured along the categories of representation accepted within that ideology'.[53] To analyse the semiotics of disease does not automatically require a collapse into post-modern solipsism: smallpox was not *just* a textual construct, and to imply so would clearly be an insult to those many generations who suffered the pain of illness and grief.[54] To make a claim for the importance of the literary imagination in framing smallpox is not to imply that the disease was merely *imagined*, but does invite acts of recovery and analysis which hopefully serve to expose the historically contingent epistemic frames – be they scientific, religious, philosophical, legal, psychological, poetic or pictorial – within which the disease was encountered, interpreted and ultimately contained.[55] While recognising that in the post-Foucaldian world of literary analysis 'there are (virtually) no limits to the ways in which disease can take on the attributes of discourse', Porter and Rousseau suggest that this is 'not necessarily a bad thing, provided that the power over the semiotics of sickness lies in the hands of sufferers and users empowered to deploy illness language in ways which are not necessarily more stigmatizing than any alternative terms of description and evalua-tion'.[56] This is perhaps no less Utopian than Sontag's desire to rid illness of metaphor, but it would seem to be a more realistic aim and one I fully endorse. Above all my own project aims at comprehending the semiotics of smallpox through the recovery of a broad range of literary texts which I seek to read in their social and historical contexts.

Scientific and mythopoetic discourse may now seem to be wholly at odds in our present age of advanced biochemical technologies and 'two cultures' when medical professionals often speak about illness and disease in a very different language to that commonly used by their patients. But the classically educated writers of the long eighteenth century inherited an ancient sense of the intimate link between poetics and therapeutics; an alliance symbolised by the mythical figure of Apollo, god of poetry and medicine.[57] Reflecting on this historic marriage of 'medicine and the muses', G. S. Rousseau has observed how the rhetoric of seventeenth and eighteenth-century physicians and poets – many, like Lluelyn, were both – was not so much a matter of distinct categories of knowledge, more a continuum of explanation in which writing itself and other forms of representation may well have served a therapeutic role.[58]

We encounter this Apollonian tradition coming under pressure in the verses 'To Richard Champneys of Orchardly, Esq; when in Danger of the Small-Pox, which raged in the Neighbourhood', by the Somerset physician

Samuel Bowden (c.1732–1761), which are offered as a substitute for the doctor's personal attendance. Bowden adapts the complimentary country-house poem to apologise for having his social round restricted by a local epidemic. Cruel smallpox does not simply threaten death, but 'makes the Living, Strangers like the Dead' for 'While Blasts contagious taint the ambient Air, / And o'er each Mind diffuse a gloomy Care', the bonds of friendship and patronage are thwarted. His reflection that 'Perpetual Absence is a Sort of Death' prompts him to examine his faith in the ability of poetry to transcend the pestilential corruption of disease:

> But tho' condemn'd an Exile from your Seat,
> Permit the Muse to visit the Retreat,
> Where once she lov'd in echoing Walks to play . . .
> She no Infection in her Presence brings,
> No dire Effluvia lurk beneath her Wings;
> Or should you fear some Venom lies unseen,
> She'll round the Air perform a Quarantine,
> Above the cloudy Regions tow'ring rise,
> In purer Climes, and unpolluted Skies . . .[59]

When 'we're Neighbours to the Dead', poetry takes over where medical knowledge fails.[60] The prophylactic muse, who can transcend the polluted regions of an earth plagued by disease and death, provides an uncontaminated substitute for direct contact, yet when 'all Creation hurries to the Tomb', Bowden finds that the best the muse can offer are nostalgic reflections on former pastoral pleasures. Moreover Bowden's choice of Latin epigram to head this poem implies an apology for cowardice; we sense a physician torn between duty and self-protection, as Bowden aligns himself with the Ovid of the *Pontic Epistles*. In English the relevant lines read: 'Who, of the timid ones, does not avoid contact with the sick man, fearing lest by this he should become infected by the disease of his neighbour? Myself, also, amid the extreme dread and alarm of my friends, and not through dislike, did some of my [former acquaintances] desert'.[61] Complaints that doctors abandoned their charges in times of smallpox epidemic were not uncommon.[62]

Bowden exemplifies how physicians and imaginative writers shared a repertoire of culturally freighted iconographic images of disease; a commonly inherited store of biblical, classical, Spenserian, Miltonic and other figurative tropes. The classical writers provided a number of vivid stock passages describing unspecified pestilential plagues for writers on smallpox to adapt. Three commonly imitated sources were the account of the plague besetting the Greek army at the opening of *The Iliad*, the 'Plague of Athens' as described by Thucydides in his *History of the Peloponnesian War* (2. 47–54), and the later adaptation of this passage by Lucretius in *De rerum natura*.[63] The poet William Thompson, a smallpox survivor discussed in Chapter 2, was one of many writers to draw upon Ovid's *Metamorphoses* when seeking to convey the trauma of finding the body monstrously transformed.[64] Professional medical commentators often employed self-consciously poetic language. When the fever expert Thomas Sydenham, writing on smallpox in the 1670s, famously likened the colour of the skin between the pustules to a damask rose and compared their fluid to a honeycomb he was invoking benign pastoral imagery to sanitise the symptoms and thereby allay fear.[65] Mead, one of the most literal of eighteenth-century medical writers, turns for supportive diagnostic proof to a descriptive passage from a Roman poet. Arguing that the horrid symptoms of 'malignant smallpox' are 'the effects of an acrid poison . . . because the same happens to those, who have been bit by the *haemorrhois*, a Lybian serpent', Mead copies Lucan's vivid description of the effects of such a bite upon the warrior Tullus which, in part, reads

> . . . And as Corycian saffron, when 'tis squeez'd,
> Pours forth its yellow juice through all the holes
> Of the hard pressing boards; so from the pours
> Of all the parts flow'd ruddy venom'd gore.
> For their own humours, were all fill'd with blood.
> Red sweats transpir'd from all the skin inflam'd.
> His body seem'd one universal wound.[66]

Borrowed clinical detail is freighted with mythopoetic meaning as Mead's heroic comparison with the bite of one of the poisonous serpents (which sprung up out of the desert soil of Libya where the Medusa's blood was spilt) serves to reinforce contemporary associations between smallpox, Africa and the feminine to which we shall repeatedly return.

Such consciously poetic usages support Gilman's important insight that 'science often understands and articulates its goals on the basis of literary or aesthetic models, measuring its reality against the form and reality that art provides', but as he warns, we should not assume that the imaginative constructs of art are simply to be measured against a medical model presenting the fixed, objective 'truth' of the disease.[67] Observing how conventional histories often seek to test older disease models against the current state of 'scientific' knowledge, Gilman suggests that such *post facto* approaches 'tend to offer a simplistic parallel between prior and existing models rather than the subtle and complex interplay of models that actually exists'; a complexity 'present in all models of disease, from those of the ancient Greeks to those of contemporary America'.[68] The largely conjectural, sometimes highly imaginative pathological models proposed by early-modern professional commentators were often inconsistent. But in noting that physicians of the post-Restoration era were far from being unanimous over the aetiology of smallpox, it is worth observing that when J. R. Smith appends a summary of the modern 'Classification and Pathogenesis of Smallpox', to his social history of the disease in eighteenth-century Essex, he feels obliged to add the qualification that 'medical opinion, even as late as the 1960s, was by no means unanimous on the subject'.[69] Without the technology to detect the existence of viruses the common observation that you could not suffer smallpox twice and that not everyone in an infected family, village or parish succumbed did not lead to a developed theory of immunity (no-one saw an individual smallpox virus until 1947). Smallpox was widely recognised as some form of particulate infection, borne in bad or putrid air – so-called miasmas, resulting from local climatic conditions or a specific source of pollution – but individual vulnerability to the disease could be attributed to a combination of external and internal factors, including the force of the imagination. As a consequence, my opening chapter explores the importance of these multiple disease models for our retrospective understanding of how smallpox came to inform the literary imagination in the post-Restoration era.

PART I

Disease

CHAPTER I

Contagion by conceit

In Henry Fielding's Lucianic satire *A Journey from this World to the Next* (1743), a voice from beyond the grave provides an ironic glimpse of how fears of smallpox had come to shape the most casual of social encounters in mid-eighteenth century Britain. After 'departing this life, at my lodgings in Cheapside', the deceased narrator recalls being directed by Mercury to join a coach leaving from Warwick Lane for 'the other world'.¹ Settled into his seat, he enters into conversation with a fellow passenger, the spirit of a gentleman who is rejoicing because, as 'one just issued forth out of an Oven', being disembodied he no longer feels any inconvenience from the frosty night air. Asked how he met his end, this second gentleman replies that he was 'murdered', or rather 'lawfully put to death' when 'a Physician set me on fire, by giving me Medicines to throw out my Distemper' with the result that 'I died of a hot Regimen . . . in the Small Pox' (10–11). This statement startles another of the dozing spirits present: 'The Small-Pox! bless me! I hope I am not in Company with that Distemper, which I have all my Life with such Caution avoided, and have happily escaped hitherto!' Amidst loud laughter from the other passengers, this agitated gentleman realises the absurdity of his continued fear of contagion, explaining that he had been dreaming that he was still alive:

'Perhaps Sir, said I, 'you died of that Distemper, which therefore made so strong an Impression on you.' 'No, Sir,' answered he, 'I never had it in my Life; but the continual and dreadful Apprehension it kept me so long under, cannot I see be so immediately eradicated. You know, Sir, I avoided coming to *London* for thirty years together, for fear of the Small-Pox, till the most urgent Business brought me thither about five days ago. I was so dreadfully afraid of this Disease, that I refused the second Night of my Arrival to sup with a Friend, whose wife had recovered of it several Months before, and the same Evening got a Surfeit by eating too many Mussels, which brought me into this good Company. (10–11)

Fielding's crowning joke is made at the expense of the man who allowed himself to worry so much about catching smallpox that he forgot to avoid over-indulging on that notoriously unreliable comestible, seafood.

The question of the extent to which we should allow the fear of smallpox to control our daily lives has suddenly taken on unexpected new relevance with the current threat of bioterrorism. In a period when everyone who survived into adulthood could expect that they would eventually contract smallpox, Fielding could justifiable mock a man who allows his fear of the disease to take control over his entire social movements. We regulate our current fears according to governmental risk assessments which draw upon accumulated scientific data concerning the pathological actions of the virus *Variola Major*, but for Fielding's original readers of the 1740s his satire rested upon a radically different understanding of the cause and contagious nature of smallpox; one in which fear was deemed to play a potentially causative role.

We can usefully approach the theoretical assumptions underpinning these early-modern conceptions of smallpox, by first considering a related, otherwise inexplicable fictional incident in which smallpox also makes a 'strong impression'. Towards the close of the sentimental novel *The Adventures of David Simple* (1753) by Sarah Fielding (Henry's sister), the eponymous hero and his wife Camilla receive a request from Mr Ratcliff, their rich but autocratic and treacherous relation, demanding a visit from their son Peter, to whom he stands god-father.[2] David's difficult decision to refuse this request at the risk of undermining his son's prospects is made easier when 'young Peter fell ill of the Small-pox'. Camilla persuades David to write Ratcliff a 'civil' letter explaining 'that the Boy was at present too ill to take a Journey, and they were apprehensive was breeding the Small-pox' (387). Affronted, Ratcliff replies with a tirade against their ingratitude and deception, to which he adds this postscript:

P.S. ... you have rewarded all my dear wife's good Offices to you, with her Destruction; for, by my being abroad, she unfortunately opened your Letter, and I found her in Fits on my return, with the Fright of seeing the name of the Small-pox in your careless letter: and you know too, she has never had that Distemper. (386)

Despite Ratcliff's 'ill-natured-insinuations' that they are lying about Peter's illness, the narrator tells us that the conscientious Camilla might have reason to be 'concerned' that 'by her Means' such 'fatal Consequences' could have arisen, because 'she had heard so many Stories, well attested, of persons being seized with the Small-pox by the Force of their Imaginations, that she would have had some fears, lest that should have been Mrs *Ratcliff's* case' (386).

Again, as modern readers looking back from a vantage point almost thirty years after a combination of virology, vaccination and isolation measures succeeded in eradicating smallpox from the global population, how are we to make sense of Camilla's concerns over her own culpability in 'Mrs Ratcliffe's Case'? Although her husband's postscript affirms that it was generally known that you can only suffer smallpox once – something modern science largely confirms – Mr Ratcliffe's problem over the infectious communication does not rest in a charge that the letter itself is contagious in the materialist, viral sense we would now understand (indeed he is insisting that David and Camilla are lying about Peter's illness). Rather it is the very word 'smallpox' and its potential effect upon Mrs Ratcliff's mind that threatens to prove fatal. Although we might readily identify with the apprehensions earlier generations felt at the mere mention of such a virulent, disfiguring and destructive disease, at the same time, like Coleridge, we are inclined to feel smug in our superior scientific understanding: *we* know that it would take more than simply fear to cause an infection by the *Variola* virus.[3] But would the original readers of Fielding's novel, itself published thirty years after the first adoption of inoculation for smallpox in England, have considered Camilla's understanding of smallpox contagion acting through fear a reasonable concern in the light of contemporary disease concepts? Was it to be taken as a sign of an ignorant adherence to an already outmoded superstition? The ensuing discussion of how such claims for the 'Force of their Imaginations' accorded with contemporary medical theory will provide the basis for addressing a wider question, underpinning the whole of my study, of how established beliefs about the origins and action of smallpox informed the imaginations of those writers who sought to represent the disease and its morbid and disfiguring effects. In particular, I draw attention to how professional medical explanations for 'contagion by conceit' were shaped by traditional, punitive cultural prejudices concerning female pollution which, as pursued in later chapters, continually underpins many imaginative representations of smallpox.

THEORIES OF CONTAGION

The belief that smallpox could be prompted by fear needs to be considered in the broad context of what Genevieve Miller, in her still standard study of *The Adoption of Inoculation for Smallpox* (1957), once called 'the confused and conflicting theories of the cause and mechanisms of smallpox which prevailed when inoculation was begun in Western Europe and the British colonies in America'.[4] Miller talks of 'the lack of orthodoxy in medical theory and the confused multiplicity of causes and underlying mechanisms which were assigned to smallpox' at a time when 'a mixture of ancient and modern thought ... resulted in a very intricate complex of ideas that cannot be reduced to a few simple statements' (242). She does however suggest that, post-1720, 'the new experience of inoculation' prompted 'a significant shift in emphasis as the eighteenth century progressed' whereby 'the material origin of the disease shifted from a location inside the body to one without' and 'the increasing conviction that smallpox is a specific disease attributable to a specific material cause' (242). Adopting the terms employed by Charles E. Rosenberg in *Explaining Epidemics* (1992), this implies a move away from a 'configuration' model pre-dating the knowledge of specific infectious agents which attributed an epidemic to 'a unique configuration of circumstances, a disturbance in the "normal" health-maintaining and health-constituting – arrangement of climate, environment, and communal life', towards what Rosenberg terms a 'contamination' model: this latter often 'reduced itself down to person-to-person contagion, of the transmission of some morbid material from one individual to another'.[5] But even as Rosenberg was describing 'contamination' as 'logically alternative' to 'configuration', he was having to concede that 'historically the two have often been found in relatively peaceful, if not logical co-existence'.[6] More recently Roy Porter, in *The Western Medical Tradition*, observed that 'it has been tempting for historians to split disease theories into two rival camps: "miasmatists" against "contagionists"', but although this 'seems a convenient division because each doctrine had a destiny ahead of it' (with the former eventually fuelling Victorian public health movements and the latter seemingly a forerunner to germ theory), 'such a polarity is anachronistic and simplistic' when 'medical thinking on epidemics was many-faceted and eclectic'.[7] With specific respect to theories of smallpox Miller herself describes a situation of 'co-existence' in which '[v]estiges of the old and elements of the new persisted side by side' (256). This accords with my own reading of pre-modern accounts of smallpox where several explanatory models are often being drawn upon, sometimes even in the one treatise. As we shall see, claims for the causative role of the imagination further confound any neat division between 'configuration' and 'contamination' explanations.

As noted in my introduction, late seventeenth-century scholars were divided over whether the classical authorities ever encountered smallpox but there was a general scholarly consensus that the first writer to offer a fully codified account of the disease was the tenth-century Arabian physician Rhazes (Abū Bakr Muhammad ibn Zakariya al Rāzi). Rhazes treated smallpox, alongside measles, as a relatively mild depuratory fever; a natural form of purgation caused by a 'ferment' of the blood producing corrupt matter analogous to the must of fermenting wine. For later commentators the drastic impact of smallpox upon native populations in the Americas, where it was previously unknown, encouraged a prevalent view that it was a disease of modern luxury; a view which persisted into the Georgian era, despite increasingly blatant evidence that smallpox impacted upon all levels of society. Mead, for example, who commissioned the first English translation of Rhazes, concluded that though 'this be naturally a dreadful disease, yet it is sometimes found to produce very good consequences' for 'in constitutions where the blood is vitiated, either from an original taint, or by the manner of living; and glandular tumours are occasioned by the viscidity of the lymph; the Small-Pox, by purifying the juices, contributes to a better state of health for the future'.[8] Orthodox treatments, based on Rhazes's 'Hot Method', were designed to assist this natural process of purification by inducing perspiration through keeping the patient wrapped in blankets in a closed room and by the use of purges, diuretics and phlebotomies aimed at drawing the disease outwards, down from the eyes and away from the vital organs.[9] As the mortal impact of the disease increased in the 1660s debates over treatment intensified, especially after the prominent English physician Thomas Sydenham, publishing in the 1670s, drew upon corpuscularian theoretical models to argue for an innovatory 'Cold Method' (hence Henry Fielding's ghostly victim's reference to dying at the hands of a physician using the discredited 'Hot' treatment method). But despite changes in medical vocabulary and this long-standing debate over treatment, largely conservative physicians were reluctant to abandon long-held authoritative theories of causation and contagion.

Girolomo Fracastoro of Verona had been the first to describe smallpox and measles as distinct disease entities in his treatise *De Contagione et Contagionis morbis et eorum curatione* (1546), as part of his influential hypothesis that specific diseases could be contracted through exposure to specific ('seeds' or 'semina') either through intimate, one-to-one contact or by breathing in particles ('fomites') lingering in bedding, clothes, or transported goods.[10] Airborne 'seeds' of disease might infect the air of sick-chambers (or linger in sealed crypts), generate local pestilential climates (miasmas and so-called 'constitutions of the air'), or be carried over long distances on the wind. But Fracastoro also acknowledged some validity in an established claim that smallpox originated as a so-called 'innate seed' of corruption implanted in the blood of the foetus during gestation as a result of the blocked menses of the mother. These seeds remain dormant until triggered by external 'contagious' conditions or by a humoral imbalance in the individual resulting from a surfeit or general bad regimen.[11] As the medical historian Vivian Nutton has shown, Fracastoro had himself adopted and adapted the apt concept of 'seeds of disease' from Galen and a number of more ancient sources because it had obvious explanatory force in positing that the object is a living entity, that its origins are very small and that it contains within itself the potentiality for growth. While later theorists often drew analogies with the action of poisons and employed different vocabularies – corpuscularian, animalculist and Newtonian – to explain the precise mechanisms at work, all these underlying resonances continued to pertain each time the seed metaphor was invoked.[12]

Examining case histories from contemporary medical treatises attributing smallpox to fearful imaginings reveals how physicians sought to accommodate the older seed model within more fashionable mechanistic models, while often still hinting at other subtle and possibly immaterial mechanisms for contagion at a distance. In doing so, we should be alert to Nutton's reminder that 'in all this we are dealing with descriptions of the invisible, with hypothetical reconstructions of how things are or act, based only on the observance of "macrophenomena" ' for 'no ancient doctor ever *saw* the seeds, animalcula, or effluvia that were said to cause the disease, or carry it from person to person'. Ancient and early-modern concepts of contagion were 'usually discussed in terms of what could be observed' yet crucially, as Nutton adds, 'the temptation was always there to seek for its invisible causes'. With his notion of seeds Fracastoro in particular had given physicians 'a whole set of fresh and striking metaphors to play with in their discussion of communicable disease'.[13] While such metaphors often made sense in the light of currently observable phenomena, they were metaphors nevertheless, and as such were inevitably informed by a given physician's own culturally biased imagination. Not least this is illustrated in the underlying Levitican concept of menstrual pollution which lay at the heart of many medieval and subsequent seventeenth-century accounts of an underlying, internal cause of smallpox.

The explanations offered by the anonymous author of *A Short Treatise of the Smallpox* (London: 1652), a somewhat typical mid-century text, illustrate how medical writers often drew upon a range of ancient and medieval authorities – in this instance primarily Veletius, Avicenna and

Fracastorius – to provide a variety of causative explanations which effectively covered all practical possibilities. Broken down into four, essentially
Galenic causative categories, all are rooted in constitutional imbalance: the
'primitive cause' is 'by alteration of the aire, in drawing some putrified and
corrupt quality unto it, which doth cause an ebullition of our bloud', while
the 'antecedent' cause is 'repletion of meats, which do easily corrupt in the
stomack, as when we eat milk and fish together at one time' or 'by neglecting
to draw bloud, in such as have become accustomed to doe every year'. The
'conjunct cause' is 'the menstruall bloud, which from the beginning in our
mothers wombs wee received, the which mixing it self with the rest of our
bloud, doth cause an Ebulition of the whole' and the finally 'efficient cause' is;

> ... heat, which by that menstruall matter mixing it self with the rest of our bloud,
> doth cause a continuall vexing and disquieting thereof, whereby an unnatural heat
> is increased in all the body, causing an Ebullition of the bloud by which this filthy
> menstrual matter is separated from our natural bloud, and the nature being
> offended and overwhelmed therewith, dost thrust it to the outward pores of the
> skin as the excrements of bloud, which matter if it be hot and slimie, then it
> produceth the Pox, but if dry and subtil, then the *Measles* or *Males*.[14]

The 'innate seed' theory clearly offered an explanation for why everyone
seemed vulnerable to smallpox and why, if they survived its eruption, it did
not appear in them again, but as the above extract illustrates, this traditional medical model was clearly informed by some deep-seated stigmas
and taboos concerning the fecund female body which found widespread
support in both classical and biblical authority. Envisioning smallpox as
symptomatic of a corrupt maternal inheritance has obvious hermeneutic
ramifications which will be explored later in this study with respect to
poetic and other imaginative accounts of the disease. For the present, in
order to comprehend how this admittedly disputed, but long-standing
prejudice informed related notions of contagion by fearful conceits it will
be useful to examine some contemporary case histories. Intriguing narratives in themselves, these stories of smallpox invite literary as much as
retrospective diagnostic analysis.

THE CASE HISTORIES

Several of the 'Case Histories' appended to Isbrand van Diemerbroeck's
A Particular Treatise of the Smallpox and Measles (1689) concern the force of
the imagination. As professor of physic and anatomy at Utrecht,
Diemerbroeck (1609–1674) taught many visiting British medical students

and the English translation of his useful overview of seventeenth-century opinion on the history, causes and treatment of smallpox was readily available as part of his popular *Anatomy of Human Bodies* (London: 1689; reprinted 1694). Diemerbroeck's 'History VI' tells of 'a certain Apothecary that was a strong man about Thirty Years of Age' who entering 'into a Citizens House, when he found and saw of a suddain his Patient all over covered with the Small Pox upon his face, he trembled a little at the sight of so much deformity and so departed'.[15] 'To drive the Whimsey out of his head' the apothecary starts to 'drink very hard', but 'nevertheless all he could do could not put the Fancy out of his thoughts, which the sight of such an Object had imprinted in his Mind'. Though he 'were otherwise a Man of undaunted Courage' within six days of this sighting 'a fever seized him' and he sank into a delirium 'attended with the red spots that usually fore-run the Small Pox'. This fever lasted a mere twenty-four hours and the patient 'being restor'd to his Health, went abroad again in three weeks' (30). Anticipating the objection that the apothecary 'might not be [already] touched with any Infection, or whether he might not contract the Distemper from some other Cause', Diemerbroeck observes that the man had often;

... visited at other times, several persons that lay Sick of the same distemper, without any prejudice; and therefore the cause seems rather to be that suddain conturbation of his Mind and Sprits, with which he was stricken upon the unexpected Sight of this same Sick Person, and continually ran in his thoughts; from which idea such a disposition arose in his Body which at length produced the Small pox. (30)

Diemerbroeck suggests that the fear actually caused the disease by prompting a disturbance to the balance of body and mind in the apothecary. As a consequence the physician advised against 'timerous' persons going 'near those that are Sick of the pestilence or Small-Pox' when 'the sight of one ill' of the disease 'could move a Man of that courage as this Apothecary was' (30).

In Thomas Fuller's *Exanthematologia, or an Attempt to Give a Rational Account of Eruptive Fevers, especially of the Measles and Smallpox* (1730), we find a related group of cases in which contagion over a distance is attributed to contact with mediating objects bearing fearful associations. A young woman is sent a gold chain 'which another had worn in the Small-Pox, to keep them ... out of their Throat' but it 'chanced to bring Terror, and caused her Fancy to work her up into a kindly Small-Pox'.[16] Fuller makes no suggestion that this talismanic chain carried infected particles, but rather the narrative curiosity is focused upon how an object that had been used to provide protection becomes a trigger. Moreover – in what now reads like a narrative chain of contagious tales – the woman in this last case in turn tells Fuller of like events, including the story of how a gentleman who 'lay sick of the Small-pox' instructed his servant to send a key 'which he had not lately touch'd and lay in a chamber far distant from him to his Mother': she then 'conceited it brought Infection' (189) and soon fell fatally ill with the disease. Again, contrary to any modern assumptions concerning infectious contamination, Fuller clearly emphasises that the mediating object had never been in direct contact with the original victim. It does not even trigger the disease at a distance by mediating between two physical touches but merely by prompting a contaminating 'conceit'. In this respect the case invites comparison with that of the frightening epistle in *David Simple*.

Some similar case histories are more specifically concerned with the triggering effect of shocking sights. Diemerbroeck's 'History V', for example, records the story of how two young sisters 'encounter a young lad . . . newly cured of the Small Pox' who 'was got abroad, and coming along in the street, at least thirty paces distant from them, having his face all spotted with red spots, the remainders of the footsteps of the disease; with which sight they were so scared that they thought themselves infected already' (29). Diemerbroeck 'endeavour'd by many arguments to dispel these idle fears', prescribing a purge and ordering them 'to walk abroad, visit Friends, and by pleasant Discourse and Conversation, and all other ways imaginable to drive those vain conceits out of their Minds'. But 'all that I could do signified nothing, so deeply had this conceit rooted itself in their Imagination' until 'at length, *without occasion of Infection*, they were both seized' (29, my emphasis). Although Diemerbroeck's phrasing here seems to draw a clear distinction between the more usual cases of external 'infection' and a case dependent upon the internal effects of the power of the imagination, yet his appended commentary is somewhat contradictory:

How wonderful the Strength of Imagination is, we have experienced in many Persons, for that by the Motions of the Mind it frequently works Miracles. . . [and] thus in these two Gentlewomen through the continual and constant Cogitation caused by the Preceding Fear, that Idea of the Small Pox, so strongly Imprinted in their Minds, and thence in their Spirits and Humours, begat therein a disposition and Aptitude to receive the Small Pox. (29)

This use of 'receive' is perhaps no more than a matter of confused translation, but it might lead one to assume that Diemerbroeck concludes that mental perturbation had left the sisters vulnerable to contagious infection from outside. The very next case however, in which smallpox is supposedly prompted by a dream, implies a particularly subtle appeal to a 'configuration' explanation resting on purely internal causes.

Diemerbroeck had once visited a 'Noble *German*, who Dreamt that he was drawn against his Will to visit one that was Sick of the Small Pox, and was very much disfigur'd' and being 'unable to drive the dream out of his thoughts', after three weeks the nobleman fell 'into a fever and was pepper'd with the Small Pox' (29). While this case in particular might invite a modern, Freudian or sociological interpretation couched in terms of hysterical or 'emotional contagion', my current concern in unearthing these puzzling histories from the archive is not with pursuing retrospective diagnoses, but rather with comprehending how these early commentators struggled to accommodate such reports within their own largely imaginative models of how the disease might act.[17] To this end, it will be important to distinguish – initially at least – between claims that fear could exacerbate a poor prognosis in an individual case and the larger – and to modern minds more 'unscientific' claim – that smallpox was actually being 'triggered' by the imagination.

TAKING FRIGHT

Fear certainly formed part of the popular understanding of smallpox. It was often put forward as a causative factor, but also thought to have an adverse impact upon an individual prognosis. When Mary Evelyn, for example, died of smallpox in 1685 her distraught father, the diarist John Evelyn, in part blamed his own over-fondness for her failure to keep to the published advice of Dr William Harvey that all young people of nineteen should be phlebotomised because 'she had so great an aversion to breathing a veine . . . we did not insist upon it as we should', but he also identified 'another accident that contributed to the fixing it in this disease':

The apprehension she had of it in particular, & which struck her but two days before she came home, by an imprudent Gentlewomans telling my Lady Faulkland (with whom my daughter went to give a Visite) that she had a servant sick of the small pox above, who died the next day; This my poore Childe acknowledged made an impression on her spirits, it being with all of a mortal & spreading kind at this time about the towne.[18]

The same assumption that fear agitates and weakens the animal spirits informed the report Jonathan Swift sent Esther Johnson ('Stella') in 1711 concerning Lady Betty Germaine's companion, 'Poor Biddy Floyd', a noted beauty to whom Swift had addressed some complimentary verses. Reporting that Biddy has lost her looks to smallpox, Swift adds that Lady Cartaret had explained to him how her cousin had taken ill with smallpox at the house of a mutual friend and since died: 'it was near Lady Betty's and I fancy Biddy took fright'.[19] When the elderly James, Earl Waldegrave contracted smallpox in 1763 he immediately made out his will but, as his anxious friend Horace Walpole reported to a mutual friend, he had also reflected that

... the great difference between having the smallpox young, or more advanced in years, consisted in the fears of the latter, but that as I had so often heard him say, and now saw, that he had none of those fears, the danger of age was considerably lessened. Dr Wilmot says, that if anything saves him, it will be this tranquillity.[20]

This widespread belief that fear could weaken one's ability to fight the disease lay behind the popular practice of removing any mirrors from the vicinity of a smallpox patient to avoid them being traumatised by the shocking sight of their own disfigurement; a cautionary measure endorsed by the many professional medical commentators who shared Wilmot's concern that a good prognosis depended upon the patient remaining calm. Indeed some doctors also felt it necessary to caution their less sensitive colleagues against the risks of frightening patients, and smallpox patients in particular, with pessimistic diagnoses.[21]

Writing on the management of smallpox in 1718, Dr John Woodward thought that the physician's 'Masterpiece, and chief Care is to raise the Fancy, steer and rightly rule the Passions, and continually keep up the Hopes of the Patient'.[22] Claiming that unless one learns this 'great Art' of calming the smallpox patient, 'the best Medicines, directed with the utmost Wisdom, in the Small-Pox ... will prove generally ineffectual', Woodward goes so far as to claim that 'tis certain there are greater Numbers hurryed out of Life by the Disorders brought on by fright, Surprize, Apprehension, the bustle and indiscreet Shew of Concern by Relations, Friends, and those about the patient, than by the Malignity of the Disease'. His brief physiological explanation for this vulnerability is couched in terms of humoral imbalance, while specifically invoking an analogy with the pyrolic spasms of nausea:

The reason of which will be evident to those who are rightly inform'd of the Contrivance of the Body of Man: and know that the Stomach, which is the Fountain of those Principles that supply, form, and raise the Small-Pox, is likewise the Seat of the Passions. Now every unseasonable Rouseing of them must needs disturb the Oeconomy, and regular Egress of those Principles; upon which Oeconomy, and Regulation, the Event of the Disease depends. (69–70)

'The Passions' – a key term in eighteenth-century psychology – formed one of the rather misleadingly termed 'six non-naturals' of the Hippocratic tradition (the others were 'airs', 'diet', 'exercise', 'repletion and evacuation', and 'sleep and wakefulness'). As such the management of the passions were an essential consideration in disease aetiology and preventive 'Regimen'.[23] As Nutton notes, Galen and all the writers in the Hippocratic tradition did not subscribe to the idea of a disease entity in its own right. Rather they took a physiological rather than ontological approach, couched in terms of 'a deviation from the normal within a patient'. As Nutton summaries, although

... these ancient authors accepted and wrote of such discrete disease entities as fever or phthisis, they insisted on always taking into account 'the peculiar nature of each individual'. The nature of disease was to be found in a man's temperament, the structure of his parts, his physiological and psychological dynamism, and could be defined very much in terms of impeded function.[24]

Seeds were not the disease itself, but merely the trigger for a situation leading to humoral disorder and bodily malfunction which, for Galen and his followers, *was* disease. Certain groups, in particular 'hysteric' women, were perceived as being more receptive than others because of their temperamental disposition. In a list of types and conditions rendering individuals vulnerable to infection by measles and smallpox Fuller, for example, includes those who have 'strong Fancies' and who are 'apt to fall into frights and Terrors' and anyone 'when the Spirits are confused, beat down, suppress'd ... by Frights, Terrors, Grief, strong Imaginations etc' (104). Fuller was claiming that 'the Hysteric and Hypochondriac' whose 'Spirits are not able to oppose the assaulting Enemy' are vulnerable to external attack from contagious 'variolous' particles carried in the air; but crucially he also asserts there 'have been very numerous Instances of people that have got the Small Pox (but not the Measles, or any other Sorts that I have heard of) by mere Fancy and Fear' (104–105). Even as smallpox was increasingly being recognised as communicable through infection by air-borne disease-specific particles, the role of the passions remained crucial since temperamental factors could still usefully account for why some individuals were more vulnerable than others.

The notion that smallpox in particular could be prompted by fear or 'conceit' no doubt owed much to the disease's particularly gruesome visual symptoms, but these case histories also betray some vestigial adherence to an earlier, related concept of contagion through *fascinatio* or occult *sympathy* (as informs the anecdote sent to Pepys reproduced in my prologue).[25]

In some early texts concepts of seeds and sympathy were linked. Writing in 1556, for example, Francisco Valles, professor of Anatomy at Alcala, seeking to explain cases of the 'evil-eye' acknowledges the power of the imagination – anyone with a sympathetic toothache is not bewitched but is genuinely suffering – but he prefers a more material explanation which brings together Galen's notion of seeds of disease and Aristotle's discussion of the 'invisible rays' of the Torpedo Fish. One cannot simply be harmed merely by a long, hard stare, Valles insists, such cases of 'sympathy', require a transfer of a substance or poison.[26] It is in the context of such fears of an infectious gaze that we should understand the common practice of encouraging smallpox victims to remain indoors or wear veils or masks in public; this was not simply a matter of personal vanity or mere politeness, but was also informed by the widespread belief that the disease could be triggered by shock or fear at the mere sight of someone affected.[27]

SMALLPOX, 'MENSTRUOSITY' AND THE FEMALE IMAGINATION

It is impossible to establish any reliable statistics, but one certainly comes away from reading early medical texts with the strong impression that the preponderance of smallpox case histories citing fear as a causative factor were specifically concerned with the vulnerability of women, especially pregnant or nursing mothers. A significant range of related literary allusions confirm that a common linkage existed in popular discourse between smallpox contagion and the specifically *female* imagination. For example, when the male narrator in Penelope Aubin's prose-romance *Charlotta Du Pont* (1739), recalls how 'My Wife was now grown great with Child, and had never had the Small-Pox, which she unfortunately caught by going to an Opera, where she saw a person newly recovered, and at her coming home was taken ill, and died of them', no further explanation is thought necessary beyond the fact that she 'saw' a recovering victim.[28] Samuel Richardson adds his usual moralising note when reporting a similar incident in *Sir Charles Grandison* (1753). In what is clearly meant to be read as a case of providential moral retribution Mrs Farnborough, a town mistress, is fatally 'struck with the small-pox, in the height of her gaiety and pleasure . . . [when] she was taken ill at the opera, on seeing a lady of her acquaintance there, whose face bore too strongly the marks of the distemper . . .'.[29] Indeed the vulnerability of a purportedly weak and overly receptive female imagination was somewhat proverbial. In William Wycherley's stage-comedy *The Country Wife* (1674), a play riddled with metaphors of disease, the misogynist fop Sparkish readily quips that 'we men of wit have amongst us a saying that cuckolding, like smallpox, comes with a fear, and you may keep your wife as much as you will out of danger of infection, but if her constitution incline her to't, she'll have it sooner or later, by the world . . .' (IV, iv). To make full sense of these novelistic assumptions and proverbial assertions we must turn back to the writings of contemporary physicians like Fuller who sought to explain the psychosomatic reciprocation at work in such cases.

For Fuller the risk of a perturbation of the passions overwhelming the imagination not only underscored concerns over the effects of fear, but clearly helped to account for some otherwise baffling cases of smallpox acting at a distance. One of 'the most unaccountable' of such cases was that of a young man, 'who being scared with seeing one that lately had it, was taken ill upon the spot . . . and had them come out upon the very next day'. Emphasising that this was not a simple case of invasive particles, Fuller thought this case 'beyond all Rule and Precedent; for there was no Time for Assimilation or Concoction of the matter before Expulsion' (188). Such rapid onset posed a challenge to Fuller's usual humoral understanding of the disease as an eruptive fever with a regular symptom pattern. Although Fuller's account attempts to reconcile old and new ideas by describing the triggering of 'innate seeds' (what he terms 'ovula') by contagious disease-specific particles using the mechanistic vocabulary of corpuscularian ('atomistic') matter theory, he is unsure whether triggering by the imagination amounts to true contagion:

. . . when a Person is taken with a thorough panic and Fright, and thinks of nothing but Infection, that extraordinary Perturbation and Terror may form the Spirits into such Species, and create such an Alteration of the Particles of the Body, as will directly and peculiarly act upon the latent *ovula* as effectively as an actual Contagion might do. (149)

Fuller suggests that the shock of seeing a confluent victim acts as the trigger for the 'ovula' lying dormant in the blood and, as if seeking to cover all possibilities, adds that 'NATURE, in the first compounding and forming of us, hath laid into the Substance and Constitution of each something, equivalent to *Ovula*, of various Kinds, productive of all the Contagions, venemous fevers, we can possibly have as long as we live' and this in turn explains why, when 'all men have in them those specific sorts of Ovula which bring forth Small pox' all are 'liable to them'. (175) Having moulded the inherited 'innate seed' theory to produce his own conjectural explanatory edifice, Fuller then buttresses this with biblical authority:[30]

... every sort of these Ovula can produce only its own proper Foetus, as it is said, 1 Corinth. xv. 38. *To Every Seed its Own Body*; and therefore the Pestilence [i.e. Bubonic Plague] can never breed the Small Pox, nor the Small-Pox the Measles ... any more than a Hen can a Duck, a Wolf a sheep, or a Thistle, Figs; and consequently, one Sort cannot be a preservative against any other. (175)

Fuller's adherence to a model of specific disease entities might invite interpretation as a small step in the direction of modern germ theory, but his typically hybrid explanations owe little to empirical microscopic observation and everything to a rhetorical embroidering of older accounts. Most striking is Fuller's imaginative elaboration upon the sexualised meanings already implicit in terms such as 'breeding', 'seminaria' or 'seeds', as he asserts that the ovula 'always lie quiet and unprolific, till impregnated, and therefore these distempers seldom come without Infection; which is as it where the Male, and the Active Cause' (175). Surely it is here, in this wholly conjectural, blatantly sexualised aetiology that we glimpse the cultural pressures shaping Fuller's otherwise arbitrary adoption of the term 'ovula' over 'seed' (or 'seminaria'): it simply reinforces the passive female origins of the innate seeds while enabling him to equate the external triggers with manly activity. Borrowing Nutton's remarks on the essentially rhetorical value of Fracastoro's contagious 'seeds' hypothesis, like many similarly fanciful explanatory accounts, Fuller's conjecture simply represented 'a philosophical luxury for the intellectual practitioner' but had no therapeutic impact.[31]

And where do the smallpox 'ovula' originate? In providing his answer Fuller simply rehearses the traditional idea of impurities derived from the maternal blood which, he argues, remain dormant in the body like other poisons such as syphilis and rabies. More tellingly, Fuller endorses the underlying religious and moral implications in this concept of 'innate seeds' by paraphrasing an 'excellent passage' from St Severinus (d. 482):[32]

DISEASES (saith he) have, as well as Plants and Animals, their proper seeds in their Way and Manner. God hath (ever since the Fall of Adam) created for the Punishment of man the seeds of evil, as well as of good things. Our Bodies are the soil where they are sown: they grow-up and bring forth certain Distempers, every one according to its several natures; each sort hath its peculiar and like symptoms; every Sort of plant hath its Fibres and Figure. (178)

While Fuller and others sought to marry a modern medical language with the established religious doctrine that disease is a postlapsarian consequence of sin, other physicians were more sceptical. Discussing the causes of smallpox in a treatise of 1696 the physician Gideon Harvey notes how it has been the 'universally received' opinion 'that there is a *labes*, or taint and impurity inherent in the Maternal Blood that gives nutrition ... to the parts of the Foetus ... of which impurity, nature, at some uncertain time after Birth, doth discharge and purify all the parts and juices of the Body, by throwing it out into Measles or Small-Pox'. It has been assumed that 'this original *labes* is synonymous to original Sin' so, as a consequence, all mankind must at some stage in their lives undergo 'that purgatory' of either measles or smallpox (or both) as 'one of the most Ancient Diseases of Lost Paradise'. But, he continues, the idea of smallpox being 'derived from the foulness of the menstruous Blood on the fluid, or solid parts of the Infant, is scarce possible' because some people do not have smallpox until they are very old by which time any active 'tainted ... particles' would have long lost their malignancy.[33]

Other prominent Restoration and early-Georgian physicians either rejected or ignored the maternal seed theory but nevertheless, as Miller observes, 'the notion ... was a very persistent one' (256). Moreover, in seeming to anticipate the putrefaction of the grave, the power of smallpox to leave permanent disfigurement was taken as a lasting emblem of the underlying corruption of a fallen human nature, responsibility for which could be traced back to a transgressive femininity. Throughout the eighteenth century smallpox was often interpreted as a pointed reminder that all disease is the direct consequence of Eve's proud and undisciplined imagination, with scarring serving as a providential cure for female vanity.[34] This pervasive structure of feeling will be discussed at length in Chapter 5, but for the present it is enough to observe that these judgemental literary configurations were supported by equally misogynistic medical theories, themselves reinforced by Classical, Judæo-Christian and Islamic taboos concerning women and blood pollution.[35] While physicians continued the debate over whether smallpox is a maternal inheritance, imaginative writers personified 'Variola' as a monstrous female. This deep-rooted association between smallpox as maternal pollution and monstrosity was in part semantic. This is made overt in *An Elenchus of Opinions Concerning the Cure of the Small Pox* (1661) by the Royal physician Tobias Whitaker. Discussing theories of the neo-natal origins of the 'seeds' of smallpox, Whitaker exploits an established, but false etymological linkage between *menstrua* and *monstrum* to create the telling neologism in the epithet 'Maternal Menstruosity'.[36] This term encapsulates a then commonplace, yet purely figurative association of ideas which, as Elaine Hobby observes, was shortly to be contested by Jane Sharp in *The Midwives Book* (1671).[37] Nevertheless the diagnostic implications of this false derivation lead us straight back to those contemporary smallpox histories invoking fear;

specifically a sub-set of cases presenting smallpox as a type of monstrous birth in which mothers reportedly 'imprint' the disease onto the foetus after being overtaken by fearful imaginings.

Again we have Fuller, this time reporting the case of a gentlewoman who was accidentally brushed by some soil when passing a Sexton digging a grave: upon returning home she was 'most terribly frighten'd, fancying some Corps that had dy'd of the Small-Pox had broke out upon her; upon which she fell in Travail, brought forth a Child full of them; both Mother and Child dy'd. So the Distemper bred upon both from nothing at all but a mistaken Conceit'. (189–90) A similar incident printed in the *Philosophical Transactions* of the Royal Society in 1749, as the 'Case of a Lady, Who Was delivered of a Child, which had the Small Pox appeared in a day or Two after its Birth', describes an incident dating back to 1700 when a pregnant woman reportedly encountered someone full of smallpox across a forty-foot courtyard. This leaves Dr Cromwell Mortimer, the case's author, baffled by 'how the Imagination only, affected by the Disagreableness of the sight, should convey the Infection to this Child in this case … especially as there was no Fright or Surprize'.[38] But Fuller thought as 'strange a Thing as breeding of the Small-Pox by the force of fear and Fancy' was no more to be wondered at than the common knowledge that 'longing-women' can 'by the pure workings of the Imagination, form the Spirits into such Ideas, figures, and Species, as to Imprint marks upon their Foetus in the Womb' (189). As G. S. Rousseau has shown, the ancient idea that the fancies and cravings of so-called 'longing women' might affect the foetus, as discussed at length in Aristotle's *De Generatione et Corruptione* and subsequent medical commentaries, was a commonplace of seventeenth-century texts on midwifery.[39] The particular need to avoid visual shocks during pregnancy was emphasised, for example, in Claude Quillet's Latin poem *Callipaedia* (1655), frequently reprinted throughout the eighteenth century in an English translation sub-headed 'The Art of Getting Pretty Children':[40]

> If then, ye Matrons, who Conceive, design
> A future Offspring, which may grace your Line:
> Let not your Fancy at all Objects fly,
> But keep strict Reins upon your roving Eye.
> Shun every Thing which Shocks your Sense, and View
> Ingenuous Looks alone of shining Hew.[41]

Such concerns were not only endorsed by early physicians concerned with the role of the imagination in causing so-called monstrous births but, as

Rousseau in particular has shown, the question of the precise physiological mechanisms at work in such so-called 'imprinting' continued to be
the subject of medico-philosophical debate until at least the 1760s.[42] The
fear of smallpox as a form of monstrous generation is encapsulated in
the use of the verb 'breeding' with respect to this disease; we have just
witnessed Fuller's professional comments on the 'breeding of the Small-
Pox by fear', a commonplace usage reflected by the novelist Sarah
Fielding when, as quoted at the opening of this, my opening chapter,
she has her characters David and Camilla report on their apprehension
that their son 'was breeding the Small-pox'. The notion of smallpox
stemming from the 'contagious' imagination is perhaps understandable
when the porosity of pustulate flesh pictured forth such a monstrous
collapse of the integrity of the normally sealed boundaries of the body.
Encouraged by existing religious prejudice and related medical precepts,
both scholarly physicians and lay-persons were tempted to blame the
ultimate source of this gross disruption on that most primal challenge to
our sense of unique bodily integrity, the umbilical linkage between the
embryo and its mother.

Traditionalist medical historians largely disregarded the early-modern
claims for contagion by fearful conceits or maternal imprinting discussed
above.[43] Rosenberg is clearly frustrated to find that 'eighteenth-century
physicians did not understand the nature of the "virus" that was passed
from individual to individual during inoculation' when 'it was clear that
the epidemics of this great killer were caused by a specific, reproducible
"matter"' (295, footnote 4). But Miller had already shown that, however
illogical in hindsight, not only did configuration explanations persist into
the age of inoculation, but moreover for many commentators the accumulative empirical evidence that inoculated smallpox left the patient free
of the disease for life merely served to confirm that it grew from an
inherited 'seed' susceptible to an artificially induced purging. Such a view
remains notably implicit in the 'Account of the Rise, Progress, and State
of the Hospital for relieving poor people afflicted with the Small-pox
and for inoculation', as it appeared regularly alongside the London
hospital's anniversary sermons published almost annually from shortly
after its foundation in 1746 until the mid 1770s, where we read how 'the
Benefits of INOCULATION appear every Year ... more certain'
whereby 'the dreadful destructive Distemper is ... rendered mild and
manageable, and becomes rather a Purgation of the Body, from the latent
Seeds of an expected Disease, than creating a Disease itself' and thus
'delivers people from those Apprehensions, with which, till they have had

the SMALL-POX, they are always haunted'.[44] At the very least the internal model accorded well with the commonplace observation that you only had smallpox once and it continued to provided a reasonable explanation for why, when smallpox became epidemic in a particular district, not everyone succumbed. Moreover the older theory also helped to allay religious scruples opposing inoculation, notably those prompted by the much-discussed claim of the Revd. Edmund Massey that Satan was the first inoculator when he inflicted Job with 'sore boils'.[45] If smallpox was merely caused by a seed already present in the body then, it could be argued, inoculation did not amount to the evil introduction of a new disease. Posing no immediate challenge to an innate seed model, inoculation did not necessarily nor immediately undermine a popular belief that smallpox could be either triggered or contracted by 'conceits'.

In Fuller's treatise of 1730 acknowledging the causative power of the imagination, old and new concerns are effectively held in tension: it bears an appendix defending inoculation against Massey's blasphemy charge, yet Fuller's list of the exceptional circumstances in which the operation is inadvisable includes 'such as are extremely fearful, fanciful, Hysteric or Hypochondriac' (414). Subsequently the inherent danger of being fright-ened by the sight of a confluent victim of natural smallpox might even form part of the pro-inoculation argument. As late as 1779, the pseudonymous author of a pamphlet supporting the philanthropic inoculationist John Coakley Lettsom argues for the advantages of inoculation by comparing the progress of the mild form of the disease amongst the inoculated – who may only bear a few pustules – with the victims of the natural, confluent form, whose 'miserable body . . . is covered with indistinguishable mil-lions'. Though it might be argued that the confluent patient is 'confined to his chamber' while the 'inoculated one is abroad in the street, obvious to the approach of every passenger', the latter case is preferable because if the confluent patient dies, his chamber must be thrown open releasing a stream of malignant particles, in their highest state of energy, dispersed at once among the neighbourhood. Moreover, if the confluent patient lives, he must inevitably 'come abroad' at some stage, usually 'much too soon, and object of disgust and terror, deformed by the violence of the distemper, and loaded with contagion'. In contrast the inoculated patient 'is almost perpetually in the air, the action of which will gradually dissipate the effluvia exhaling from his body, and prevent their accumulating in his garments'. Thus the natural, confluent patient 'might communicate the disease by the most instantaneous interview' whereas the inoculated patient 'could communicate it only by an approximation of some considerable duration':

ADMITTING what has often been asserted, that fear, by acting on the nervous system, sometimes produces the smallpox, the natural disease must be infinitely more mischievous than inoculation; the confluent subject walks the streets, as before hinted, imprinted with alarming tokens of his dangerous condition, so visible and peculiar as not to be mistaken; the inoculated subject has at most only a few pustules not to be distinguished from common pimples but by close examination, and often has none.[46]

Here the explanation for the mechanism of contamination by conceit has now accrued a fashionable explanation in terms of nervous sensibility, but in keeping with Rosenberg's 'illogical' juxtaposition, the account as a whole moves comfortably between an explanation resting on external contagion from airborne 'reproducible matter' and one which acknowledges the risk of contagion by fear. Tellingly both are proffered in defence of what the anonymous writer terms the 'modern regimen' of inoculation, thus confirming Rosenberg's own comment on how the equilibrium model of health active in the eighteenth century, in which 'the idea of specific disease entities played a relatively small role', continued to dominate 'even when a disease seemed not only to have a characteristic course but (as in the case of smallpox), a specific causative "virus" '.[47] Indeed by the 1760s entrepreneurial inoculators like Suttons were establishing isolation houses in the countryside where, for those who could afford it, regulated sociability with fellow risk-takers formed an inherent part of a pre-inoculation regimen designed to quell individual fears over the risks of the procedure.[48] In *The Practice of Inoculation Justified* (1767) one advocate reassures us that here 'is no confinement' and all 'is mirth' since 'this fortnight-visit to Mr. Sutton's abounds with real pleasure and satisfaction' as 'the pleasing conversation of the company, added to their various amusements, makes the time glide way imperceptibly'.[49]

Faced with the synchronic co-existence of multiple explanations of smallpox, we might refine Rosenberg's somewhat bifurcated schema by borrowing the model of dominant, residual and emergent 'structures of feeling' proposed by the cultural historian Raymond Williams.[50] Thus the contagion by fear theory survives, as in my last quoted example, as a residual, yet still active structure of feeling articulated alongside what was rapidly becoming the more dominant external contagion model. Rather than push for a coherent and purely 'progressive' narrative of smallpox, we need to extend the methodological framework, to embrace and explore the wide and complex range of meanings generated by the disease during this crucial period. As this discussion has shown, Sarah Fielding's 1753 portrayal of Camilla's concerns that her disturbing letter may have put Mrs Ratcliff's life in jeopardy was entirely in keeping with popular belief as buttressed by traditional linguistic formulas, if not fully coherent medical models; beliefs which continued to find support from some professional commentators into the age of inoculation. In the event Camilla had no need to feel responsible because we are told that 'she knew that Mrs Ratcliff had long ago had that Distemper, and had visible marks of it on her face; though, in order to have an Opportunity of making herself of Consequence by her affected Frights and Fears, she insisted . . . that they were only the Marks of the Chicken-pox' (386). 'Mrs Ratcliff's case', it emerges, is simply a selfish ploy to ensure that her husband does not become attached to his god-son Peter and make him his heir. Fielding exposes Mrs Ratcliffe's fear that she will contract smallpox through the mere words in a letter as socially manipulative affectation, but this satirical depiction relied for its reach upon the novelist's ironic manipulation of what she can assume are her reader's own morally freighted associations between the imagination, femininity and the risk of contagion by conceit. The fictional Mrs Ratcliff had acquisitive motives for pretending that she had never suffered smallpox. In Chapter 2 we turn to the writings of genuine survivors of the disease.

CHAPTER 2

'What odious change . . .?': smallpox autopathography

Few writers tried to imagine the horror of contracting smallpox quite so resonantly as Restoration elegist Henry Bold who castigated a disease which is so loathsome '. . . the Soul would hardly, own / The Body, at the Resurrection!'[1] In Bold's vision of dualism as ultimate self-alienation smallpox renders the bodies of its victims so unrecognisable that, despite the best hopes of Christian eschatology, reparative reintegration might not even be possible. We are left wondering how actual survivors of the disease gave shape and meaning to such a traumatic experience of self-estrangement.

The theories of medical professionals only give us part of the historical picture of how smallpox was comprehended and narrated. The past twenty years have seen a shift of focus in approaches to medical history, away from creating a narrative of progressive 'breakthroughs' associated with an heroic cast of clinicians towards a more inclusive consideration of the embodied experience of the actual sufferers of a given disease. Addressing these other 'stories of sickness', Howard Brody goes so far as to assert that he 'would rather see physicians as part of the general landscape of illness – a foreign species of animal, perhaps, that sick people encounter on their journey – than as the main characters of the narrative'.[2] An exclusively 'top-down' perspective on the making of medical meaning is gradually giving way to one willing to consider the role of what one-time clinician Arthur F. Kleinman influentially termed 'illness narratives' to the extent that the recognition that storytelling plays an essential and therapeutically significant part in shaping medical understanding has begun to shape practical reforms in the actual conduct of the clinical encounter.[3]

For Kleinman such narratives create a 'symbolic bridge that connects body, self and society' in a network which 'interconnects physiological processes, meanings and relationships so that our social world is linked recursively to our inner experience'.[4] In a similar vein Brody observes how stories of sickness enable the individual concerned to label their own experience in relation to those of others (for example, when *bravely* facing

40

up to disease can be construed as a form of religious devotion). In this sense, each sickness narrative 'partakes of both these individual and socio-cultural dimensions'.[5] Writing from their complementary perspective as social and literary historians, Porter and Rousseau open their cultural history of gout by observing that 'literary scholars, biographers, psycho-historians and other humanists have been drawing attention to illness experience and body awareness as facets of identity and the thread of the narration of one's own life'. 'Pathography' they conclude 'may be the key to biography'.[6]

The literary scholar Anne Hunsaker Hawkins usefully defines 'patho-graphy' as 'an autobiographical or biographical narrative about an experience of illness', distinguishing the former as 'autopathography'.[7] While insisting upon the importance of studying such narratives in 'res-toring the patient's voice to the medical enterprise', Hawkins claims that this is overwhelmingly a modern genre emerging in the late nineteenth century; since 'pathography is used to construct a framework of meaning to understand and thereby control a frightening experience' there was less need for it in earlier periods when religion provided that framework 'ready-made' and, moreover, the threat of serious or fatal illness striking at any time was omnipresent.[8] As Hawkins shows, modern pathographies offer cautionary tales of unpredicted physical collapse to a popular readership cushioned into thinking that the orderly world of the healthy is secure and natural, but her historical explanation may prove over-simplified: she herself addresses such precedents as John Donne's *Devotions Upon Emergent Occasions* (1624). Indeed her work on modern pathography grew directly out of a previous study of Calvinist conversion narratives in which she finds earlier 'paradigms of religious sickness' con-gruent with 'the patterns of experiencing illness and recovery today'.[9] Nonetheless she alerts us to the importance of recovering and analysing older examples of pathographical writing for arriving at any adequate historical understanding of the cultural codes shaping the embodied experi-ence of disease.[10]

The early-modern archive provides many accounts of smallpox by professional clinical observers but where are the *autopathographies*? Where are the first-hand accounts of succumbing to the disease which might reveal to us what it felt like to endure the socially isolating ordeal of contracting smallpox and how this self-alienating trauma actually impacted upon the survivor's sense of their own identity? Such neglected accounts are understandably scarce. Fortunately the two most substantial examples presented for discussion below, a labouring-class woman's personal prose narrative and a long, allusive poem by a literary scholar, offer usefully contrasting viewpoints in terms of gender, class and genre.

Frances Flood's disturbing autopathography appeared around 1723–1724 in the form of a short, cheaply produced pamphlet bearing a sensational descriptive title: *The Devonshire Woman: Or, A Wonderful Narrative of FRANCES FLOOD, Shewing how she was taken by the Small-pox in the street of Saltford, near Bath, in the Year 1723; and having no Place of Abode (being a stranger) she got to a Barn in the said Town, where her Legs broke short off in the Small; and was healed without the Help of Physician or Surgeon.* This descriptive title suggests a popular style of 'wondrous tale' aimed at feeding a hunger for news of curious events. Often the spurious fabrications of opportunistic hacks, such ephemeral narratives nevertheless suggest the reception context for the emergent novel.[11] In placing the experience of illness and healing within a divine providential framework, Flood's auto-biographical *Narrative* belongs to the same protestant tradition of spiritual autobiography upon which Defoe was also drawing in such purportedly 'True' first-person narratives as *Robinson Crusoe* (1719) and *Roxana* (1724). Sickness crises leading to a conversion or revival of faith are a common plot element in these early autobiographical fictions which follow the patterns of moral reckoning and spiritual awakening characteristic of puritan testa-mentary writing.[12] Flood's shocking Narrative has particular thematic affinities with Defoe's contemporaneous *Journal of the Plague Year* (1722), narrated by 'H. D.', ostensibly a first-hand witness.

Defoe scholars are still debating whether, as he claimed, he was acting as the editor of a genuine document or if he simply fabricated the *Journal*. In Flood's case the fact that a stone memorial mentioned in her text is still extant confirms her historical existence, but we cannot assume that Flood had ultimate editorial control over her own narrative. It seems more likely that she dictated her story to her charitable benefactor, the clergyman from Keinsham mentioned in the text itself, who probably arranged publi-cation. Certainly the colophon, 'Printed for FRANCES FLOOD, and Sold by No-body but her self' implies that Flood marketed her disturbing illness narrative not only to advertise the providential workings of God, but also to raise funds to subsist. In either case, the literary primitivism of Flood's text usefully lays bare how the attempt to convey the subjective experience of smallpox (or indeed any illness) takes place within pre-established, explanatory cultural paradigms concerning the meaning of disease and physical suffering.

Flood's opening account offers some precise matters of time and location which play an authenticating function with respect to the text's claims to be factual reportage:

I *Frances Flood* was born in *Gitson*, near *Honiton* in *Devonshire*; being on the 22nd of *January*, 1723, being 23 Years of Age, I went from *Philips Norton* to the Town of *Saltford*, where I paid for lodging at an Inn. I arose well in the Morning thinking to go about my Business; but being come out of the Door, I was taken very ill [and] was forced to hold by the Wall as I went along.[3]

Flood was taken ill while travelling outside her native county, but she never specifies the nature of her business, nor does she give many clues as to her social background, making no mention of any husband nor of being reunited with her family back in Devon (the fact that she affords an inn indicates that she was not wholly indigent). Initially her tale concerns the unkindness of strangers after the onset of an illness which suddenly turns her into a stigmatised pariah:

With great Difficulty I got to the Overseer's House, and desir'd him to get me a Lodging but he denied me; whereupon I went up the Street and lay in a Hog-Sty; where many people came to see me. I lay there till Evening in a sad Condition, when the Overseer's Wife of that Place led me to the Overseer's again, but he still denied me Relief; and, not being very sensible, I return'd again to the same Place, but they had been so inhuman as to put some Dung into it, to prevent my lodging there again; but at last I got into another which had no Cover over it as the other had. In the Morning when I awoke, I went into the Street, and with Weakness fell down, so that Streams of Water run over me, till helped by the Clerk of the Parish'd Wife, who led me till I came to the Wall, by which I held, and with great trouble got to the Barn, and Stranger let me in, but the Owner of the Barn, was so barbarous as to unhang the Door the next day; a young Man, out of Compassion hung the Door again; the Owner was so displeased, that he came a second Time, and unhung it. (2–3)

The next day 'the Small-Pox appeared on me, and was noised about' (3). She is again visited by the 'Overseer' who 'put up the Door' and provides her with food and drink she receives no further care for fourteen days.

Such exclusionary practices, prompted by obvious fears of contagion, might be sanctioned by Old Testament laws concerning the ritual removal of 'unclean' lepers from the tribe (notably Leviticus 13: 6). In Flood's case 'the Small-Pox appeared very-kind and favourable' and she hoped to be recovered after two weeks, but then 'I was taken in the Calfs, which turned black and cold, and looked much like Scalds, and broke out'. These signs of gangrene indicate blood-poisoning or a related opportunistic secondary infection. Though she was brought some ointment by the Overseer, she received no help in dressing her own wounds and when she bathed the affected parts 'the Flesh speedily parted from the small of my Legs to the Bones'. Her 'pains increased to a wonderful degree, and my Legs grew worse, and [I] was driven to dismal Extremety [sic], and lay in that Condition three Weeks'. (3–4)

Flood's disturbing tale is far from over. With further exactitude, Flood records how she was visited 'on March 18th at 8 o'clock in the evening' by a woman enquiring of her well-being. Flood was showing her the wounds, but '. . . leaning a little harder than ordinary upon my left Leg, it broke off as though it were a rotten stick. A little below the Calf; the Woman left me and I was surpriz'd, but God enabled me to bind up my Leg again with the same Medicines as before'. (4) That evening a man living nearby brings her some beer before leaving her alone for the night:

I submitted myself to God, and after some time fell asleep, and slept till Morning, and, as soon as 'twas Light, dressed the Wound before any came to me, and the Flesh covered the Bone, but had no Loss of Marrow, and but little of Blood, nor hardly any pain; the Mercies then received at the Hands of God, exceeded all the Punishment was due to me thro' Sin, and his Mercy I never did deserve. I was visited by abundance of People, and amongst them God sent me the minister of *Keinsham*, and Mr. Brown of the same Town came along with him, and they afforded me Comfort; they told me they never saw the like, and it was God's handy Work, and not Man's, so taking leave of me they wished that the God of Heaven might be my Physician, and it gave me both a Merry Heart and cheerful Countenance, and gave me Thanks for what favours I had received from them, and my pains still ceased. (4–5)

A tale of social ostracism turns into one of divine intervention. If the first part of Flood's story does not reflect very favourably upon the people of Saltford, it is noticeable that the narrative voice awkwardly pulls back from any blatant criticism of the parochial authorities in their moral obligations towards the sick or from entering into any larger debate over the appro-priate civic measures to be taken in the containment of a communicable disease. Deliberately deflecting the charge of being an ungrateful, burden-some guest, Flood assures her readers that 'I freely forgive all the parish; and as for the Overseers, they did to the utmost of their Power, when my Flesh was separated; and, whatever I desired of them they sent me, so I desire that all may be blameless of my Misfortunes'(3). The *Narrative* closes with orthodox religious reflections on the place of sickness and physical suffer-ing within a pattern of personal, spiritual redemption.

One suspects that this marked shift of tone from complaint to contrition betrays the point where Flood's, possibly dictated, first-person narration ends and the framing, controlling discourse of her clergyman benefactor takes over. Once identified by the church authorities as the subject of divine assistance, Flood becomes a legitimate public spectacle: 'Abundance came from far and near all the week to see me; but upon Sunday I had scores of people to visit me, and amongst the rest was a Surgeon, who persuaded me to have the bone of my right Leg taken off, to which I gave Consent' (5). Early on the morning of 25 March, just a week after her lower left leg had snapped off, Flood removed her dressings to find that both stumps had stopped bleeding, the flesh had healed over and she was almost free from pain, 'so I had great Reason to praise the Lord for all his Mercies and Favours' (5).

This distressing, if compelling prose-narrative ends on this note of religious acceptance. Appended to it is a short 'Epitaph in Saltford Church-Yard, where the Legs were buried' (6). Epitaphs for severed limbs were not so unusual in a period when church doctrine broadly held that the body would be resurrected whole and uncorrupted on the Day of Judgement.[14] Accidental or surgical amputations posed something of a challenge to theologians concerned with explaining the actual mechanics of post-mortem bodily integrity.[15] Such anxieties inform the message on the stone originally erected over the place where Flood's lower legs were interred; a memorial since removed into the protective porch of St Mary's Church, Saltford:

> Stop reader, and a Wonder see,
> As strange as e-er was known,
> My Feet drop'd off from my Body
> In the Middle of the Bone:
> I had no Surgeon for my Help,
> But God Almighty's Aid,
> In whom I ever will rely,
> And never be afraid.
> Tho' here beneath they lie
> Corruption for to see;
> Yet they shall one Day re-unite
> To all Eternity. (6)

Flood's *Narrative* ends with a prayer based upon some appropriate lines from the Old Testament, prompted when God punishes the errant Ephraim with a 'wound' that King Jereb cannot heal: 'Come and let us return unto the Lord, for he hath torn and will heal us, he hath smitten and will binds us up' (Hosea, 6. 1). As a sinful supplicant Flood asks God to be merciful in bringing about amendment through sickness. The prayer exploits metaphors of healing central to Christian doctrine: 'Apply, Oh lord, the only and

wholesome medicines of thy Son's Passion, death, and resurrection unto my
Soul, against Fear, Faintness, Doubts and Desperation . . . Be merciful unto
me who, as a seeing Member of one Body, adore thy holy Name . . .' (7).
Though smallpox has led to physical dismemberment, Flood's epitaph and
prayer look forward to the restoration of a more expansive wholeness beyond
the grave within the risen 'Body' of Christ as symbolized through the
spiritual communion of the church.

POETIC AUTOPATHOGRAPHY: WILLIAM THOMPSON'S *SICKNESS*

In marked contrast to the humble Frances Flood, William Thompson
(c.1712–c.1766) the author of *Sickness; a Poem in Three Books* (1745), was
educationally equipped to turn his own personal trauma of surviving smallpox into a sophisticated, richly allusive literary composition.[16] (Illustration 2)
An Oxford fellow with a scholarly interest in Renaissance literature,
Thompson employs Miltonic blank verse and Spenserian allegory to present
his sudden fall into the deadly chaos of smallpox as an epic testing of personal
faith. In the present context *Sickness* clearly invites close scrutiny, not least
when we consider how the very act of composition must in itself have played
a therapeutic role in the poet's own recovery. Internal evidence confirms that
Sickness was written during the months of Thompson's immediate recovery,
but what little we know of the poem's precise inception is limited to a few
authorial comments in the original annotations:

A Recovery from the Small-pox the last spring [i.e. 1744], gave occasion to the
following poem. I only at first (in gratitude to the great physician of souls and
bodies) designed to have published the Hymn to the Trinity upon a recovery from
sickness; which concludes the third book. But the subject being very extensive, and
capable of admitting serious reflections on the frail state of humanity; I expatiated
upon it as far as it came within the bounds of my following design.[17]

Versified thanksgiving prayers by smallpox survivors are not uncommon; a
typically ecstatic example appeared in the posthumous works of the popular dissenter poet Elizabeth Rowe and two similar first-person prayers of
'Thanksgiving after Recovery from the Small-Pox' were included amongst
the exemplary 'Hymns for the use of Families' by Charles Wesley, the
Methodist founder.[18] Wesley's supplicatory hymns recall how 'O'er my
weak flesh from foot to head / The loathsome leprosy was spread' and
figure enduring the fire of smallpox – the 'foulest plague our race can feel, /
The deadliest fruit of sin and hell' – as a form of physical purgation and

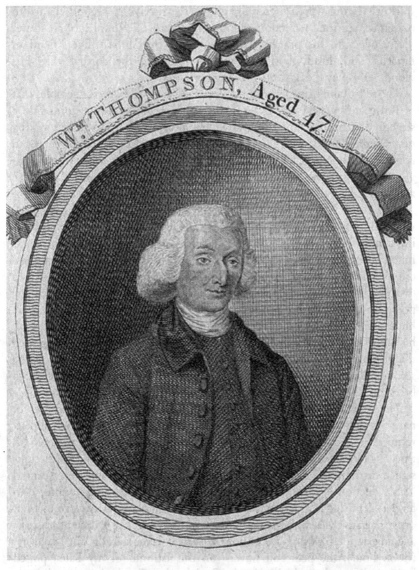

2. Engraved portrait of the poet 'William Thompson aet 47'. A rare example of a contemporary portrait which includes the type of pock-marks characteristically left on the faces of survivors of smallpox.

spiritual testing which mercifully allows the survivor a second chance to undertake spiritual reflection and moral reform. The supplicant attributes his recovery to his prayers being answered by Christ, 'The Friend of Lazarus' and 'kind physician' who, by mixing 'the cordial with His blood, / Display'd His dead-reviving art'[19] (94–5).

The self-dramatising, emotionally charged tone of *Sickness* resembles that of Rowe and Wesley but by expanding this short devotional form into a structurally complex illness narrative Thompson was consciously breaking new poetic ground.[20] In doing so he would have found encouragement to consider sickness a viable theme in the critical success of John Armstrong's *The Art of Preserving Health* (1744), which also employs Miltonic blank verse and appeared in the very year of Thompson's recovery. Edward Young's *The Complaint; or Night Thoughts on Life, Death, and Immortality* (1742–1745), which Thompson commends in *Sickness*, also provided a model for addressing a morbid psychological theme. There were obvious formal problems inherent to this popular, if unwieldy eighteenth-century genre of long descriptive and didactic poetry, but Thompson was particularly self-conscious over tackling such an innovative topic: 'I do not remember to have seen any poem on the same subject to lead me on the way, and therefore it is to be hoped, the good natur'd reader will more readily excuse its blemishes'. With his health permanently undermined, Thompson's protracted tinkering with the original three-part sub-division of *Sickness* to create five books for the second edition of 1757 is indicative of a struggle to find the right structure to bring his disorienting experience under suitable narrative control.[21]

The medical sociologist A. W. Frank identifies three typical types of narrative pattern in the stories of patients who have suffered a chronic illness: restitution, chaos, and quest narratives.[22] *Sickness* has characteristics of all three. Book One announces the poet's theme before recounting the circumstance surrounding the onset of his illness, but it is noticeable that a central 'chaos' section in which he describes the crazed visions he encountered in fever is kept under retrospective control by being placed between a form of quest narrative describing an allegorical journey to 'The Palace of Disease' and an extended, closing 'restitution' narrative. At the start of 'The Recovery' (Book Four), the poet still wavers 'on this Isthmus of my Fate', poised between life and death, but in the final book, 'Thanksgiving', a didactic passage on the therapeutic limitations of ancient philosophy when compared with the superior consolations of Christianity leads directly into a concluding 'Hymn to the Trinity', the devotional germ of the whole piece.

Unlike modern restitution narratives celebrating the 'miraculous' powers of medical science, *Sickness* affirms the healing power of Christ, presenting surviving smallpox as a stern reminder of mortality and a doctrinal lesson in the redemptive purpose of suffering. Recounting his fears that 'the Lustre of the Eyes is fled', Thompson finds retrospective solace in the thought that even if he had been left blind, we are all destined for the darkness of the grave where 'these Tunicles of Flesh' will be destroyed by worms and where 'e'er long, the Filial-light himself shall shine' (247–8). By drawing upon traditional biblical tropes linking light with salvific enlightenment, Thompson exploits the symbolic potential of his own temporary blindness; sickness, the poem implies, can prompt a Pauline conversion.

The resolution of a Manichean struggle, which often features in modern illness narratives, exemplifies what Hawkins terms 'mythic thinking' (in which she includes religious belief) whose narrative function is ultimately 'integrative, connective, and . . . analogical'. Hawkins alerts us to both the therapeutic and 'dynamic' nature of such admittedly 'fictive' myths which 'not only reflect experience, but . . . also determine its actual shape': such 'myths about illness must also be seen as profound truth in that they describe the inner configuration of the ill person's experience'. The trauma of illness results in a counter-impulse towards creation and order; what Robert Jay Lifton, in a celebrated study of the survivors of Hiroshima, terms 'formulation'. In so far as this reparative process involves narrative 'mastery', Hawkins suggests that pathography 'can be seen as re-formulation of the experience of illness, as the artistic product and continuation of the instinctive psychological act of formulation'.[23] She identifies three prevalent narrative archetypes or 'sickness myths': 'battle', 'journey', and 'death and rebirth' (her last two closely correlate with Frank's 'quest' and 'restitution' patterns).[24] All three archetypes have relevance to a closer structural analysis of *Sickness*.

Thompson's personal sense of battling with smallpox is conveyed through numerous heroic allusions to Homeric and Virgilian epic. Equally Hawkins's account of how the 'journey myth uses metaphors of travel and entry into a strange world to address the experience of sickness', is exemplified in Thompson's 'The Palace of Disease' episode, portraying a recursive visit to the netherworld of disease where the poet re-encounters and remonstrates against a personified 'Variola'. Finally, having portrayed smallpox delirium in terms of an heroic struggle against despair and death, *Sickness* emphasises the need for spiritual as much as physical restitution.

Thompson is what Frank terms a 'wounded storyteller'. Examining the motivations behind modern pathographies, Frank encounters a pressing need for the survivors of chronic illness to stand as witnesses before the wider community.[25] Thus Thompson puts himself forward as moral exemplar, self-dramatising his sense of having to fulfil a burdensome, but necessary duty in testifying to the horrors of smallpox: 'What heavy Scenes / Hang o'er My heart to feel the Theme is Mine! / But providence commands; His Will is done!' (229) The result is what Hawkins terms a 'testimonial pathography', yet as a fastidious neo-classicist poet Thompson expresses concerns over the literary decorum of addressing such a potentially disgusting theme:[26]

It cannot be suppos'd that I should treat upon sickness in a medicinal, but only in a descriptive, a moral, and a religious manner: the versification is varied accordingly; the descriptive parts being more poetical; the moral, more plain; and the religious, for the most part drawn from the holy scriptures. I have just taken notice of the progress of the Small-pox, as may give the reader some small idea of it, without offending his imagination. (310)

This anxiety over giving offence resurfaces in an annotation to Book One where he explains that he intrudes a lyrical paean to St Valentine, patron of the Spring, because sickness 'being a subject so disagreeable, in itself, to human Nature, it was thought necessary, as Fable is the soul of Poetry, to relieve the imagination with the following, and some other Episodes' for 'to describe the anguish of a distemper without a mixture of some more pleasing incidents, would, no doubt, disgust every good natur'd and tender reader' (202). Thompson was faced with a dilemma identified by modern medical sociologists: the patient needs to find a shared and acceptable language with which to convey their felt experience, but this immediately creates a distance between themselves and that experience. Thompson feared alienating his readers, but as Brody observes with respect to modern illness narratives, for the 'sick individual this degree of reflective distance may be a tool for relieving suffering and anxiety by coming to feel more in control of the sickness' (116). Presenting himself as an 'example', Thompson is able to impose retrospective didactic meaning onto the experience of a now barely recognisable former self; a carefree youth who was unexpectedly, yet not arbitrarily confronted with likely death or, at the very least, permanent blindness. As he puts it in the 'Argument' heading Book One, the 'suddenness of the first Attacks of a Distemper, in particular the Small Pox' serves as a lesson in the 'Frailness of Youth, Beauty and Health' (196). In Book One proper Thompson looks back upon his own naivety when his muse had 'too long, a Libertine, diffus'd / On Pleasure's rosy Lap' while his now wiser self must sing of 'Dust'; for 'What is man, who proudly lifts / His Brow audacious, as confronting Heav'n, / And Tramples, with Disdain, his Mother-Earth / But moulded Clay?' (198).

Thompson makes much of the fact that the first onset of his illness had interrupted a scene of naïve pastoral bliss. The poet recalls listening to a female companion dubbed Ianthe, singing on St Valentine's Day (14 February):[27]

> To my heart I prest
> Her spotless Sweetness: when (with wonder, hear!)
> Tho' She shone smiling by, the torpid Pow'rs
> Of Heaviness weigh'd down my beamless Eyes,
> And press'd them into Night. The Dews of Death
> Hung, clammy, on my Forehead, like the Damps
> Of midnight Sepulchres; which, silent, op'd
> By weeping Widows, or by Friendship's Hand,
> Yawn hideous on the Moon, and blast the Stars
> With pestilential Reek. My Head is torn
> With Pangs insufferable, pulsive Starts,
> And pungent Aches, grinding thro' the Brain,
> To Madness hurrying the tormented Sense,
> And hate of Being. (204)

A weeping Ianthe takes his hand to ask 'What sudden Change is this?', to which the poet stammers a 'fault'ring' reply before 'a lethargick Stupor steeps my Sense / In dull Oblivion'. His vivid recollections of being in a fever now serve as a reminder that 'Pleasure is a Dream', as he employs Homeric analogies to lend his sufferings elevated, heroic proportions:

> . . . the rapid Flood
> Of throbbing Life, excursive from the Laws
> Of sober Nature, and harmonious Health,
> Boils in tumultuary Eddies round
> Its bursting Channels. Parching Thirst, anon,
> Drinks up the vital Maze, as Simois dry,
> Or Zanthus, by the Arm-ignipotent,
> With a Torrent of involving Flames
> Exhausted, when Achilles with their Floods
> Wag'd more than mortal War; [. . .]
>   O! ye Rivers, roll
> Your cooling Crystal o'er my burning Breast,
> For Ætna rages here! (204–205)

Thompson is moved to ask God directly why he was plunged into such agony: 'Good Heav'n! what Hoards of unrepented Guilt / Have drawn this Vengeance down, have rais'd this Fiend / To lash me with his Flames?' (206) But like Wesley, in retrospect Thompson kisses-the-rod, recognising that sickness serves as a 'School of Virtue'; smallpox is designed to 'save us as by

Fire' by 'purifying off the Dross of Sin', until we are swept up 'On Wings of Meditation, to the Skies' (206). Regretting the time he once wasted upon 'ye dear deluders' of Greece and Rome, Thompson now realises that an unchallenged state of health acts like a 'disease' on our morals because it encourages us vainly to neglect 'the Volumes which will make us Wise' (206). Book One, which concludes with more stern reminders that we can only depend upon the rock of Christian 'Virtue', is designed to ensure that the subsequent allegorical account of Thompson's journey into what Sontag once memorably called 'the kingdom of the ill', is to be interpreted within a sound theological model of redemptive, providential suffering.[28]

REVISITING 'THE PALACE OF DISEASE'

Like Dante journeying through Hell, Thompson does not revisit 'The Palace of Disease' unaccompanied: he opens Book Two with an invitation to Lady Hertford 'in all the Beauty of Distress, / To take a silent walk among the Tombs' (219). The poet's friend in sorrow was Frances Seymour, (née Thynne) Countess of Hertford, later Duchess of Somerset (d. 1754), an ardent Christian and influential literary patroness whose other associates included James Thomson, Elizabeth Rowe, Isaac Watts and William Shenstone. Thompson's choice of companion is in part explained towards the close of this section of the poem, where a list of those whose worthy lives have been cruelly cut short by smallpox dwells upon 'our recent Grief' over the loss of Hertford's son George, Lord Beauchamp who had died of the disease on 11 September 1744, while staying at Bologna during an Italian tour. The death of Hertford's only son on the evening of his nineteenth birthday marked the start of 'a long series of pain and infirmity' for the mother from which, despite the consolations of religious retirement and poetry, 'she never afterwards perfectly recovered'.[29] Thompson, who had probably taught Beauchamp, asks rhetorically 'are the Muses, with their Hertford Dumb?', before concluding Book Two with his own eulogy to Beauchamp's beauty, intelligence, purity, benevolence and patriotism. Exploiting the family anecdote that the Italians had dubbed Beauchamp 'the English Angel', this monody culminates in a reassuring vision of the apotheosis of this 'spotless Youth of Heaven' (234).

Beauchamp's premature death in the autumn immediately after Thompson had himself almost succumbed to smallpox is enough to explain the inclusion of this set-piece (Thompson also dedicated his 1757 volume, containing the final version of *Sickness*, to Hertford).[30] An invitation to accompany the poet as he confronts 'Variola' could be construed as rubbing salt into a bereft mother's wounds, but Thompson's declared purpose was to 'Lend Charm to sorrow' and 'smooth her Brow'; an act of restitution which he symbolically compares with that of the dove (Hertford's family emblem) which flew out of the ark and 'Spread all its Colours oe'r the boundless Deep / . . . Chaos reform'd, and bade Distraction smile!' (219)

Thompson's imaginative confrontation with Variola aims at calming the waters of grief, but the visit to 'The Palace of Disease' presents a theology which insists on associating disease with sin. Book Two bears an epigraph taken from the Archangel Michael's visionary revelation to Adam in *Paradise Lost* Book XI of the ways in which death will ravish fallen mankind through fire, flood, famine, intemperance and disease. In full Milton's lines read 'Diseases dire, of which a monstrous crew / Before thee shall appear; that thou may'st know / What misery th'inabstinence of Eve / Shall bring on men' (l. 474). This equation between disease, sin and female transgression is immediately reiterated in Thompson's opening argument where he insists that death was not intended as 'man's inheritance' until 'monstrous Sin, / The motly Child of Satan and Hell, / Invited dire Disease into the World, / And her distorted Brood of ugly Shapes, / Echidna's Brood!' (217) The allusion is to Spenser's description of a monster with a woman's torso and a serpent's tail:

> Echidna is a Monster direfull dred,
> Whom Gods doe hate, and heavens abhor to see;
> So hideous is her shape, so huge her hed,
> That euen the hellish fiends affrighted bee
> At sight thereof, and from her presence flee:
> Yet her face and former parts professe
> A faire young Mayden, full of comely glee;
> But all her hinder parts did plane express
> A Monstrous Dragon, full of fearful ugliness.
>
> (*The Faerie Queene* VI. 6. x)

Offended by 'her so dreadful face' the Gods cast Echidna 'furthest from the skie' to live in 'hideous horour and obscurity' among 'rocks and caues' (VI. 6. xi). Spencer's references to Echidna's ugly 'hinder parts', with the added implication that she represents the punitive outcome of female sexual transgression, reinforce the pervasive air of misogynist disgust. Thompson's comparison therefore prepares us for the similarly gendered figure of Variola as monstrous female which we are about to encounter in 'The Mansion of Despair' at the symbolic heart of Book Two's allegorical landscape.

To reach this Gothic mansion the poet takes Hertford through a 'Desert Vale' untouched by the seasons, inhabited only by night-birds, serpents and toads; a macabre place of 'Eternal Damps, deadly Humours, drawn / In pois'nous Exhalations from the Deep' (221) where only the kind of noxious plants gathered by Medea thrive.[31] The palace itself stands in 'sad magnificence', its frontage of 'ruinous Design' bearing a central, emblematic entablature on which appears the very opening of *Paradise Lost*, Book I, 'In Gold the Apple rose "Whose mortal Taste / Brought Death into the World, and all our Woe".':

> Malignantly delighted, dire Disease
> Surveys the glittering Pest, and grimly smiles
> With hellish Glee. Beneath, totters her Throne,
> Of jarring Elements; Earth, Water, Fire;
> Where hot, and cold; and moist, and dry maintain
> Unnatural War. Shapeless her frightful Form,
> (A Chaos of distemper'd Limbs in one)
> Huge as Megæra, cruel as the Grave,
> Her Eyes, two Comets; and her Breath, a Storm.
> High in her wither'd Arms, she wields her Rod,
> With Adders curl'd, and dropping Gore ... (222)

'Disease' points to 'the dead Walls, besmear'd with cursed Tales' depicting red-spotted plagues and 'blue Pestilence' with 'Havock at their Heels' and 'Lean Famine, gnawing in Despight her Arm' (222–3). Thompson describes these murals, presenting a litany of human disasters down through history illustrating how famine is the inevitable attendant of epidemic, as displaying more of 'the Distresses and Agonies of human Nature' than even 'Spagnolet cou'd paint' (223). Jusepe de Ribera (known as 'lo Spagnoletto', 'the little Spaniard', 1591–1652) was famous for his explicit depictions of martyrdom and torture. Ribera's 'Apollo Flaying Marysas', widely available in print form certainly provides a particularly potent image for conveying the symptoms of smallpox. Given the implicit critique of the violent excesses of the Inquisition in much of the artist's output, Thompson's comparison also feeds into a thread of conventional anti-Catholic bias felt throughout *Sickness*.[32]

Some of the grotesque wall-paintings in Disease's throne-room specifically portray the 'execrable Crew / Which Michael, in Vision strange disclos'd, / To Adam, in the Lazar-house of woe; a Colony from Hell'. This is yet another reference to Michael's revelation of the consequences of the Fall in *Paradise Lost*, IX (lines 474–89), but in composing his own catalogue of ailments – the 'knotted Gout', the 'bloated Dropsy', the 'racking Stone' and

'Lepra foul', the 'Strangling Angina', 'Ephialtick starts', 'Unnerv'd Paralysis' and 'murderous Apoplexy' (223) – Thompson was also influenced by a precedent passage describing 'Sicknes' as one of 'The Furies' in the *Le Semaine* (1578; 1584) of Guillaume de Saluste Sieur du Bartas (widely available after 1605 as *The Divine Weeks and Days* in Joshua Sylvester's English translation). Sylvester's intrusion of a passage recounting his own protracted sufferings from fever must have also inspired Thompson.[33]

Neither Milton nor du Bartas specifically name smallpox in their galleries of disease, but Thompson readily reconfigures their iconography to portray the six 'Furies' inhabiting his own 'Palace of Despair'; the personifications of 'War', 'Intemperance', 'Melancholy', 'Fever', 'Consumption' and finally 'Variola':

> The last, so turpid to the View, affrights
> Her Neighbour Hags, Happy Herself is blind,
> Or Madness wou'd ensue; so bloated-black,
> So loathsome to each Sense, the Sight or Smell,
> Such foul Corruption on this side the Grave;
> Variola yclep'd; ragged and rough,
> Her Couch perplex'd with Thorns. (229)

Variola is imagined as a 'Fury' the very sight of which has the potential to kill. While Thompson's mythic portrait encapsulates all the clinical symptoms typically found in severe cases of smallpox – the blackening and bloating of the skin from confluent haemorrphagic blistering, the noxious, putrid smell and, of course, blindness – this Medusa-like figure also encapsulates those images of femininity as the root of smallpox corruption discussed in my opening chapter.

More broadly, *Sickness* places an archaic, mythological understanding of disease as a malign force alongside more modern conceptions of the sick body as a hydraulic machine subject to erosive friction. Initially Thompson talks of his encounter with smallpox in terms of being possessed by a malicious anima invading his blood and consuming his vitality from within: 'She rushes through my Blood; she runs along, / And riots on my Life' (229). But the questioning voice with which he finally confronts 'Variola' belongs to the project of enlightenment science; a voice demanding that she reveals the secret of how and why she restricts her harmful actions to humans:

> 'Variola, what art thou? Whence proceeds
> This Virulence, which all, but We, escape;
> Thou nauseous Enemy to human-kind:
> In Man and Man alone, thy mystick Seeds,
> Quiet, and in their secret Windings hid,

> Lie unprolifick; till infection rouze
> Her poisn'ous particles, of proper Size,
> Figure, and Measure, to exert their pow'r
> Of Impregnation . . . (229)

Thompson cites no specific medical sources, but these rhetorical speculations on the pathology not only invoke the theory of a dormant seed, but also betray his exposure to the mechanistic vocabularies of Descartes and his corpuscularian followers. In particular, when Thompson refers to 'Atoms subtle, barb'd / Infrangible, and active to destroy / By Geometrick or Mechanick Rules / Yet undiscover'd', we catch the fashionable iatro-mathematical language of Newtonian matter-theory which was currently being adopted by such physicians as William Hillary, the author of *A Rational and Mechanical Essay on the Small-Pox* (London: 1735).[34] Seeing how readily Thompson intrudes this new vocabulary into his largely religio-mythic poetics, we might apply the observation made by Hawkins that 'the metaphor of the body as a machine, a metaphor basic to contemporary biomedicine, is itself a kind of mythic thinking'.[35] In *Sickness* both the mythic and mechanistic understandings of illness inform a cataclysmic vision of smallpox as evidence of invasive corruption and universal disorder: 'quick the Leaven runs, / Destructive of the Solids, Spirits, Blood / Of mortal Man, and agitates the whole / In general Conflagration and Misrule' (229).

'OVIDIAN REALMS'

Such disorder is pictured forth in Book Three, where Thompson employs an array of mythological allusions to convey the monstrous transformation of his own body at the height of the disease:

> But am I wake? Or in Ovidian Realms,
> And Circè holds the Glass? What odious Change,
> What Metamorphose strikes the dubious Eye?
> Ah, wither is retir'd the scarlet Wave,
> Mantling with Health, which floated through the Cheek,
> From the strong Summer-beam imbib'd? (246)

This moment of shock when the smallpox victim catches a first, self-alienating sight of their transformed features in a mirror was already an established pivotal moment in imaginative smallpox narratives, more especially in those concerning the disfiguring impact of the disease upon female beauty (addressed in Chapter 5). Adapting a pictorial trope of self-reflection more traditionally associated with the vanity of Venus, Thompson avoids the risk of seeming to indulge in an effeminate narcissism through his rhetorical insistence that it must be the witch Circè who holds the mirror.

Circè was the Goddess of the Sun, the daughter of a Titan, whose palace, as described by Ovid, thronged with victims she had transformed into beasts (*Metamorphoses*, XIV, l. 300 ff.) Though best known for transforming Odysseus's men into swine, Thompson was also invoking Ovid's account of how Circè was asked by Polyphemus for a love potion that would make Scylla reciprocate his affections (in *Metamorphoses*, XIV). Circè, acting out of her own sexual jealousy, uses skills learnt from Hecate to cast a spell over the pool where Scylla bathes. As described in Arthur Golding's 1567 English translation, 'This plash did Circe then infect against that Scylla came / And with her poisons, which had power most monstrous shapes to frame, / Defilèd it'.[36] The ensuing scene of transformation was often isolated for pictorial illustration in contemporary editions of Ovid. (Illustration 3) In the popular 1717 English translation added emphasis is placed upon Scylla's self-estrangement:

> Soon as the nymph wades in, her nether parts
> Turn into dogs; then, at her self she starts.
> A ghastly horror in her eyes appears;
> But yet she knows not, who it is she fears;
> In vain she offers from her self to run,
> And drags about her what she strives to shun.[37]

This translation is the work of the famous physician Sir Samuel Garth. Whether or not Garth consciously chose his phrasing with the effects of smallpox in mind this graphic episode struck a chord with Thompson who later draws upon another Ovidian tale of bodily transformation to convey the specific sensation of discovering that one is covered with pustules:

> The Forehead roughens to the wonder'ing hand
> Wide o'er the Human-field, the Body, spreads
> Contagious War, and lays its Beauties waste.
> As once the breathing Harvest, Cadmus, sprung,
> Sudden, a Serpent-brood! an armed Crop
> Of growing Chiefs, and fought Themselves to death. (246)

This rather forced comparison with a battle-field puts an heroic gloss on sordid symptoms.[38] Finally Thompson turns to a not wholly unrelated Ovidian story in a later passage describing the pain inflicted by smallpox:

> Pain emptys all her Vials on my Head,
> And steeps me o'er and o'er'. The envenom'd Shirt

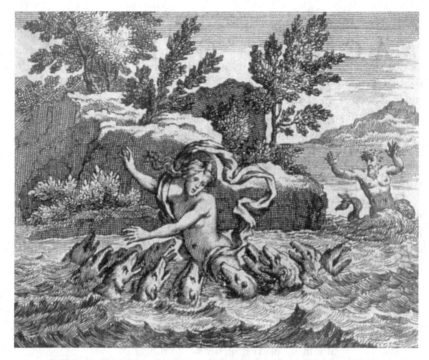

3. Scylla's monstrous transformation, from *Metamorphoses d'Ovide en Rondeaux*
(Amsterdam, 1679). Ovidian images of bodily transformation are frequently employed
by writers seeking to convey the self-alienating impact of smallpox.

> Of Hercules enwraps my burning Limbs,
> With Dragon's Blood: I rave and roar like him,
> Writing in Agony. Devouring Fires
> Eat up the Marrow, frying my Bones.
> Oh wither, wither shall I turn for Aid? (252)

Thompson has chosen another tale of male heroism in the face of bodily
torment and, if the full story is followed through, one in which such
torment is implicitly associated with a revengeful, sexually jealous
woman. As recounted in *Metamorphoses* Book IX, the poisoned shirt was
originally given to Hercules' wife Deianera by the centaur Nessus, after he
has been hit by an arrow fired by her husband (the centaur had tried to
abduct Hercules's wife). Nessus tells Deianera that his bloodstained shirt
will act as a love-philtre. When she later becomes jealous over rumours of
her absent husband's love affair with Iole, Deianera sends the shirt of
Nessus to Hercules hoping to secure his love but when he wears it to

make a sacrifice at an altar-flame the heat releases the poison. Thompson
clearly identified with Ovid's ensuing description as a suitable comparison
through which to convey his own symptoms:

> Where'er he plucks the vest, the skin he tears,
> The mangled muscles, and huge bone he bares
> (A ghastly sight!), or raging with his pain,
> To rend the sticking plague he tugs in vain.
> As the red iron hisses in the flood.
> So boils the venom in his curdling blood.
> Now with the greedy flames his entrails glow.
> And livid sweats down all his body flow;
> The cracking nerves burnt up are burst in twain,
> The lurking venom melts his swimming brain.[39]

These interlinked Ovidian allusions provide Thompson with some suitably
vivid, yet familiar accounts of physical transformation and torment, lending elevated poetic and mythic dignity to what he knows is a disturbing
catalogue of horrific symptoms. They provide him with a distancing form
of descriptive short-hand through which to convey the more gruesome
aspects of his personal encounter with 'Variola'.

In Book Three Thompson turns to the psychological effects of this
trauma. He recounts his disturbing experience of sinking into the delirium
of fever while reflecting on the irony that the loss of his outward sight had
thrown him into a 'Wilderness of Dreams':

> Tho' at their visual Entrance, quite shut out
> External Forms, forbidden, mount the Winds,
> Retire to Chaos, or with Night commix;
> Yet Fancy's mimick Work, ten thousand Shapes,
> Antick and wild, rush sweeping o'er my Dreams,
> Irregular and new; as pain or ease
> The Spirits teach to flow, and in the Brain
> Directions diverse hold . . . (248)

The convoluted syntax betrays the poet's confused resistance to this uncon-
trollable plunge into his own chaotic unconscious, but an authorial footnote
explains that although 'the following Lines upon delirious Dreams may
appear very extravagant to a Reader, who never experienc'd the Disorders
which Sickness causes in the Brain . . . the Author thinks that he has rather
softened than exaggerated the real Description, as he found them operate on
his own Imagination at that Time' (248). In fact Thompson's attempts to
describe his descent into this semiotic Maelstrom as sublimely peaceful,
ecstatically beautiful visions of an Elysium or Eden suddenly give way to

fearful encounters with hellish, murderous 'Haggs', produces some of the poem's most intriguing passages as he reconstructs his feverish delusions as a series of disorientating episodic shifts between 'Pain or Ease'. Thompson draws heavily upon literary allusion in these hallucinatory episodes: a passage in which he dreams of being cast down into 'Vulcan's shop', then holding 'the reins of Phlegon', before being blasted by 'Astolpho's Horn' combines imagery from the *Iliad* and Ariosto's *Orlando Furioso*, while his memories of spatial delusions, notably a sense of being thrown across a vast gulf between Heaven and Hell, are informed by the cosmic topography of *Paradise Lost*. After imagining a line of bards processing through the grounds of Queen's College Oxford, his *alma mater*, he suddenly finds himself being propelled down a burning mountainside as his skeleton is racked in the chain-like grip of pain. Further references to scents and tastes imply that these were not merely visual delusions.

But there was some ambivalence attached to the revelatory value of a smallpox fever so obviously rooted in the body. We can usefully compare Thompson's carefully wrought, elevating poetic recollections of his fevered hallucinations with the deliberate bathos of the journalist John Dunton's quotidian, sarcastic description of his own descent into delirium when he succumbed to smallpox as an apprentice bookseller:

Instead of those *sage and grave Notions* that used to fill my Head, 'twas cramm'd top full of *Whimseys and Whirligigs*, by the vehement agitation of my *distemper'd Fancy*, as ever a Carkase-shell with Instruments of Death and Murder. I was nothing but *all Flame* and *Fire*, and the red-hot Thoughts glared about my Brains at such a rate, and if visible, wou'd, I fancy, have made just such a dreadful Appearance as the *Window of a Glass-House* discovers in a dark Night – *viz.*, a parcel of straggling *fiery Globes* marching about and hizzing, appearing and vanishing high and low, transverse, and every where [. . .] What a multitude of *Visions, Raptures* and *Revelations* did I then see and enjoy! and could I but have manag'd my *Pen* then as well as now, I might have clapt down Matter enough for *a Book of four and twenty times as long as all these Rambles* – But they're Lost to the World, and there's an end on't; 'tho neither *Rice Evans*, who foresaw the blessed holy Christian Court of K[ing] *Ch[arles]* the II, nor Mrs. *James*, who prophesies as fine things for his brother's, cou'd ever have pretended to higher flights than the *young Evander*. I foresaw Things that never *was, are, or will be* – *The Restauration of K[ing] James*, and the religion of his Friends, the Courage of the *Irish* – with twenty thousand things more too tedious and strange to instance in.[40]

These mocking references to contemporary visionaries and prophets betrays Dunton's scepticism towards religious enthusiasts and their diseased imaginations. Thompson displays a serious desire to exploit the dramatic potential of his own 'delerious dreams', but it is notable that ultimately he also understands these deranged imaginings in purely materialist terms as symptomatic responses to bodily extremes of pleasure and pain rooted in the 'brain'.[41]

The remainder of *Sickness* Book Three describes a protracted state of semi-delirium in the form of a dramatic dialogue between three conflicting voices: 'Patience', ('That Panacea of the Mind' who shows him the patient sufferings of Christ on the Cross and various holy martyrs) accompanied by her daughter 'Hope', and the countervailing voice of 'Despair . . . the sole Disease of which the damn'd are Sick' (255). Like a wavering believer in a morality play, Thompson transforms his illness experience into a battle between competing external forces who struggle over possession of his very soul. This agonistic use of these externalised poetic personifications suggests a retrospective attempt to create a distance between a core, surviving self and the painful memories of a disorientating and harrowing ordeal (Dunton's flippant descriptions of 'young Evander's' torments serve the same function). When the exhausted Thompson wonders where to seek aid a seraphic voice instructs him to 'Turn to God; So peace shall be thy Pillow' (255). With angelic attendants rallying forces to encourage him to find strength and solace in religious faith, the poet turns what had been a private ordeal into a universal lesson in humility.

'MY SKIN IS BLACK UPON ME . . .'

Thompson's illness prompted him to address the wider ethical issue of pain as undeserved punishment. The representation of pain has been a contentious issue in recent literary criticism. In one of the most profound modern meditations on this theme, Virginia's Woolf's 'On Being Ill' (1926), the novelist considers why the 'daily drama' of illness and pain has not been a more dominant literary topic.[42] As Lucy Bending has recently examined, through selective readings of Woolf's remarks, many of her recent followers, most notably Elaine Scarry in her influential study *The Body In Pain: the Making and Unmaking of the World* (1985), have insisted upon the utter ineffability of pain, rooting this in a supposed failure of language.[43] Physical pain, Scarry insists 'unlike any other state of consciousness – has no referential content. It is not of or for anything. It is precisely because it takes no object that it, more than any other phenomenon, resists objectification in language'.[44] But as Bending notes, while Woolf identifies barriers of taste, decorum and fear facing the illness writer, she does not suggest that pain lies wholly beyond words: 'To look these things squarely in the face', Woolf writes, 'would need the courage of a lion tamer; a robust philosophy; a reason rooted in the bowels of the earth. Short of these, this monster, the body, this miracle, its pain, will soon make us taper into mysticism, or rise, with rapid beats of the wings, into the raptures of transcendentalism'.[45] Here Bending observes that while Woolf acknowledges the writer's need for courage, yet she recognises that language 'is compelled to move outwards from the direct description of pain itself into a metaphorical and explanatory realm in which pain is fitted into another and distinct frame of reference'. As Bending vigorously demonstrates, contrary to Scarry's often self-contradictory claims, which rely upon exaggeration and category confusions, pain is 'always' referential; having no 'innate meaning'.[46]

It will already be evident how the entire structure and metaphoric reach of Thompson's poem wholly supports Bending's counter-claim that pain 'is given meaning – has meaning imposed upon it – when the sufferer . . . draws suffering into association with something else'.[47] Faced with describing and comprehending the intense pain of smallpox, the tormented voice of *Sickness* identifies itself closely with 'Job's Punishment'. Thompson hopes that,

> With Patience like his own,
> O may I exercise my wounded Soul,
> And cast myself upon his healing Hand,
> Who bruiseth at his Will, and maketh whole. (246)

At the very start of Book One, he compares the muse Urania's powers of heavenly inspiration with those felt when 'from the Whirlwind, God's all-glorious voice / Bursts on the tingling Ears of Job':

> My humble Hopes
> Aspire but to the Alpha of his Song;
> Where, roll'd in Ashes, digging for a Grave,
> More earnest than the Covetous for Gold
> Or hidden Treasures, crusted o'er with Boils,
> And roaring in the Bitterness of Soul,
> And heart-sick Pain, the Man of Uz, complains.
> Themes correspondent to thy Servant's Theme. (199)

This identification is made again at the head of Book Three with the placing of a pointed biblical epigraph from Job 30. 30–31: 'When I waited for Light there came Darkness. / My skin is black upon me; and my Bones are burnt with heat. / My harp is tuned to Mourning' (244). The comparison is rendered even more visually explicit in Thompson's account of finding his body turning into 'One black-incrusted Bark of gory

Boils, / One undistinguish'd Blister, from the Soal / Of the sore Foot, to the Head's sorer Crown', which adapts the biblical lines 'So went forth Satan from the presence of the Lord, and smote JOB with sore boils from the sole of his foot unto his crown' (Job 2. 7). Thompson's tormented outbursts mimic both Job's cry that 'My flesh is clothed with worms and clods of dust; my skin is broken, and become loathsome' and his complaint to Yahweh that 'thou scarest me with dreams, and terrifiest me through visions: So that my soul chooseth strangling, and death rather than life' (Job 7. 5 and 14–15).

The sick have traditionally identified with Job. The original Hebrew text does not give Job's eruptive disease a specific name but, as noted in my introduction, several early eighteenth-century theologians published retrospective diagnoses claiming it was smallpox. It is unclear if Thompson was implicitly endorsing this modern medical exegesis, but certainly by the time he wrote *Sickness*, the association between Job's boils and smallpox had received heightened publicity after Edmund Massey delivered his controversial *Sermon Against the Dangerous and Sinful Practice of Inoculation* (1722), based on Job II, VII, which argues that the biblical account of how 'the Devil by some venomous Infusion into the Body of Job, might raise Confluence of inflammatory Pustules, all over him' implies that the disease was 'conveyed to him by . . . Inoculation'.[48] Massey's denunciations of inoculation as 'a Diabolical Operation' attracted mockery from less literal-minded theologians and physicians alike, but nonetheless fuelled an ethical debate over the morality of a physician deliberately infecting his patient.[49]

Sickness is glaringly silent over inoculation. Thompson may have shared Massey's religious objections, but when he does address the morality of medical intervention in general his comments are in keeping with the orthodox line taken by most early-modern commentators on sickness. Donne, for example, who Thompson studied, insists that the sick person is in error who 'neglects the spiritual physic . . . instituted in thy Church', but also knew God 'hast made . . . the man, and the art; and I go not from thee when I go to the Physician'.[50] Thompson himself observes that even 'pagan Wisdom' associated healing with an eternal divinity in the figure of Apollo, while insisting that the 'aids inferior' available to mortal physicians are the gifts through which 'God our Great Physician' providentially compensates mankind for the consequences of the Fall. The human body is an organised 'Instrument of various Pipes and Tubes / Veins, Arteries, and Sinews' which when healthy breathes forth melody, but to 'refit this shatter'd Frame' requires an 'Art divine' beyond the reach of humans.

Thompson observes that no mortal doctor can do much when faced with smallpox: '... something yet, beyond the kindly Skill / Of Pæan's Sons, Disease, like mine, demands; / Nepenthe to the Soul, as well as Life (259–60). Like Wesley, the recovering Thompson emphasises the need to address 'the festers of the wounded Soul', more than those of the ravished flesh (276). Thompson reiterates this need for spiritual as much as physical healing throughout the latter part of *Sickness* at the same time as exalting the therapeutic power of friendship and faith over the limited skills of physicians who only focus on the body.

'THE PROGRESS OF SICKNESS'

Thompson's poetic reconstruction gives smallpox temporal dimensions wholly absent from the usual medical accounts. There is a radical difference between the conception of a given disease as defined by professional clinicians and the subjective experience of illness. As Brody notes, a patient will tell of their sickness with a logic *internal* to the experience; one that does not necessarily conform to the purely *external*, medically meaningful logic of the physician.[51] In this context Hawkins even talks of 'two quite distinct realities, the one grounded in experience and the other in abstraction'.[52] An aside confirms that Thompson's smallpox episode lasted fifteen (sleepless) days, but otherwise his poetic account does not conform to the neatly ordered chronology typically encountered in the diagnostic writings of contemporary physicians. They typically reduce the 'progress' of smallpox down to a series of readily recognisable 'stages' conceived in terms of a febrile process of onset, crisis and elimination which served the purposes of recognition, intervention and hoped-for regulation. Fuller, for example, talks of 'assimilation, concoction, eruption, augmentation and maturation'.[53] William Cullen, in his influential Edinburgh University lectures on the 'First Lines of The Practice of Physic', subsequently gave extraordinarily detailed attention to the precise duration of the stages of smallpox depending on the precise time of day the first symptoms present themselves.[54] But as the physician Walter Lynn discovered when he succumbed to smallpox himself, such stages, being based upon the supposed actions of *the* disease as indicated by external bodily signs, did not necessarily conform with the patient's own sense of the 'progress' of *their illness*. Lynn was left admitting that the 'whole Progress of my Distemper, and my recovery out of it, seems difficult for me to relate'.[55]

Discussing this dichotomy between clinical and experiential perspectives, Hawkins refers to the recent observational work of the medical phenomenologist S. Kay Toombs – herself an MS sufferer – who places emphasis upon illness as a disruption of the 'lived body'; a phrase which echoes Kleinman's earlier insistence that chronic illness episodes are 'embodied in a particular life trajectory, environed in a concrete life world'.[56] Reflecting on her own 'embodied' experience, Toombs observes how illness is often first felt as being 'out of time' or 'rather, part of one's subjective or inner, time' which does not necessarily correlate with objective time as measured by clocks and calendars (hence we commonly say time 'stands still' when we are frightened or 'zooms by' when we are happily absorbed).[57]

The tendency for illness to make time drag as the attention turns inwards and isolates the sufferer is exacerbated and complicated in cases concerning diseases which are contagious and cause delirium. Hence Donne, writing of his own experience of a severe fever in his *Devotions*, recalled '*daies* and *nights*, so long, as that *Nature* her selfe shall seeme to be *perverted*, and to have put the *longest day*, and the longest night, which should be *six monthes* asunder, into one *naturall, unnaturall day*'.[58] Thompson probably recalled this passage when representing the 'progress' of his own illness as a disruption of the seasonal cycle. In particular he exploits the ironic circumstance of being suddenly taken ill at the start of spring, on St Valentine's day; the 'Festival of Youth' when 'Lover's Wounds / Afresh begin to bleed' (202). These metaphorical 'wounds' of frivolous pastoral lovers turn into the all-too-real symptoms of smallpox, as Thompson reminds his readers that disease can strike 'in all the Portions of the Year' (246–7). When Thompson finally celebrates his recovery, he writes rapturously of how 'The Winter of Disease all pass'd away' while 'The Spring of Health, in bloomy Pride, calls forth / Embosom'd Bliss' (290). For the smallpox sufferer a whole year has been condensed into two weeks. For his reader – who has vicariously shared Thompson's disorientating experience of what Donne tellingly terms 'perverted time' – vernal imagery reassuringly re-imposes a natural, restorative order. The effect is ultimately optimistic; recovery is presented as inherent to a providential cycle as Thompson casts his individual illness within universalising images of rebirth.[59]

At least one modern reader has recoiled from *Sickness* for what they term its mannered 'pseudo-Jacobean decadence'.[60] Given the subject matter, it is perhaps understandable that Thompson's poem was never popular but it was 'favourably received by the polite and religious world' and continued to be anthologised into the nineteenth century.[61] In 1794 Robert Anderson heaped praise on *Sickness* while introducing Thompson as a neglected but 'ingenious poet' and in 1810 Alexander Chalmers thought it his best poem in which, having chosen 'a new subject', he 'discovers considerable powers of invention'.[62] It is surely no coincidence that both these editors were medically trained and isolate for praise 'the Palace of Disease', the 'Delerious Dreams' and 'the Recovery' sections, the key passages conveying the subjective experience of smallpox. We can endorse Chalmers's observation that *Sickness* 'abounds in original, or at least uncommon thoughts' through which Thompson 'evinces real feeling, the consequence of having suffered what he describes, and having been alternately depressed, or elevated by the vicissitudes of a long and dangerous illness'. *Sickness* still warrants historical interest as an early exercise in the Spenserian gothic, but more particularly as a rare example of a highly literary smallpox autopathography which anticipates the pathological concerns of later romantics, notably Coleridge and De Quincy who were fascinated by the diseased imagination. Alongside Flood's *Narrative* and the other autobiographical writings addressed in this chapter it represents an attempt at restitution. Addressing the motives fuelling modern pathographies, Hawkins remarks on how 'the need to communicate a painful, disorientating, and isolating experience . . . often involves the need to project it outwards – to talk or write about it'.[63] For Hawkins the 'task of the author of a pathography' is not merely to describe the 'disordering process' of illness 'but also to restore to reality its lost coherence and to discover, or create, a meaning that can bind it together again'.[64] Crucially that meaning must be one that the patient finds acceptable within their existing belief system and worldview. Unsurprising, with the exception of two brief autobiographical case studies by physicians, all the survival writing recoverable from this period interprets the personal experience of surviving smallpox within a redemptive Christian framework.[65]

PART II

Death

CHAPTER 3

Smallpox elegy

With mortality rates of anything from 15 up to 90 per cent for the most virulent strains, it is unsurprising to find that the literary legacy of smallpox is dominated by elegies. The present chapter addresses the efforts of those seventeenth-century poets who strove to comprehend the tragic impact of this sudden-onset disease, to commemorate its victims and reconcile the living to their loss. When Dryden composed his verses 'On the Death of Lord Hastings' in 1649 he was working within an established form, the aristocratic elegy, in which grief for an individual is given public, if not national meaning. Dryden pointedly presents the ravages of smallpox in terms of divine retribution for collective transgression: 'The nation's sin hath drawn that veil, which shrouds / Our day-spring in so sad benighting clouds' (lines 49–50). Describing pustules in terms of a bodily 'insurrection' against the heroic Hastings, Dryden even makes an albeit incongruous comparison between the weeping pustules and the tears of repentant rebels:

> Each little pimple had a tear in it,
> To wail the fault its rising did commit;
> Which, rebel-like, with its own lord at strife,
> Thus made an insurrection 'gainst his life. (lines 59–64)

Modern critics have disagreed over whether this forced simile amounts to a candid declaration of the young poet's political loyalties.[1] Most recently John McWilliams, accepting that Dryden's contribution has royalist resonances, offers a contextual argument for reading the whole of *Lachrymae Musarum* as 'a project shot through with precisely the conflict between defeatism and defiance that the critical debate . . . suggests'.[2] More broadly this memorial volume illustrates how Hasting's fellow-pupils sought to find poetic and political meaning in his otherwise meaningless, ugly death. Dryden struggled to accommodate the symptoms of smallpox to a poetics in which the body personal and the body political are implicitly allied, but as in so many similar examples, a question-mark lingers over whether the disease is a sign of corruption stemming from outside or within that body. This issue became all the more pressing in 1660 when the disease started to strike at the restored House of Stuart. Faced with the task of finding images to accommodate such unforeseen depredations, loyalist poets were to draw out the political metaphors implicit in several of the *Lachrymae Musarum* elegies to develop a convincing rhetoric through which to explain and contain this outbreak of visible corruption at the heart of the body politic.

In the first part of this chapter I consider how pro-monarchist Restoration poets and physicians were compelled to interpret and thus contain this potential challenge to providential royalist claims of divine right and the gift of healing through recourse to politicised conceptions of lingering pollution. Attention to the conflicted gaze cast by many elegiac poets upon the desecrated body of the smallpox victim prompts a discussion of how this fierce disease challenged the therapeutic claims of the elegiac muse. The chapter concludes with an account of how some acclaimed commemorative verses prompted by the deaths of the two women poets, Katherine Philips and Anne Killigrew, served to establish a figurative link in the literary imaginary between smallpox and the thwarting of female power and ambition.

'GREAT GLOUCESTER'S DEAD'

A perception that smallpox was the peculiar scourge of the Stuarts, to be confirmed by the death of Queen Mary in 1694, had first begun to gain force in 1660 when it killed two of Charles II's siblings within months of the Restoration.[3] The first sign of weakness came with the untimely death of the twenty-one-year-old Prince Henry, Duke of Gloucester in September 1660, a mere four months after he had accompanied his elder brother Charles out of exile and attended his Restoration coronation that May. Accounts of the progress of Gloucester's illness record a period of temporary remission with his subsequent death from haemorrhaging within ten days of the first appearance of symptoms prompting public accusations of misdiagnosis and medical mismanagement. Samuel Pepys ends his diary entry for 13 September with the blunt statement that 'this day the Duke of Glocester dyed of the small-pox – by the great negligence of the Doctors'.[4] Writing a year later, the royal biographer Thomas Marley summarised public opinion when he wrote that '... the disease under which he laboured was common to this English nation and very seldom if ever mortal; curable for the most part by the attendant care of some knowing Nurse, but became mortal to the Duke by the over-nice and too severe rules of the Learned Physitian, who contrary to the nature of the disease did several times let him blood'.[5] Taking an alternative tack, the royalist poet Katherine Philips represented Gloucester's death as a 'wise and just' act of divine retribution designed to teach a sinful, ungrateful post-Restoration nation a lesson in humility:

> We have so long and yet so ill endur'd
> The Woes which our offences had procur'd,
> That this new shock would all our strength destroy,
> Had we not knowne an interval of joy.
> And yet perhaps this stroke had been excus'd.
> If we this interval had not abus'd.
> But our ingratitude and discontent
> Deserv'd to know our mercies are but lent;
> And those complaints heaven in this rigid fate
> Doth first chastise and then legitimate.
> By this it our divisions doth reprove,
> And makes us joine in griefe, if not in love.[6]

Philips exploits an orthodox Christian concept that disease is ultimately under the control of an all-wise creator to insist that Gloucester's death stands as a providential lesson to his erring subjects who have not shown enough gratitude for the blessings bestowed through the restoration of the Stuarts.

The need for national 'penance' is also invoked at the opening of the 'Elegie on the Death of the Most Illustrious Prince, Duke of Glocester [sic]' (1660), written by one of the attendant physicians, Martin Lluelyn.[7] Seeking to deflect blame away from his profession, Lluelyn's poetic diagnosis is even more overtly rooted in the political upheavals of the Interregnum and Restoration. Arguing that young Gloucester's death was a well-earned release from an unbearable burden of suffering at the hands of rebel subjects, Lluelyn implies that smallpox has performed what the cowardly 'Cromwell wisht' but 'trembled to performe':

> When pawzing here after Thy slaughter'd Sire,
> He seem'd to fear this was to murder High'r.
> And bathing his black soule, ith'sacred flood,
> He durst gorge Royal, but not tender blood.
> Where then shall Innocence in safety sit?
> When a disease it selfe doth Cromwell it.[8]

Lluelyn's notably clinical account of the symptoms of the disease, cited in my introductory chapter, closes with him returning to his political metaphor as he draws out the irony that the prince – having not only survived the rebellion but also the assassination of his father and deprivations of exile – was to return to England only to die. Lluelyn even exploits the controversial progress of Gloucester's illness – at one stage he had been declared out of danger by his physicians – to imply that the prince was double-crossed by a treacherous disease working as Cromwell's posthumous agent:

> She slew against the Augury of Art.
> No adversary could worse spight display.
> Since it is lesse to Kill, then to betray.
> Twas savage beyond fate; for others lie,
> Dead off Disease, you of Recovery.
>
> . . . Affronts, plots, scandals, false friends, cold Allyes,
> Exiles, wants, tempests, battails, rebels, spies,
> Restraints, temptations, strange aires: in all these
> Was there no Feaver, no maligne Disease?[9]

Pursuing these pathological analogies, Gloucester is likened to the Phoenix which flies through 'each distemper'd region of the Aire' only to be consumed by fire in his own nest. If he had died earlier, in the dark days of the commonwealth, Lluelyn argues, 'our greedy Interests' might have been justifiably tempted not to call our prince back from the grave where he has justly escaped the buffetings of an unworthy world. But for him to die now, when sequestered goods and land have been returned to their rightful owners, when the houses of cavalier widows are no longer occupied by hungry troops, when churches are no longer being spoiled out of zeal and when his 'just Brothers equal Government' has brought peace and order, is like being 'satiated' by 'so rich an odour to Your sense'. Playing upon the notion of a noxious miasma, Lluelyn implies that Gloucester died after being overcome by the sensual overload and sheer delight of witnessing the Restoration.

Lluelyn's politicised conceit of smallpox as a symptom of lingering social corruption also informs loyalist medical texts like Tobias Whitaker's 1661 treatise *An Elenchus of Opinions Concerning the Cure of the Small Pox*, published in defensive response to the ignominy being cast on the medical profession over Gloucester's death.[10] As his title-page declares, Whitaker had just been made 'physician in ordinary to his majesty and House-hold' and in an 'Epistle to the Reader' he intimately aligns himself and his medical endeavours with the fate of Charles II: 'It is not as yet a complete year since my Landing with His Majesty in England, and in this short time have observed as strange a difference in this subject of my present discourse, as in the variety of opinions and dispositions of this Nation . . .'.[11] Whitaker even invokes a quasi-messianic image of his own resurrection from the grave of political exile: it 'is well known I have been buryed in Exile from my own Country the major part of three Lives, and by the same providence am raised and restored again'.[12] Moreover, in offering 'this short direction of Government in this disease', he equates the physician's role with that of a strong ruler bringing potentially disruptive bodies under due control.[13] The conceit was commonplace, but when Whitaker attributes the increased virulence of smallpox to something in the 'present constitution of the ayre' and compares this physical alteration in the atmosphere with the perceived change in the socio-political climate he implies more than just a figurative linkage. His pointed wording implies obvious ideological motives: 'The contagion that infected rebellious Spirits, is known to come, and be received from the malicious breath of some venene [i.e. poisonous] Natures; and hath been permanent for many yeares, and conveyed to severall parts of this region (not extinct at this day.).[14] The phrase 'malicious breath' clearly functions here as a metonym for the rebellious speech of republican usurpers.

Whitaker's entire analysis of smallpox – part of a broad move by newly restored conservative members of the now 'Royal' College of Physicians to denigrate parliamentarian professional rivals – sought to draw attention away from the potential for concluding that there must be a taint of corruption infecting the Stuart bloodline.[15] It also aimed at countering the verdict of oppositional, critical voices, summarised in the retrospective comment of the Whig memoirist Bishop Gilbert Burnet when he observed of Gloucester's premature death that 'the mirth and entertainments of that time raised his blood so high, that he took the small-pox; of which he died'.[16] Burnet simply attributes Gloucester's death from smallpox to a sanguine plethora brought on by over-indulgence in the excesses of the Stuart court.[17] But Whitaker's ink was barely dry before the fatal association between the Stuarts and smallpox was strengthened further when Charles II's sister, Princess Mary of Orange also died of the disease in December 1660, just three months after she had come over from the Hague to join the English Court.

'. . . THE BANE OF GREATNESS'

Princess Mary, eldest daughter of Charles I, had already been deeply affected by smallpox. Her husband, William II of Orange, had succumbed to the disease in November 1650, just a week before she gave birth to a son, the future William III. Mary's own death from the same disease, coming so soon after that of her brother Henry, left the Stuarts vulnerable to further charges of excess. Another outpouring of loyal elegies once again sought to interpret this increasingly virulent disease as further divine punishment for the nation's unexpiated sin in rebelling against her father.

In Henry Bold's 'Elegy on the Death of Mary Princess Dowager of Aurange', for example, we are urged to accept that this further death is yet another sign of 'the Nations sins': 'But must (Oh Times!) more Royal Blood be Spilt / To make atonement for the Subjects Guilt? / Thus the Lamb suffers, while the Fox still thrives, / Heaven's Kingdome's near! 'tis time t'amend our lives / Curst be that Bane of Greatness!'[18] The elegy turns Mary's death into a sacrificial offering in expiation of national transgression. What might easily be taken as further evidence of Stuart weakness is turned into a compliment to a 'Greatness' that bears the brunt of such a burdensome 'Bane' on behalf of the people. Anticipating any charges that the Stuarts are vulnerable to smallpox because they are weakened by their own domestic dissipation, Bold implies that these deaths are evidence of their dutifulness in standing as sacrifices for a people who have themselves failed to 'amend'. He relocates the ultimate source of 'Disease' in the continued disobedience of their subjects: 'Tis, for the Nation sins, a Punishment / When Princes falls, they'd live, if wee'd Repent'. Mary's 'goodness needs no gloss to set it off, / Say but – 'twas Charles his Daughter, that's enough'.

Mary's loss is also 'allied' to that of 'Great Charles' in Thomas Shipman's poem 'Beauty's Enemy, Upon the Death of M. Princess of Orange, by the Small pox, 1660', which also compares this 'Fatal Disease' with the destructive, criminal activities of the Parliamentarians during the interregnum and Cromwell's compulsory appropriations of royalist owned property; just like its 'damn'd Masters' who out of mere 'spite' acted like 'Sequestrators, on the Eminent', smallpox has now 'ruin'st England with a blow'.[19] These general charges of national sin were to reappear in some of the tributes to Queen Mary II when she also succumbed to smallpox at Christmas 1694, but it was not until the 1790s, when Jenner's promotion of vaccination coincided with the national emergency of the Napoleonic wars, that smallpox was to accrue such overtly politicised meanings as it did immediately after the Restoration.[20]

For the Stuarts, whose dynastic claims on power drew heavily upon the concept of primogeniture, charges of *mala stamina vitæ* or tainted blood posed a genuine threat to their political authority.[21] This risk was not lost on the author of 'The Muses Tears for the Loss of the Illustrious Prince, HENRY Duke of Glocester' (1660), when he asked rhetorically 'Must that disease which does so ill be-friend / The *Noble Blood* conduct him to his End? / His Ermines drink new spots that he may lie / In his own *Purples* and more *Princely Die*'.[22] Despite such loyal efforts to transmute the signs of such a blatantly corrupting disease into the sartorial symbols of nobility, the failure of the Stuarts to resist smallpox was never lost on their political opponents. Writing in 1724, responding to claims from some High-Church pulpits that inoculation was originally the devil's work, the Whig satirist Nicholas Amhurst challenges the exiled James Stuart, the Old Pretender, to build a stage in the Roman Forum and 'By this grand secret prove the Stuart line / And let thy cures confirm thy right divine'. With pointed irony, Amhurst hails that '... sacred art! the priesthood's darling theme, / Unlike our late inoculating scheme'.[23] By the time Amhurst was making these sectarian jibes, smallpox had already gone some way towards extinguishing the entire house of Stuart. After the death of Queen Mary in 1694 John Glanvill was already castigating a 'Tyrant Disease, that may'st, with rude Success, / Boast now the death of half a Royal Race', while one 'J. S.' deplores 'an Inexorable and Pittyless Disease, too too Fatal to the Royal Family'.[24] Viewed in retrospect, Gloucester's death in 1660 can be said to have had profound political consequences. Had he survived as an acceptable protestant heir to Charles II, then the Exclusion Crisis and other sectarian plots which marked the reign of the Catholic James VII (II) and culminated in the Whig coup of 1688–1689, might have never occurred. It was certainly the subsequent death from smallpox of Queen Anne's only surviving child, the twelve-year-old William, Duke of Gloucester, in 1700 which left the British throne open to the Hanoverians.

'...SO MANY WOUNDS'

These royal elegies are just the most prominent contributions to a subgenre of occasional poetry revealing a cathartic, angry need to confront smallpox. Despite ample evidence of the popular adherence to internal concepts of smallpox as an inherited seed, smallpox elegists more frequently display recourse to ideas of external attack through tropes of bodily violation drawn from human warfare. The medical sociologist Brody observes how militaristic metaphors of invasion and wounding have been a commonplace of the rhetoric of disease and illness in any age, but given the immediate context of the English Civil War it is no surprise to find later seventeenth-century writers readily equating the physical symptoms of smallpox with battle wounds.[25] Whitaker's 1660 treatise, for example, is replete with images of battle. Invoking a blatantly pro-Stuart inflection of the traditional analogy between the body politic and the body personal, he declares that 'diseases are as mutineers against natural government', casts smallpox as a enemy to be routed, and compares himself with an army commander whose role is to protect against the 'various Affects which besiege the body of man, and are continually storming or laying battery to it'.[26]

Neo-classical poets inherited mythic precedents for employing such combat imagery. Drawing upon the darker aspect of the myth of Apollo as the archer-god whose arrows not only heal but may also inflict sudden illness, smallpox becomes a poisonous tool or agent of death. Thus Thomas Jordan's verses 'On the Death of the Most Worthily Honour'd Mr. John Sidney, who dyed full of the Smallpox' (1643) upbraid 'Death' for its 'cruel Office' which could only separate Sidney's body from his mind by resorting to a 'fatal *sicknesse*, that confounds / The beauteous *Patient*, with so many *wounds*':

> But by Sure when thou mad'st his *Fabrick* to shiver,
> Thou could'st not chuse but empty all thy Quiver.
> What man (to all odds open) in the Wars,
> Dies with such Solemnity of Scarrs?[27]

Jordan invites a flattering comparison between Sidney's death from smallpox and cavalier heroics. In a similar vein, William Strode's epitaph 'On Sir Thomas Savill Dying of the Small Pox' (1655), talks of 'greedy death' and 'a body here entomb'd / That by a thousand stroakes was made one wound'. It took 'fifty wounds' before Caesar, like a whole 'troop of men', allowed death into the fortress of his body, but in Savill's case,

> ... though each wound did reach
> The very heart, yet none could make a breach
> Into his soule, a soule more fully drest
> With vertuous gemmes than was his body prest
> With hateful spots, and therefore every scarr
> When death itselfe is dead shall be a starre.[28]

Wishing to lend heroic status to a domestic death, Strode not only employs the familiar spots-gems analogy to turn pustules into noble battle-scars, but in so doing places an impregnable *cordon sanitaire* around Savill's virtuous soul.

This conception of smallpox as an unprovoked military assault was most influentially developed in John Oldham's very substantial Pindaric verses

'To the Memory of My Dear Friend, Mr. Charles Morwent'.[29] Morwent had been Oldham's close friend at Wooton-under-Edge grammar school but after taking his BA in 1674 he 'retir'd to Gloucester' where, only twenty, he died of smallpox on 25 August 1675. Oldham's poem is addressed directly to the departed friend who, by way of compliment, is presented as one not destined to linger long in a corrupt world but whose soul, unlike 'thy mortal Frame' will remain 'Free from Contagion' (Stanza XXVI, 433–7). Morwent nobly bore being 'fetter'd here in brittle Clay', but his spirit longed for 'dear Enlargement' and 'wish't to disengage and fly away . . . to the sweet Freedom of Eternity' (577–85):

> XXXIII
> Nor were its Wishes long unheard,
> Fate soon at its desire appear'd,
> And strait for an Assault prepar'd.
> A suddain and a swift Disease
> First on thy Heart Life's chiefest Fort does seize,
> And then on all the Suburb-vitals preys:
> Next it corrupts thy tainted Blood.
> And scatters Poyson thro' its purple Flood.
> Sharp Aches in thick Troops it sends,
> And Pain, which like Rack the Nerves extends.
> Anguish through every Member flies,
> And all those inward *Gemonies*
> Whereby frail Flesh in Torture dies. (595)

The Gemonies – being used here in the figurative sense of 'tortures' – is a telling reference to the steps on the Aventine at Rome to which the bodies of executed criminals were dragged by the use of a hook in the mouth before being thrown in the Tiber. For Oldham's educated readership the reference offers a suitably gruesome image of bodily desecration. Oldham also invokes the emotional impact of seeing engraved illustrations of other acts of physical violation: those 'Shapes of Torture, which to view in Paint / Would make another faint; / Thou could'st endure in true reality, / And feel what some could hardly bear to see' (636–39). Oldham's comparisons with scenes of torture are probably what prompted William Thompson's subsequent allusions, as discussed in Chapter 2, to graphic depictions of the cruelties of the Inquisition when recounting his own painful experience of smallpox.

The personification of smallpox as a rapacious assailant is even more prevalent in the many poems mourning female victims penned by men. These are dominated by romanticised, if often retributive images of

wounding enabled through the appropriation of Petrarchan conceits which
rest upon heroic conceptions of the *femme fatale* or beautiful woman as a
dangerous conqueror of men's hearts. One such extended analogy forms
the central conceit in Samuel Holland's elegy 'On the Untimely and Much
Lamented Death of Mrs Anne Gray, the Daughter of the Learnedly
Accomplist Doctor Nicholas Gray of Tunbridge in Kent, who dyed of
the Small Pox', published as a broadsheet dated 24 March 1656. Holland
argues that 'Death' who boasts of his 'high Prerogative' and 'hourly
Conquests over all alive',

> Did here begin the startle and did seeme
> To fear her Beauties would now conquer him
> Therefore a danger to prevent so nigh,
> Drew forth at once all his Artillery,
> And so direct a Battery laid,
> So full the Charge, so fast the Case-shot play'd,
> That the poore Body fell upon the place,
> A thousand wounds being printed on her face . . .[30]

The punitive strain in these early elegies anticipates that encountered in a
large number of eighteenth-century verses and other writing focusing upon
the scarring of female survivors to be discussed in Chapter 5. Here it is
sufficient to note that such texts frequently betray a vicious note rooted in a
desire for revenge. For example, in verses 'Upon Madam A. C. a fair Lady
that dyed of the Small-Pox' by the cavalier wit Matthew Stevenson, the
poet's main concern is again the destruction of female beauty, but having
first tried to draw an unconvincing analogy between the heat of smallpox
fever and the warm glow of heaven, he falls back on a familiar rhetoric of
female conquest and masculine captivation. His purportedly consolatory
sentiments, cast in terms of divine justice, carry a distinctly vindictive
undertone:

> So the unruly Blood did over-boil,
> That Beauty is it self become a foil.
> The furious feaver all advantage takes,
> And thus a shadow of a Sun-beam makes.
> Her crystal cheeks, that challeng'd once all praise
> Are now berainbow'd with refracted Rayes.
> Forme! yet forbear, and not a reason ask,
> Since Heaven is pleas'd to put thee on this mask;
> Let no repining open any Lips,
> Shall Heaven the Sun, and not thy face Eclipse?
> Heaven has revok'd the radiance that he gave,
> Where Love had once his Throne, has now his grave.

Not but her Soul, that Spark Immortal, burns
Bright in Dark-Lanthorns, or obscurer Urnes.
Whose forme, though faded, and her face uneven,
Through this red-lattice found the way to heaven.
What though distempers moulder the Mud-wall,
Captives are ransom'd where the Prisons fall.
Was it not time to quit that batter'd Fort,
Where every Pimple was a Sally-port?
But she has ended now her Christian wars,
And thus in triumph carrys off her scars.[31]

After shutting down any avenue of complaint on the woman's part, this closing couplet struggles to adopt the usual Crusader imagery to wrest back a compliment. In this context Anselment rightly observes that while 'the metaphoric rainbow and lattice' do at least have some basis 'in the actual red and varicolored eruptions', Stevenson's 'image of sallyports or fortress gates upsets the connection between the figurative and the literal'; nothing 'sallies forth' from oozing pustules 'except a vile smelling suppuration'.[32]

For Anselment, Stevenson's elegy exemplifies a certain failure of poetic sensibility found in the work of other minor seventeenth-century elegists writing on smallpox amongst whom such free associations tend to become 'a mere poetic exercise' in 'laboured originality'; the worst examples, he observes, 'develop a strained wit even more disconcerting than the grotesque and ironic reaction to venereal disease'.[33] Desperate to salvage something of the body's lost integrity, for such poets 'the noisomeness of smallpox must be confronted . . . yet it also has to be denied or transformed'. Anselment does acknowledge however that their repeated insistence upon a resemblance between pustules and jewels or stars was not simply unrestrained wit but part of a bid for 'intellectual control over the destruction wrought by the smallpox' as they 'struggled to find purpose and even beauty in the appalling disease'. Death from smallpox, Anselment concludes, presented elegists with a distinctive problem in aesthetics in which the 'figurative and the literal are indeed ambivalently bound together'.[34]

Such ambivalences open up wider questions with regard to the ontology of the body. Writing on 'disease and disorder', the social theorist Bryan Turner notes that while 'questions concerning birth, dying, personhood and social membership are indications of a generic issue which hinges on the relationship between nature and culture, the concept of 'disease' is the most sensitive indicator of the problematic quality of the nature / culture division'.[35] Considered in these terms smallpox presented a challenge to established distinctions between the body social and the body natural.

Largely unresponsive to the cultural intervention of medical praxis, the
smallpox victim suffered a loss of bodily integrity as the epidermis became
semi-porous through the eruption of suppurating, foul smelling pustules.
Suggestive of the premature, accelerated putrescence of the grave, this
pocked and putrid body seemed to confront any observer with traumatic
visible evidence of the often repudiated, but nevertheless inevitable fact
that all bodies eventually return to nature. Such foul symptoms represented
a breakdown of the boundary between the body's inner, threateningly fluid
interior and the established public contours of an individuated, social self.
Characterised by porosity and protuberance, the smallpoxed body presented the helpless onlooker with what Bakhtin, in his influential account
of Rabelais, considered 'the artistic logic of the grotesque image' for it
'ignores the closed, smooth impenetrable surface of the body and retains
only its excrescences (sprouts, buds) and orifices' and thus 'leads beyond
the body's limited space or into the body's depths'.[36] Bakhtin himself notes
that in the early modern period, when putrefaction and fecundity were
often conflated, the grotesque body was as much associated with death and
decay as with sexuality, birth and becoming. The elegists used the mythopoetic symbolism of stars and flowers to rescue the body of the smallpox
victim, lending it the life-affirmative, if not carnivalesque qualities the
Russian theorist claimed for some popular invocations of the grotesque
(though the latter term, with its more comic implications, does describe the
tone of some of the more irreverent, facetious responses to facial scarring
discussed in a later chapter). Poems concerned with the disfigurement of
both victims and survivors can all be read as efforts to comprehend and
thus contain the disease's ultimately deadly powers of disruption; attempts
to recall and rescue what Bakhtin terms the individual's 'closed, smooth,
and impenetrable' social body from a sudden monstrous transformation
that renders once firm flesh permeable.

However, in presenting such a drastic erosion of the boundaries between
inside and outside, nature and culture, the body of the smallpox victim
becomes a site of conflicted desires for, as Anselment also observes,
seventeenth-century smallpox elegies frequently betray an ambivalent
gaze. Compelled by the need to remember and celebrate the smallpox
victim for what they so recently were and yet recoiling in horror at their
transformation into something monstrous and alien, the gaze of the poet
oscillates between attraction and repulsion, fascination and disgust. This is
surely the Freudian 'vortex of summons and repulsion' described in Julia
Kristeva's 'Essay on Abjection'.[37] As a gross disruption of the normally non-
porous boundary between the solid – and thus definable – external surface of

the body and its fluid inside, suppurating pustules exposed what Kristeva calls 'The Horror Within'; in the smallpox corpse we 'behold the breaking down of a world that has erased borders'.[38] Smallpox presented a particularly intensified site of disruption, where the stabilising distinction between the governable body cultural and the disruptive body natural breaks down.[39]

Death, of course, carries varied cultural meanings. For seventeenth-century neo-classicist poets, as Christians they usually present it as a merely physical, transitional state since the soul of a person was considered immortal. As we saw in Thompson's *Sickness*, in their poetic bids to rescue the smallpox victim from gross decay they were able to draw upon both an Ovidian tradition of mythic bodily metamorphosis as well as the Christian concept of transfiguration. This is well illustrated in *Uraniæ Metamorphosis in Sydus; or, The Transfiguration of our Late Gracious Sovereign Queen Mary, Discover'd in a Miraculous Vision, since the Celebration of her Funeral* (1695), which bears on its title page the epigraph 'In nova fert animus mutatas dicere formas corpora . . .', taken from the very opening of the *Metamorphoses*. The anonymous elegist writes as 'a Doctor of Physic' who personally witnessed the symptomatic progress of the Queen's small-pox and 'waited at her Death / And saw Her vent Her utmost panting Breath'. He was by her side when the destroying angel, 'Which gave th'Infection to the Royal Blood', dipped his arrow in poison, and anxiously attended as '. . . *struggling Nature labour'd* tho in vain, / The *'imprison'd Venome* to discharge again':

> I saw when it at first with angry Face
> *Lurk'd* undistinguish'd in the *tainted Mass*;
> And *blooming Spots* appearing from within,
> *Creep'd* through the little *crannies* of the Skin.
> A skin so charming, so wonderous Fair,
> That I want words its Beauty to declare. [. . .]
> The *livid spots* now o'er her Body range,
> The sure forerunners of the Tragick change.
> These give the signal of approaching Death,
> And *curdling* Blood *thick'd* her Sighs and Breath;
> For now the florid rubies shone no more,
> But back retir'd into the putrid Gore;
> The languid Spirits, now few, together throng,
> And slowly drive the Circulation on.
> Or (as Flocks hurri'ed promiscuously stray)
> Through the *Convulsive Channels* fly away. [. . .]
> How wan! How strangely chang'd she seem'd to me
> That knew her in Her Youth and Bravery!

This makes quite a show of rendering symptoms into suitably vivid verse until we reach the unconvincing comparison between a racing pulse and startled sheep. But more crucial to the present discussion is the fact that this attention to corporeal detail is later offset by the poet's vision of a heavenly Mary in which 'her Body now grew EMINENTLY bright..'. No doubt conscious of professional failure, this visionary doctor does not avoid giving us the clinical facts, but enacts a poetic transfiguration which insists upon the miraculous recuperation of an unsullied queen from a 'tainted mass' of 'putrid gore'.

'SOME TEARES DROPT ON THE HERSE . . .'

Alongside the psychological struggles to comprehend, contain and transform the horrors of smallpox revealed in the work of individual elegists we also need to consider the wider social function the production of such memorial verses held within the rituals of mourning. As modern readers encountering such verses in scholarly editions or as on-screen 'texts', we are apt to forget the performative function such poetic tributes originally played in actual funerary rites. Anthropological and sociological studies of the fundamental rituals associated with both births and deaths emphasise how these are designed to subject the individual to acts of social inclusion and exclusion. Structuralist approaches in particular have been alert to the way cultural meanings attached to embodiment reveal how individuals as bodies are understood within a categorical distinction between 'Nature' and 'Culture' (though this dichotomy is of course itself culturally defined). Religious rituals of initiation typically demand cultural work upon the body, such as the washing, cutting and burning involved in baptism, circumcision and scarification. These serve to transform the natural body into a social subject with a name and status. In this context Turner observes how, in traditional societies, 'the fact of birth is not an immediate guarantee of social membership; one had to be transferred from nature to culture by rituals of social inclusion' while adding that likewise the 'transfer of culture back to nature is equally ritualised by exclusionary practices' for 'the dead are buried, cremated or embalmed: their persons are deconstructed by rituals which indicate that they are now to some extent once more "natural" '.[40] As a funeral song, the classical elegy had originally played a participatory part in this process.

Discussing the specific role of 'the lament by a poet for a poet' within the neo-classical tradition of pastoral elegy, Eric Smith remarks that it 'seems as if the flowers strewn on a hearse or tomb in earlier days are in part replaced by the poem itself'.[41] A similar act of substitution is hinted at in Bishop King's 'Elegy on Donne', which talks of how 'Each quill can drop his tributary verse, / And pin it, like a hatchment to his hearse'.[42] This act of somatic substitution implied in a typical title such as *Some Teares Dropt on the Herse of the Incomparable Prince Henry, Duke of Gloucester*, a broadsheet poem of 1660, and reinforced in the elegy's closing claim that 'these Loyal Drops fall'n into Verse / Shall wash the Cypress on his Royal Herse'. But this is not just a figurative embodiment of the act of mourning; such broadsheet poems were designed to be pinned onto the hearse or coffin.[43] By 1700 this practice was ceasing to form part of the rites at upper-class Anglican funerals, but further down the social scale, particularly amongst non-conformists the practice seems to have continued into the next century.[44] Certainly as late as 1716 we find the schoolboy Robert Cotesworth reporting to his father that, 'our seat is to-day making Latin verses upon one of our Scholars who is dead of the small pox; they are to be pinn'd upon the Pall'.[45] As in the contribution of the Westminster School pupils to *Lachrymae Musarum*, the actual writing and anthologised publication of elegies functioned as a therapeutic, collective social activity integral to the mourning process. Drawing attention to the several poems in *Lachrymae Musarum* making direct analogies between imprinting and the tears of the mourners, John McWilliams remarks how 'in this way the ideas of physical, public gathering, and a gathering of print become intertwined'.[46] With its elaborate, black-bordered title-page and engraved frontispiece, *Lachrymae Musarum* was a costly example of a wider phenomenon represented by the survival of numerous individual elegies cheaply printed as single-sided broadsheets.

The ritualistic meanings attached to the transformation of death are strikingly emblematised in the frontispiece to *Lachrymae Musarum* (Illustration 4).[47] At the centre of this engraving we are presented with the image of an upright corpse wrapped in a winding sheet ascending heavenwards out of an embalming tub. A resemblance to the iconography of the risen Christ is clearly deliberate. Largely veiled by the draped sheet, this image of a body with its recognisable contours partially occluded as if already undergoing a process of transformation encapsulates the hope expressed in many of the verses that Hastings's soul remains untouched by the ravages of the disease. But the engraving also emblematises the faith of a seventeenth-century neo-classical tradition in the restorative, redemptive power of poetry motivating all such memorial works.[48] Hastings's apotheosis is witnessed by an astonished group of nine, classical dressed

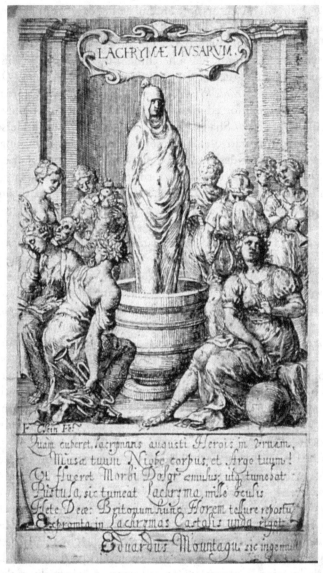

4. Frontispiece to *Lachrymæ Musarum; the Tears of the Muses ... upon the Death of Henry, Lord Hastings* (London, 1649). Smallpox prompted poets to question this image of Apollonian healing in which the muses serve to ease the work of mourning.

female attendants whose various attributes, including musical instruments and theatrical masks, immediately identify them as the nine muses of Apollo. Through the visible connection to the waters of the Castalian spring, the muses are being linked to the purification rituals of actually washing the dead and the healing powers of poetic inspiration. Horace's lines, translating as 'The Muses forbid the man worthy of praise to die', appearing on the opposite title-page serve as a reminder of this memorial-ising function.

Anselment suggests that the primary intention of most early smallpox elegists was not so much 'witty exhibitionism nor clinical objectivity' but what he terms 'a therapeutic fancy'.[49] The implications of this last phrase are worth pursuing. As indicated by the wording in some of their titles, the presentation of elegies as 'cordials' against grief was rooted in a contemporary adherence to an Apollonian notion of the 'profound and mysterious union between the healing powers of language and medicine'.[50] But despite their conventional appeals to the Apollonian muse, early-modern smallpox elegists display no consensus of faith over the adequacy of language when confronted by the ravages of this peculiarly corrupting disease. Certainly the Hasting's frontispiece is accompanied by six lines of Latin verse which seek to forge an analogy between 'the pustule swelled' and the prophylactic 'weeping' of the grief-stricken muses. But while the poet, Edward Montague, offers up these lamentations as 'a rival of the sickness', it is notable however that to do so leaves the 'Castalian stream ... dry' and requires the body of a Niobe and the eyes of an Argus.[51] More confidently the scholar-poet Joshua Barnes begins his tribute to Mary II, by invoking the power of the muse 'whose sweet *Nepenthean* tongue / Can charm the Pangs of Death with Deathless Song / Can stinging Plagues with easie thoughts beguile, / Make Flames and Torments objects of a smile ...'.[52] But it is with less assurance, that the anonymous 'Young Lady' writing her own 'Ode Ocassion'd by the Death of her Sacred Majesty' (1695), asks an 'insolent' smallpox: 'Could not languages of that charming Tongue per-suade, / That ne'er Commanded, but was still Obey'd?' In presenting the snatching of the queen as a failure in due obedience to the all-powerful charms of a woman's tongue, this unidentified poetess puts in question any claims for the prophylactic power of language *per se*.

Thomas Shipman had already cast serious doubt over the power and appropriateness of using poetry to ameliorate the impact of smallpox in his tributary verses 'BEAUTY'S ENEMY. Upon the Death of M. Princess of Orange, by the Small pox, 1660'. He begins by distancing himself from 'those hard Wits, who name the Scars / Upon her Face, Ennamel, and bright Stars' for ''tis a Sin to be / A witty praiser of a Misery'. Such wits, he charges, are in effect crowning themselves with 'Garlands of Flow'rs, which they from Coffins take'. Shipman's strictures against the self-indulgent use of stock tropes to transfigure pock-marks into constellations anticipate those of Johnson a century later yet by the end of this poem Shipman seems to forget his own warning. Declaring that 'Her Eyes, amidst her torments, sparkled beams: / Thus martyred Saints smil'd in their hottest flames', he has to admit that this is undeniably a suitable 'paralel' for one who died 'Beauty's Martyr'. And by the last stanza Shipman is resorting to those very tropes he at first condemns: 'Most cruel Death! could not one wound suffice? / Must she as many have as Heav'n has Eyes? / Each Spot upon her Face a Comet show'd, / Which did, alas, this fatal ruine bode! . . .'[53]

Anselment attributes Shipman's glaring failure to find any more appropriate images to individual artistic weakness, but it also illustrates a problem faced by any poet who, being moved to record the ravages of smallpox, nonetheless felt constrained to keep within the acceptable bounds of literary propriety. If we abandon pursuing an aesthetics of coherence for a critical approach open to such dissonances, any purported weaknesses in Shipman's self-contradictory poem become all the more revealing as evidence of a profounder tension than that suggested in the purely formalist charge of a failure of technique. The poem's self-defeating looping back upon its own desire to avoid cliché not only lays bare the degree to which the language of smallpox elegies had quickly sunk into the rehearsal of a number of predictable codified conventions, but also exposes the limitations on any poet's hopes for the restorative power of words. For all its Apollonian claims, poetry proved no ultimate protection against smallpox. Indeed, like monarchs, many poets also famously fell prey to the disease.

'HOW MANY LIVING LYRES, BY THEE UNSTRUNG . . .?'

> As Adders deaf to Beauty, Wit, and Youth,
> How many living Lyres, by Thee unstrung,
> E'er half their Tunes are ended, cease to charm
> Th' admiring World?   from William Thompson, *Sickness*.[54]

Reflecting upon his own good fortune in surviving smallpox, in 1745 William Thompson could readily answer his own rhetorical question by reciting a mournful catalogue of less fortunate fellow poets whose literary careers had been cruelly curtailed by the disease. He includes the names of Katherine Philips – 'By Cowley honour'd, by Roscommon lov'd' – who died in 1664 aged thirty-three, John Oldham, who died of smallpox in 1683 at the age of twenty-nine and the painter and poet Anne Killigrew who was barely twenty-five when she died in the London epidemic of 1685.[55] A full list of post-Restoration poets lost to smallpox would also have to include John Pomfret who succumbed in 1702, Octavia Walsh who died in 1706 and William Pattison who was only twenty when he died of smallpox in 1727.

With so many literary lives prematurely thwarted, it is understandable that Thompson imagined smallpox as a disease with specific designs on poets but rather than evidence of a professional predisposition, such prominence is, of course, merely the illusory effect of the very process of accumulative literary memorialising to which *Sickness* itself contributes. Philips's sudden death in particular, coloured by the irony that this came just a few weeks after she penned her elegy to another smallpox victim Lord Rich, was to prompt some influential poetic responses. Indeed Thompson's own phrasing echoes the opening of Cowley's famous verses *On the death of Mrs. Katherine Philips* composed as personal address to the 'Cruel Disease!'[56] Cowley's poem pursues an extended argument structured around six rhetorical questions challenging an unchivalrous disease, a familiar enemy who, in destroying 'The Matchless Orinda' out of 'old and constant spight', tyrannically oversteps the limits of just warfare. Smallpox is not actually named – Cowley assumes his readers know how Philips died – but it is pointedly addressed here as a male aggressor whose 'Depredations' are rooted in 'Thy Malice or thy Lust'. Smallpox especially likes to vex 'the fairest Sex' and 'in them most assault the fairest place, / The Throne of Empress Beauty, ev'n the Face',

> There was enough of that here to asswage,
> (One would have thought) either thy Lust or Rage,
> Was't not enough, when thou, prophane Disease.
>   Dids't on this Glorious Temple seize.
> Was't not enough, like a wild Zealot, there,
> All the rich outward Ornaments to tear,
> Deface the innocent pride of beauteous Images?
> Was't not enough thus rudely the goodly Pile?
> And thy unbounded Sacriledge commit
> On th'inward Holiest Holy of her Wit?[57]

Exploiting the traditional Christian trope of the body as a temple of the soul, Cowley presents this assault upon the body of the female poet as an act of blasphemous iconoclasm. The overt allusion to the sacking of the Temple of Jerusalem is prompted by the usual assumption that smallpox originates in the Middle East, but coming from the pen of such a staunch royalist as Cowley, the extended image of smallpox as an enthusiastic fanatic is surely yet another barely coded reminder of puritan depredations on church monuments during the Civil War and Commonwealth. But Cowley defiantly asserts that there are limits to the disease's destructive power:

> Cruel disease! There thou mistook'st thy power;
>   No Mine of Death can that devour,
> On her embalmed Name it will abide
>   An everlasting Pyramide
> As high as Heav'n, the top, as Earth, the Basis wide.[58]

Philips's 'Wit', as represented in the abiding body of her poetry comes to serve in the place traditionally ascribed to the soul. It represents the transcendental part of the self that escapes diminishment by a disease which can only destroy the body physical.

Cowley's emphasis upon Philips's physical beauty illustrates how it proves impossible for a contemporary male commentator to compliment a woman's literary achievements without first dwelling upon her physical appearance. The same applies to Dryden's famous ode 'To the Pious Memory of the Accomplisht Young Lady Mrs Anne Killigrew, Excellent in the two Sister-Arts of Poësie, and Painting' in which he praises his female counterpart's beauty as much as her artistic accomplishments.[59] Dryden, a family associate, originally wrote this poetic tribute to serve as a preface to a legacy volume of Killigrew's poems published at the family's instigation within three months of her death.[60] A Maid of Honour, Killigrew was known in court circles as an accomplished painter, but her poetry had only been circulated in manuscript.[61] In what is often acknowledged to be Dryden's most accomplished use of the loose Pindaric stanza-form, he only alludes to smallpox as the cause of Killigrew's death towards the close (in stanza VIII). Echoing the imagery of Cowley's elegy to Philips, Dryden directly links the loss of Killigrew with that of Philips, whose work was familiar to the younger poet, and whose sobriquet 'The Matchless Orinda' encapsulated her posthumous role in being held up as a chaste moral *exempla* for the next generation of women poets.[62] Complaining that Killigrew's beauty and grace will never be seen again by mortals, and that smallpox has acted like a 'hard'nd Fellon' who does not simply murder, but also defaces his victim, Dryden employs the established metaphor of a violated temple:

> O double Sacriledge on things Divine,
> To rob the Relique, and deface the Shrine!

> But thus *Orinda* dy'd:
> Heav'n, by the same Disease, did both translate,
> As equal were their Souls, so equal was their Fate.[63]

Dryden's modern editors suggest that his closing use of this metaphor of literary translation to equate the premature curtailment of the careers of both poets by the same disfiguring disease may be a specific borrowing from Sir Charles Cotterell's preface to *Poems by the most deserved Admired Mrs. Katherine Philips The Matchless Orinda* (1667).

Writing as Philips's literary executor, Cotterell regrets that she did not live long enough to revise her own poetry for the press. In so doing he employs a telling extended metaphor to denounce the piratical printing of an unauthorised edition of Philips's poems in 1664:

But the small Pox, that malicious disease (as knowing how little she would have been concern'd for her handsomeness, when at the best) was not satisfied to be as injurious a Printer of her face, as the other had been of her Poems, but treated her with a more fatal cruelty than the Stationer had them; for though he to her most sensible affliction surreptitiously possess'd himself of a false Copy, and sent those children of her Fancy into the World, so martyred, that they were more unlike themselves than she could have been made had she escaped; that murtherous Tyrant, with greater barbarity seiz'd unexpectedly upon her, the true Original, and to the much juster affliction of all the world, violently tore her out of it, and hurried her untimely to her Grave, upon the 22. of June 1664. she being then but 31 years of age.

But he could not bury her in Oblivion, for this Monument which she erected for her self, will for ever make her to be honoured as the honour of her Sex . . .[64]

Cotterell's comparison between the disfigurement of Philips's poetry by pirate booksellers and the premature disfigurement of her beauty by the disease forges an arresting metaphoric link between female textual and sexual reproduction. In his role as Philips's heroic champion Cotterell makes flattering claims for her lack of personal vanity in her physical appearance, yet the rhetorical force of his analogy relies upon the woman poet's reproductive body and literary productions being seen as inextricably linked together in terms of male admiration and violation. Philips's poems are the abused 'children of her Fancy'; unwillingly thrust out into the world after being disfigured by an unauthorised editor, they are as alienated from themselves as their mother would have been had she survived but left disfigured by the smallpox which killed her. In turn Cotterell takes on the role of executive guardian to these literary orphans: her 'once transformed, or rather deformed Poems, which, are here in some measure restor'd to their native Shape and Beauty and therefore certainly cannot fail of a welcome reception now, since they wanted it not before, when they appeared in that strange disguise'.[65] Professional male intervention purports to rescue Philips's poetry from a mortal disfigurement she herself proved unable to avoid. Dryden's adoption of a similar stance of chivalrous recuperation in his subsequent composition of a double-elegy to Philips and Killigrew served to reinforce the literary image of smallpox as the peculiar nemesis of female beauty, virtue and wit. We shall return to examine these continued associations between women and disfigurement by smallpox in Chapter 5, but first I consider how the mortuary tradition developed in the eighteenth century.

CHAPTER 4

Sentimental smallpox

With smallpox remaining endemic and frequently epidemic throughout eighteenth-century Britain, elegists were far from being left redundant, but inevitably their responses show signs of stylistic transformation in keeping with changing attitudes to death.[1] As noted earlier, for Samuel Johnson writing in the 1760s, the attempts by an earlier generation of poets to wittily transform pustules into rose-buds or gems smacked of metaphysical 'wit' rather than true poetry.[2] Johnson was recoiling from an overly-intellectual poetics of death dependent upon the kind of mortuary detail we typically encounter in earlier seventeenth-century smallpox elegies. In this context Draper notes that of all Dryden's many elegiac poems Johnson favoured that to Killigrew 'which barely mentions the tomb and only in connection with the Resurrection'.[3] Fed by the increasingly more optimistic religiosity of low-church dissenters the literary response to death gradually abandons the type of horrid detail hitherto prompted by smallpox in favour of a far greater emphasis upon spiritual transcendence. Moreover, as Draper observes, the emotionalism of the post-Restoration puritan elegy furnished 'a fertile field for the cultivation of Sentimentalism', as mortuary realism gives way to a heightened psychological interest in the pathos of grief.[4] Summarising this shift of aesthetic focus Elisabeth Bronfen talks of how 'the emergence of the modern family, of a new spiritualization of human experience, of the new emphasis on personal affections, sentiments and the imagination brought about a new welcoming of death, but with the attention on the surviving family not on the dying individual'.[5] With the consolidation of the bourgeois economic and cultural revolution of 1689 this shift of tone becomes all the more pronounced from mid-century onwards, not least in the narrative context of the emergent novel, a principal vehicle for the promotion of the sentimental values underpinning what G. J. Barker-Benfield has influentially termed 'the culture of sensibility'.[6] As a particularly horrifying cause of domestic tragedy, smallpox plays an ambiguous role within this culture; the great enemy of family harmony, it nonetheless provides writers with a suitably familiar motif of the unifying power of shared grief with which to touch the reader.

Anselment's account of smallpox elegies ends around 1700, so I begin below by outlining the subsequent pietist and romantic developments in this sub-genre, focusing in on the work of the popular dissenter, poet, hymnologist and educationalist Isaac Watts (1674–1748). After pausing over the tale of colonial misadventure portrayed in Robert Gould's rather exceptional verses 'To the Memory of Mr. James Margetts' appearing in 1709, I address some of the highly sentimental narrative representations of smallpox as domestic tragedy to be found in early novels. The chapter concludes with an analysis of the popular narrative of the tragic fate of the South-Sea Islander, 'Prince Lee Boo' and considers its political function as a cautionary tale of imperial ingratitude.

THE SENTIMENTAL ELEGISTS

For a convenient measure of the shift in poetic responses to death from smallpox we might compare Dryden's elegy on Hastings with the elegy 'On the Death of a Favourite Schoolfellow. Phillip Bonafous, who died of small pox, in 1785', to be found amongst the poetic *juvenilia* of John Thelwall, better known as the leading reformist orator of the 1790s and an early associate of the young Coleridge and Wordsworth. Written a hundred and thirty years apart, both poems were prompted by the loss of a school-friend to smallpox, but where Dryden's elegy contrives to recover stellar knowledge and florid beauty out of the defiled corpse of dead youth, Thelwall's verses, with their repetition of the opening phrase 'I grieve to think . . .', draw attention to the feelings of the mourner and the loss of friendship. Printed in 1801, under the telling sub-heading 'Effusions of Social and Relative Affection', the elegy mourns Bonafous as having himself been an exemplary sentimentalist:

> How fraught with tender feelings was his mind!
> O'oerflowing font of sensibility!
> To friend's how true! to relatives how kind!
> In generous zeal, how boundless and how free![7]

Although Thelwall abstractedly mourns how 'O'er his fair form the noxious pest prevail'd', this is the only reference to disease and while he indulges pastoral conventions to compare his 'heart's elected friend' to some neglected 'hedge-row flower' whose virtue will yet continue to 'blossom in my view', there are no witty attempts to transform pustules into florets.

As already seen in the elegies to Killigrew and Philips, the poetic shift away from contrived, corporeal puns has particular significance with respect to the commemoration of women victims in a culture in which the female body already risks attracting the added burden of sexual sin; a tension highlighted in John Tutchin's verses 'On the Death of Mrs E. P. Who died of the Small-Pox' appearing in 1685. Tutchin's primary focus is upon the failure of the deceased woman's friends to recognise her innate divinity as a 'Sacred Maid'. The poet's gaze barely lingers upon her pocked body in any search for recuperative analogies, but passes right through it to the incorruptible soul within: 'thou hadst a Body, but it was / Clearer than transparent Glass; / Through which thy Virtue did appear'. Tutchin draws out a comparison with a hero dressed in 'homely weeds' who has roamed anonymously amongst 'th'illiterate crowd', 'unprais'd' and 'unevy'd'. Such flattery would be unremarkable were it not for Tutchin's conclusion:

> The Monster man long since has worn out
> His rags of Virtue, which he did retain:
> In Goodness weak, in Villanies grown stout;
> He vows he'll ne'er be good again.
> Stupid he lyes, and senseless in his Vice;
> He shar'd the Fall in Sin, but not in Virtues Rise.
> Woman alone does climb the Holy Hill;
> But Man below remains a Devil still:
> They ne're expect in Heaven a room,
> Only good poets and good Women thither come.[8]

This elevation of the virtuous woman may reflect the influence of Tutchin's dissenter background: his father and grandfather were both non-conformist ministers and the poet supported the Duke of Monmouth's attempted coup, before becoming a Whig pamphleteer and journalist.[9] But while the non-conformist tradition tended to accord women significant social status as spiritual oracles and moral exemplars, as Tutchin's poem suggests, this required that they conformed to a reductive stereotype of chaste, disembodied virtue. In this respect it differs little from an older cult of the Assumption of the Virgin Mary in which, as Bronfen notes 'the feminisation of the ideal, the glorified substance, is representative of alterity, of Woman as ethereal being, to be venerated in her intact splendour' (68). The figure of the Virgin 'functions as an epitome of timelessness, of undifferentiated, immortal beauty and bliss, and an allegory for the defeat of death and the promise of eternal life, precisely because in her mythic construction the materiality or body is missing from the

start' (68). With smallpox so readily appropriated as a sign of Eve's legacy
of sinfulness, death and decay as rooted in the animal body and sexuality,
the image of a sacred virgin provided an alternative strategy for the writer
seeking to protect the reputation of a female victim. Although elegies to
women dying of smallpox had always tended to portray a process of
transfiguration from one form of disembodiment to another, with the
cultural consolidation of the Whig revolution of 1689 placing added weight
upon reforming values hitherto defined as feminine – chastity, piety,
politeness, charity, benevolence and sympathy – flattering elegies to real
women, like those to Killigrew and Philips, increasingly cast them as
wholly disembodied, angelic beings who were simply too good for this
world.

ISAAC WATTS ON SMALLPOX

The ideal of disembodied female virtue is pronounced in the popular verses
of the influential dissenter Isaac Watts. For example, in 'An Elegiac
Thought on Mrs. Anne Warner, Who died of the Small-pox, Dec. 18,
1707, at one O'clock in the Morning, a few Days after the Birth and Death
of her first Child', Watt's seeks the aid of the Miltonic muse Urania to offer
a reassuring, uplifting vision of Warner's death as an entry into paradise
where she will be happily reunited with her short-lived baby and her
ancestors, 'a pious race'.[10] Watts presents Warner in terms of her familial
duties to her earthly and spiritual fathers as he portrays her dwelling
in angelic proximity to her maker while anticipating the arrival of her
dear husband. In its emphasis upon familial re-union beyond the grave,
Watts's vision accords with a broader trend, identified by Bronfen, in
which death 'became a private event, assuring continuity in the form of a
family unity and an androcentric domestication of heaven that saw it as a
continuation of repetition of earthly existence, not as a completely other
sphere' (87). The historian Phillipe Ariès called the eighteenth century 'the
age of the beautiful death'.[11] Such beautification, in Bronfen's summary
'was used to hide the physical sins of mortality and decay and to overcome
any sense of separation or loss of individualism' (87). But when the poet's
vision of a blissful, heavenly family reunion required an act of beautification, then clearly death from smallpox, with its power to wholly alienate
the dying from their prematurely putrescent loved ones, posed a peculiar
challenge.

Returning to Watts's elegy to Warner, we notice that the elegist's sights
only very briefly stray back down from his patriarchal vision of a domestic

'circle of love' to the morbid details of a smallpox death, and even then, he only looks back with reluctance:

> . . .O stamp upon my soul
> Some blissful image of the fair deceas'd
> To call my passions and my eyes aside
> From the dear breathless clay, distressing sight![12]

Calling for divine aid in this need to retain a beatified image of Warner, Watts struggles to avoid having this obliterated by the more immediate facts of physical defilement:

> I look and mourn and gaze with greedy view
> Of melancholy fondness: Tears bedewing
> That form so late desir'd, so late belov'd,
> Now loathsome and unlovely. Base disease,
> That leagu'd with nature's sharpest pains, and spoil'd
> So sweet a structure! The impoisoning taint
> O'erspreads the building wrought with skill divine,
> And ruins the rich temple to the dust!
>
> Was this the countenance, where the world admir'd
> Features of wit and virtue? This the face
> Where love triumph'd? and beauty on these cheeks,
> As on a throne, beneath her radiant eyes
>
> Was seated to advantage; mild, serene,
> Reflecting rosy light?[13]

Though this passage echoes many earlier elegies to beautiful women, when it comes to answering his own rhetorical questions Watts avoids trying to draw cosmic analogies out of gruesome details. He simply returns to an image replete with the promise of re-illumination by comparing Warner's eclipse to that of the setting sun. In this context John Hoyles notes that being a Cartesian, 'Watts was incapable of taking the microcosmic world of correspondences seriously' and largely avoided metaphysical conceits.[14]

In the surviving cover letter Watts sent to Warner's father with a copy of this elegy, the poet explains that when recollecting deceased friends 'I frequently rove the world of spirits, and search them out there' so when 'the verse breaks off abruptly' this is partly because 'when I was fallen upon the dark side of death, I had no mind to tarry there'.[15] Watts humbly claimed to write merely to ease his own grief as the 'thoughts came crowding fast upon me', but the resulting optimistic effusions convey a fresh, impassioned directness of feeling. This made them readily accessible to non-educated readers and they proved very popular with collected editions being reprinted by the thousands throughout the eighteenth century.[16] Draper, for one, in tracing the emergence of the romantic elegy, highlights Watts's bereavement poems as significant examples of the move away from a seventeenth-century 'horror of death' towards an eighteenth-century 'fondness for the pensive sadness of lingering memories'.[17] With such direct emotional appeal, Watt's memorial verses broke the mould of Calvinist austerity in church worship assuring that elegiac song remained a respectable part of dissenting funerary practice.

Watts penned at least five poems prompted by the trauma of smallpox. Such engagement is a reflection of the ubiquity of the disease, but it also had a more personal motivation. An autobiographical 'Table of Coincidents' records that Watts had himself survived smallpox in 1683 at the age of nine when he would not have been too young to remember the experience. The physical and mental after-effects are undoubtedly registered in the weak health he suffered throughout adulthood which is often a cause for spiritual reflection in his writing.[18] Hoyles, in his unduly neglected study of the 'waning of the Renaissance' in post-Restoration poetics, specifically isolates the hymnologist's 'treatment of the theme of smallpox' for discussion, but only to find that the horror is 'merely coated with the rather nauseous varnish of eighteenth-century indulgence'.[19] Taking issue with Draper, and citing the very same lines from the Warner tribute I quoted earlier, Hoyles talks of how this 'varnish is laid on thick' such that 'the precise symptoms of smallpox barely show'. But he allows that 'the result maintains a basic element of precocity such as is to be found *par excellence* in Dryden's "Upon the Death of Lord Hastings"' even though this is partly 'obscured by layers of sublimity and sentiment'.[20] However one responds to this process of occlusion, Watts's smallpox poems occupy an important transitional place in the history of this sub-genre.

Hoyle's prefers Watts's slightly later 'Elegy on Sophronia, who died of the small-pox, 1711' in which 'the physical symptoms . . . are given more attention, but their horror is covered by the elegant poetic diction and smooth syntax'.[21] In this more dramatic poem Watts adopts the voice of 'Sophron' a bereaved, unconsolable lover, but characteristic emphasis is placed upon Sophronia's exemplary life of pious retirement away from the corrupting influences of court society: 'Devotion was her work', while her soul was made of 'Celestial dew, / And angels' food were her repast.[22] Although this elegy relies upon a well-worn comparison between the beautiful, but red-faced smallpox victim and the short-lived bloom of roses, the poem does carry a certain simple dignity in confronting the symptoms:

> III.
> Unkind disease, to veil that rosy face
> With tumours of a mortal pale,
> While mortal purples with their dismal grace
> And double horror spot the veil.
>
> IV.
> Uncomely veil, and most unkind disease!
> Is this Sophronia, once the fair?
> Are these the features that were born to please?
> And beauty spread her ensigns there?[23]

This displays literary ambition in rendering private tragedy as conventional pastoral drama, but other verses such as his prayer 'For a Child in the Smallpox', clearly arose even more immediately out of Watts's practical duties and evangelical concerns as a lay minister.

In this poetic prayer Watts makes a personal supplication to Christ that he will manifest his 'saving love' and he tries to justify suffering as part of a redemptive plan, for 'Love inflicts the plague severe, / Love the dire distemper sends', and it is Christ who also gives us the power to cope with suffering if we 'Tear our hearts from earth away' and 'Nail them to Thy bleeding cross'.[24] Pleading for merciful divine intervention, Watts draws a comparison between a parent's fears for the loss of their son in the smallpox and the sufferings of God when his own son became a sacrifice on Calvary. In a similar sacrificial vein Watts's 'A Prayer for Mrs. Vigor, When her Son Was in the Small-Pox' draws upon the Christian notion that children are God's gifts and as such can be taken back into his keeping. The speaker asks Jesus to 'regard a mother's sighs' while 'Isaac on the altar lies, / Her loved and only son', as she meekly waits to discover 'If Thou her son demand'. These same reassurances are offered in Samuel Wesley's verses 'On the RECOVERY of Lady Margaret Harley (now Duchess of Portland) from the Small-Pox' where placating parental anxiety is once again the central concern.[25]

Looking back from our more secular age of medical materialism such reassurances might appear alien, if not cruelly glib, but they remind us of the framework of faith in doctrines of providential wisdom and expiatory sacrifice within which the pains of smallpox and disease in general were framed, endured and understood. For all their literary simplicity, the mode of sentimental devotional verse employed by Watts and his religious associate Elizabeth Rowe, and further popularised by the Wesleys, provided a psychologically supportive explanatory framework within which the afflicted sought to come to terms with the sudden threat of losing loved-ones and the apparently arbitrary patterns of survival.[26]

The identity of 'Mrs Vigor' remains obscure, but amongst those to whom Watts gave spiritual succour as minister and poet was his devotee Frances Seymour. The countess's surviving letters to Watts and to others in their pious circle reveal how she never fully recovered from the loss of her only son, Lord Beauchamp, to smallpox in 1744.[27] Writing to a friend in 1746 Hertford explains that 'when I lost my dear, and by me, ever-lamented Son, every faculty to please ... died with him ... the Joy and Pride of my heart withers in his Grave' and 'my Mind is continually haunting those Mansions of the Dead ... for, after my dear Beauchamp, what human Things can appear permanent? Youth, Beauty, Virtue, health, were not sufficient to save him from the Hand of Death! And who can then think themselves secure'.[28] Alongside her Bible, the grief-stricken Hertford turned to poetry for consolation, but when she came to read Shenstone's 'Ode to Autumn' she was sorry not to share his sentiments:

... he hates it as a Season which deprived him of a Friend; I love it because the latest Days my heart could boast of Happiness, in the best and most beloved of Sons ... Every thing around me seemed to sympathize with my distress, and still every melancholy Anniversary of my ever-to-be lamented Loss, put on the same friendly Appearance of social Sorrow.[29]

Hertford's evocation of the pathetic fallacy registers the emergence of the romantic literary sensibility I have been mapping above, though regrettably her response to Thompson's direct tribute to her son in *Sickness* appears to be lost.[30]

THE FATE OF JAMES MARGETTS

Thompson was not the first poet to write a memorial to a young man who died of smallpox while venturing abroad. Robert Gould's 'To the memory of Mr. James Margetts who died of the Small Pox in his voyage to Pensilvania', published in his posthumous *Works* of 1709, occupies a rather unique place in this history. Stylistically Gould's substantial memorial poem aspires to a restrained, neo-classicism but unusually it offers a narrative account of the circumstances surrounding Margetts's death at sea; a structure more suggestive of a popular ballad.[31] This aesthetic hybridity may be accounted for by the fact that Gould was a self-educated servant who later found patronage as a poet and playwright in the employ of James, Earl of Abingdon. Margetts remains obscure, though internal evidence implies that Gould witnessed the youth's parting moments with his parents.

Gould's poem relates what would have been a common tale of colonialist misadventure in a period when the risks of contracting contagious diseases on any sea passage were high. Later in the century, in the wider context of British colonial expansion, calls were to be made for the mass inoculation or vaccination of naval personnel on the grounds of military contingency. More specifically Gould's poem dates from a period when smallpox was starting to take hold amongst the increasingly urbanised white New England settlers who had previously attributed their apparent immunity to God's special providence.[32] By 1709, as minister of Boston's Old Church, Cotton Mather – who eventually promoted mass inoculations – was speculating as to why God appeared to have deserted his chosen people. Mather had recently learnt about the West African folk practice of inoculating for smallpox from the slave he named Onesimus.[33] By 1717 Boston was to establish a quarantine hospital on Spectacle Island as part of wider moves to prevent the introduction of smallpox into the East Coast ports.[34]

Gould opens his tribute to Margetts by pointing-up the irony that when this hopeful youth had courageously left the 'Albion Shore' who 'wou'd have thought, in this delightful Scene, / Secur'd without, they'd find a Foe within, / Worst than the wildest Tempest cou'd have been?' The poem closes on the irony that a certain 'Blake' (unidentified), who has accompanied Margetts had been spared from contracting smallpox on board ship, but 'in vain' for no sooner had he reached 'the Pensilvania Air', he succumbed to a 'lean Consumption' and 'but liv'd to mourn his Loss, and dyed!' In between Gould upbraids smallpox, wondering why is it not enough that 'at land you reign' without erecting 'Trophies on the Main'? It is a 'Leprous Fury' with a quiver-full of arrows loaded with 'Ghastly Bane' who aimed 'the pestilential Blast' at everyone on board and like a hungry lion who 'sullenly devours, and grumbles while he's pleas'd'. Medicine proves useless:

> In vain alas! the Aid that Drugs wou'd lend!
> Not Art, nor nature cou'd their Charge defend;
> Th'Assistants soon like the assisted grew,
> And then as fast infected others too.
> All Hands aloft had now been heard in vain;
> The barbar'ous Ill had so decreas'd the Train,
> The Ship as if unman'd, lay floating on the Main. (252)

Gould shows no compunction in expressing his regret that the disease did not settle with 'Lives we can cheaply Sell, / A vulgar Heard, who Spite and

Nonsense rules, / The Grin of Wit, and Proselytes of Fools'. Like the Israelites with the Massacre of the Innocents, he would have happily seen a thousand more sacrificed if heaven had seen fit to save 'the Youth'. He only finds comfort in the fact that Margetts 'had lost all Sense of Pain' because by the time he died on the ninth day of his illness he had long lain in a 'Death-like Silence':

> For, (as it were it self too mild a Fate,)
> A Fever still does on this Fury wait,
> Which with the Blood a Raging Venom blends,
> And then in wayward Fumes up to the Brain ascends,
> From whence a Thousand Fantoms take their Birth;
> But, Tyrant like, they're fatal in their Mirth:
> Thus lay the Youth, and in these last Extremes
> Was forming to himself delightful Schemes
> Of various things, but all without offence;
> Reason was gone, but not his Innocence.
> Ah! better, better far, than 'tis to be
> At our last Gasp of Perfect Memory,
> With all our Friends (as they were dying too)
> Pale with Affright, and shrieking at the view . . .
> Thus in a fatal Calm he Life resign'd,
> But left a Tempest of Despair behind! (253)

Gould goes on to express regret over the need for a burial at sea, for 'Ev'n yet, deform'd as 'tis, too sweet a Prey / For the remorseless Monsters of the Sea', but he finds some succour in the fact that this contingency did save Margetts' parents the additional pain of seeing his disfigured corpse: 'O Sight! well from his Parents Eyes with-held! / A Sight where Death was by himself excell'd!' (255)

Gould moves on to recall the grieved reactions of Margetts' mother, father, sisters, and brother as each in turn hears the news of the death. Bishop Richard Kidder, a relative through marriage, is 'emasculated' by the news (Kidder's 'Collate'ral Grief' was no doubt fuelled by the fact, not made explicit in the actual poem, that the Bishop had himself lost three children to smallpox in 1680).[35] Gould reassures the family that death marks 'the end of Fear' and suggests that they take some solace from the fact that their young son did not live long enough to be corrupted by a venal and irreligious world. They are to consider that they were spared prior knowledge of their son's illness, as Gould recalls the 'Train of Agonies' they recently went through with their other, younger son 'When in the same Distemper, late, he lay, / Delerious, and gasping Life away'. That son survived smallpox. Although their eldest did not, Gould assures them that this is merely the 'shunning' of a longer 'stay' for he has 'gone to the regions of Eternal Day'.

The multiple impact of smallpox upon the Margetts family was very typical. Gould's attempts at reassurance risk sounding platitudinous, but there is some literary originality in his dramatic invocation of the ship-board setting. In Gould's images of an infected ship we catch a crude precedent for the depiction of a death-ship in the 'Rime of the Ancient Mariner' which, it has been suggested, was itself shaped by Coleridge's own close-encounters with smallpox. His notable failure to write an elegy to his son Berkeley may have stemmed from guilt over his absence in Germany, but other fathers did attempt to express their feelings over the loss of children to smallpox.

FAMILIAL LOSSES

The autobiographical 'Elegy on a Favourite Child Who Died of the Small-pox' by the largely self-educated, so-called 'yeoman poet' James Woodhouse, is one of the more substantial later Georgian smallpox elegies. Woodhouse (1735–1820), an associate of his neighbour and fellow poet William Shenstone, was at times farmer, landscape gardener, steward and bookseller.[36] Composed in 1779 in what by this date are rather over-used heroic couplets, Woodhouse's heart-felt monody on the death of his young daughter Martha conveys a sense of stoic sincerity which rescues it from sinking into crude mawkishness. The bereaved father, his religious faith challenged, reflects in shock and bitterness upon the unexpected misfortune of outliving his own child: 'I little thought the Lord of all our bliss, / Would thus tear out the threads his pow'r had wove'.[37] It is this vulnerable autobiographical voice which gives genuine force to some potentially commonplace reflections on the cruelty of smallpox:

> The flinty tyrant, wrapp'd in loathsome air,
> Mix'd with her fragrant breath, in secret, stole;
> Dar'd first her lovely form with filth impair,
> Then, snatch'd away her pure seraphic soul!
> With all his marks of malice chequer'd o'er,
> Oh! had he deign'd her priceless life to spare!
> The tarnish'd casket I should scarce deplore,
> Did it but still contain the gem so rare! (153)

The poem's overall sincerity of purpose is also underpinned by the avoidance of pastoral cliché. We are hearing a true countryman's voice as

Woodhouse – who had once been paraded before Samuel Johnson as a 'wild beast from the country' – summons up a thwarted parent's recollections of the shared pleasures of a rural childhood:

> I hop'd, again, to bend the hazel boughs,
> To yield their clusters to her velvet hand,
> To range, on grassy bent, the crimson rows,
> Of ripen'd strawberries, at her mild command.
> The bramble-berry, now, may keep its bush;
> The sloe may perish on its native thorn:
> No more the field-flow'r at her lip shall blush;
> Distend her lap, or fairer breast adorn! (154)

Such genuine recollections contribute to the sense of authenticity in a long, painful poem in which the sheer rawness of feeling is well-served by Woodhouse's relative lack of urbane literary sophistication. Though Martha's death prompts her father to question the ways of heaven, he closes by insisting that we 'Urge on our steps the way our Saviour trod; / Spurn the dull earth; make heavenly views our choice; / And strive to live with Martha, and with God!' Such heartfelt devotion is all the more understandable when we consider that, as the poet himself quietly reveals in a footnote, Martha 'was the only child born alive out of sixteen, at the time'.[38]

If the tone of Woodhouse's elegy anticipates Wordsworthian simplicity, 'To the Memory of a Young Gentleman, who died of the Small Pox', by the Scottish poet and songwriter Rev. John Skinner (1721–1807), could conceivably have been directly influenced by *The Lyrical Ballads*, though efforts to establish a precise date of composition have been unsuccessful. Skinner's poem presents an exchange between the poet and a distressed young man encountered by the wayside who, when questioned, explains that he is mourning the sudden loss of his musically gifted, younger brother:

> 'But now no more his notes shall charm the fair,
> No more his Numbers soothe th' attentive Swain,
> With Tullochgorum's dance-inspiring air,
> Or Roslin-castle's sweet, but solemn strain.
> In early dawn of merit and of fame,
> To wish'd-for health, from sickness just restor'd;
> The loathsome pustules seiz'd his tender frame,
> And sudden gave the stroke that's now deplor'd!
>
> 'Tis this that grieves me, – this the loss I mourn,
> Excuse a sorrowing brother's heavy tale;

No more shall he to earth and me return,
Nor sighs, nor tears, nor love, can now prevail!'
He stopt, the tears again began to flow,
And sigh on sigh burst from his throbbing breast;
My feeling heart soon catch'd the poor man's woe,
And soon my eye the rising tear confest.[39]

Skinner's sentimental use of a chance, wayside conversation – an act of exchange in which an affecting tale of woe is, in effect, reciprocally paid for in kind by the poet-listener's own sympathetic tear – employs a tableaux-like narrative trope commonly found in contemporary novels of sensibility. To take an obvious, canonical example, in Laurence Sterne's *A Sentimental Journey* (1768), one finds the famous incident of 'The Dead Ass' in which Parson Yorick and his servant La Fleur stop to hear the tale of a man mourning the loss of the faithful beast that has carried him on his own sentimental journey: 'it had pleased heaven, he said, to bless him with three sons, the finest lads in all Germany; but having in one week lost two of the eldest of them by the smallpox, and the youngest falling ill of the same distemper' he 'made a vow, if Heaven would not take him from him also, he would go in gratitude to St. Iago of Spain'.[40] Such concordances between poetic and fictional responses to smallpox deaths alert us to the fact that the emergence of smallpox in Britain coincided almost exactly with what the last generation of literary scholars often termed 'the rise of the novel'.[41] The next section considers how the early novelists absorbed the tragic scene of smallpox into their extended social narratives.

SMALLPOX IN THE SENTIMENTAL NOVEL

Sudden death from smallpox is employed as a simple plot-device in the earliest post-Restoration novels. The active presence of the disease, or simply the ever-present risk it poses is frequently mentioned throughout the canon of early prose-fiction from Aphra Behn through Daniel Defoe, Eliza Haywood, Samuel Richardson, Henry and Sarah Fielding, Sarah Scott, Frances Burney to Jane Austen, Walter Scott and beyond. In immediate post-Restoration examples, as in the stage-dramas of the same era, such deaths often take place 'in-the-wings', safely out of the reader's immediate sight, yet smallpox often lurks in the shadows of the novel, circling around the site of domestic stability, posing an ever-present threat to parental happiness and, as discussed at length in Chapter 5, female beauty. In many instances smallpox merely serves as a convenient, though wholly familiar and hence realistic motivation for the sudden removal of superfluous characters from the narrative; a commonplace cause of sudden reversals in family fortunes.[42] The more sentimental presentation of the domestic scene of death can be traced back to the popular accounts of the last days of Queen Mary in 1694.

The circumstances surrounding Mary II's fatal illness were particularly well documented thanks to the published disclaimers of the court physicians, the outpourings of a myriad elegists, the memorials of loyal biographers like Defoe, and the memoirs of her Bishop, Gilbert Burnet.[43] These varied accounts eventually provided the Whig historian Lord Macaulay with the materials for painting a particularly sentimental death-scene in his once standard *History of England* (1849–1855). A number of key narrative elements quickly ossified in the hagiography of the queen's fatal illness. We are told how the nurses and physicians first thought the queen only had measles, but when Dr Ratcliffe recognised smallpox she was undisturbed. Emphasis is also given to how her bishops were humbled when they witnessed how the devout and charitable queen was spiritually prepared and faced death with such resigned composure. We are also informed how she left her husband a letter privately rebuking him for an adulterous liaison at court and asking him to reform; and finally we have the image of the soldierly king, who slept in her chamber on a camp-bed, weeping openly when she died. With their emphasis upon piety, spiritual resignation and a woman's domestic role as religious and moral exemplar, these iconic accounts of the death of Mary contain all the seeds of a sentimental mode of representation which, particularly after the mid-century successes of Samuel Richardson, came to dominate eighteenth-century fiction. With the consolidation of this literary fashion for the depiction of virtue in distress, by the 1760s the domestic tragedy of smallpox comes more fully to the narrative fore, providing a prompt for melodramatic displays of pathos in emotionally voyeuristic set-pieces deliberately designed to invite a sympathetic response in the reader.[44]

It was left to the Irish writer Henry Brooke to fully exploit this emotive potential in his once popular novel *The Fool of Quality* (1765–1770). Since there is no readily available modern edition, the exemplary episode in question warrants a brief summary. Recounting his personal history to a female cousin, the character Harry Clinton describes his early business successes and his happy marriage to a devoted, if over-anxious wife, but suddenly 'the Small-pox, that capital Enemy to Youth and Beauty, became epidemical in the City'; the children catch 'the Contagion' and, despite the employment of 'all possible Art', the 'Distemper took a sudden and malignant Turn and, in one and the same Minute, both my Babes expired in the Arms of their Mother':

... as I knew the extreme Tenderness of my *Matty's* nature, all my Concern, as well as Attention, was turned upon her. I took her fondly by the Hand, and, looking up to her Face, I was instantly alarmed and shocked by that placid serenity which appeared in her countenance, and which I expected to be quickly changed into some frantic Eruption. But, first dropping a smiling tear on her Infants, and then lifting her glistening eyes to Heaven, I thank thee, I thank thee, O my master, she cried, thou hast made me of some use, I have not been born in vain; thou hast ordained me the humble vehicle of two safe and certain Angels, living Attendants on thy Throne, and sweet singers of thy praises in the Kingdom of Little Children, for ever, and for ever ... So saying, she suddenly cast herself into my Bosom, and grasping my Neck, and gushing a Flood of Anguish, we mingled our Sobs and Tears together till no more were left to shed. You are affected, my dearest Cousin. I had better stop. If you are moved by small matters ... I must not venture to proceed. Go on, cried the Countess, go on, I insist upon it. I love to weep, I joy to grieve, it is my happiness, my delight to have my heart broken to pieces.[45]

The cousin's masochistic response might now appear absurd, but it is that of the ideal witness to this type of sentimental narration which was designed to invoke an immediate sympathetic emotional reaction in the reader. Encouraged by his cousin's indulgent empathy, Clinton carries on recounting the equally alarming reaction when the servants abruptly announce the news of the children's deaths to their devoted grandfather, who 'casting himself into a Chair, remained without Sense and Motion'. He has to be attended by the physicians and a surgeon who calm him with opiates. Feeling 'sick, and ready to faint under the oppression of his lamentations', Clinton withdraws to an adjoining chamber 'and there plentifully vented the contagious Shower'. With Brooke striving to wring out every last ounce of reciprocal sentiment from this pathetic episode, tears have become as contagious as smallpox.

The moral of Clinton's story lies in the fact that the grandfather, who had hitherto devoted his entire life to commerce realises that no amount of money can compensate for the loss of his grandchildren. This reflects the broad concern of sentimentalist writers who celebrated a circumscribed domestic world as the crucible of emotional authenticity providing a sanctuary from the falsity and corruption of a public world of business and commodity culture. A very similar tragic scenario is made to bear the same moral message in Henry Mackenzie's lesser-known novel *The Man of the World* (1773) where, early in the story, smallpox kills a 'doubly endeared' baby whose mother had died giving birth. As in Brooke, a child's death propels an already bereft grandfather to abandon his commercial interests.[46]

While infant deaths offered a readily exploitable motif for furthering the domestic and philanthropic concerns of the sentimental writer – the

Dickens who created 'Little Nell' comes immediately to mind – these eighteenth-century novelistic episodes may in fact amount to a reasonable reflection of the medical facts: evidence of mortality rates for this period suggest that the overwhelming majority of smallpox victims were indeed infants because adults were becoming increasingly immune in part as a result of more widespread inoculation.[47] But smallpox remained endemic, especially amongst urban populations (in more static rural populations it tended to flare-up in sporadic epidemics). In London, out of an estimated population of three-quarters of a million, well over a thousand deaths from the disease were reported in 1773, but this was considered an average year; in the severe epidemic of 1752 3,500 deaths were reported, over 17 per cent of all deaths in London recorded that year.[48] By this date the initial religious objections to inoculation had largely abated and in 1755 the London Royal College of Physicians endorsed the procedure, but although there were calls for government intervention to promote inoculation amongst the urban poor this movement only gained momentum in the 1760s, with the development of safer methods.[49] The response of imaginative writers to the ethical debate over inoculation is a concern of a later chapter, but one narrative depiction of a tragic failure to inoculate invites attention here for its sentimental treatment, its significant colonial context and its abiding resonance in the popular imagination.

THE DEATH OF 'PRINCE LEE BOO'

One of the most widely circulated narratives of an avoidable death from smallpox was that of Prince Lee Boo [Lebuu], the second son of Abba Thulle [Ibedeul], King of the Pelew Islands in the Western Pacific.[50] (Illustration 5) This twenty-year-old native prince sailed to England under the care of Captain Henry Wilson but succumbed to smallpox on 27 December 1784 only five months after first landing.[51] Wilson had been in command of a British East India packet-boat, 'The Antelope', when it was wrecked on the Ulong reef off Koror. He had lent armed support in a native war while his men built a replacement boat which enabled them to leave the island with Lebuu as guest. Upon first reaching England Lebuu was

... introduced to several Directors of the East India Company, taken to visit many of the captain's friends, and gradually shown most of the public buildings in the different quarters of town; but his prudent conductor [Wilson] had the caution to avoid taking him to any places of public entertainment, lest he might accidentally, in those heated resorts, catch the small-pox, a disease which he purposed to

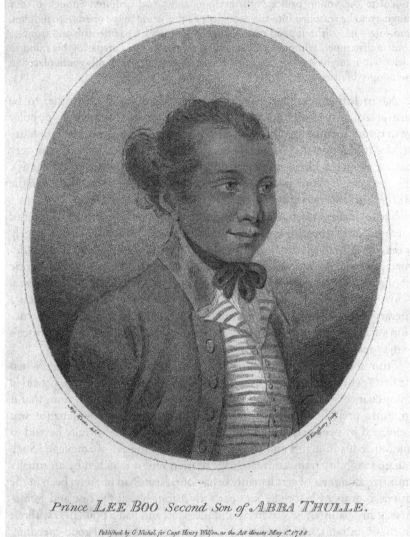

Prince LEE BOO Second Son of ABBA THULLE.

Published by G Nichol, for Capt Henry Wilson, as the Act directs May 1st 1788.

5. Portrait of 'Prince Lee Boo', engraved by H. Kingsbury, from George Keate, *An Account of the Pelew Islands* (1788). A native of the Pelew Islands, Lebuu died of smallpox within five months of landing in England in 1784.

inoculate the young prince with, as soon as he had acquired enough of our language to be reasoned into the necessity of submitting to the operation; judging, and surely not without good reason, that by giving him so offensive and troublesome a distemper, without first explaining its nature, and preparing his mind to yield to it, it might weaken that unbounded confidence which this youth placed in his adopted father. (260)

Eager to learn, Lebuu was sent to 'an Academy at Rotherhithe, to be instructed in reading and writing' where he proved immensely popular with tutors and pupils alike (260). But just as 'he was proceeding with hasty strides in gaining the English language' he was 'overtaken with the very disease, which with so much caution he had been guarded against' (265). The East India Company later paid for a commemorative tombstone in the Rotherhithe graveyard where the native prince was interred.

    These details of Lebuu's story are all derived from the closing chapter of George Keate's much-reprinted *Account of the Pelew Islands* (1788), largely based on Wilson's journals. Keate was no adventurer himself, but a gentleman poet and the author of a sentimental novel that reveals him as a critic of slave-conditions who imitated the Laurence Sterne of *A Sentimental Journey* in adopting the discourse of sensibility for ameliorist purposes; a literary influence discernible throughout Keate's personalised reconstruction of Lebuu's time in England and his pathetic account of the prince's actual death.

    From the outset Keate portrays Lebuu as a natural man of feeling. When he first met the prince in Wilson's charge at a dinner party, Keate beheld 'a countenance, so strongly marked with sensibility and good-humour, that it instantly prejudiced every one in his favour; and his countenance was enlivened by eyes so quick and intelligent, that they might really be said to announce his thoughts and conceptions without the aid of language'. Such innate sensibility transcends language barriers and is matched by an equally intuitive awareness of gentlemanly behaviour: Keate had not long been in the prince's company before he 'was perfectly astonished at the ease and gentleness of his manners; he was lively and pleasant, and had a politeness without form, or restraint, which appeared to be the result of natural good-breeding' (259). Lebuu also embodies generous qualities peculiar to his tribe: his 'temper was very mild and compassionate, discovering, in various instances, that he brought from his father's territories that spirit of philanthropy, which we have seen reigned there'. But such innate benevolence is balanced by 'good sense' and an inborn application of a distinctly protestant work ethic: 'if he saw the *young* asking relief, he would rebuke them with what little English he was master of, telling them, it was shame to beg when they were able to work; but the intreaties of *old age* he could never withstand saying, *must give poor old man – old man no able to work*' (262).

In support of this image of Lebuu as consummate man of feeling, Keate carefully constructs a series of affecting domestic incidents which, by eliciting Lebuu's 'tears of sensibility', are designed to convey the depth of the young man's affectionate regard for Wilson in his official role as surrogate father and for the captain's wife, who Lebuu insists on calling 'Mother' (263). When Wilson was 'sometimes incommoded with severe headaches' Keate records how 'the feelings of Lee Boo were ever alarmed' and he 'would creep up softly to his protector's chamber, and sit silently by his bedside for a long time together, without moving, peeping gently from time to time between the curtains, to see if he sleep or lay easy' (262–3). This scene of bedside devotion comes to function ironically in so far as it prefigures Keate's subsequent account of the vigil at Lebuu's own death bed.

Lebuu had taken ill on 16 December. Keate was himself at Rotherhithe a few days later when the royal physician Dr Carmichael Smyth, who had published on smallpox, confirmed the diagnosis, but the death bed descriptions largely rely upon the physician's subsequent account of the progress of the illness. It is only at this point in the story that Keate explains that Wilson 'had never had smallpox himself' so he 'was now precluded from going into Lee Boo's room', though by agreement he dutifully remained close-by.[52] (265) Since this makes it clear that Wilson had never been inoculated, it casts doubt on the earlier explanation for why Lebuu had not been protected upon arrival which can now be read as Keate's retrospective attempt to justify what was in fact Wilson's negligence in not insisting that the prince was inoculated upon first landing.

Detailing Lebuu's last days Keate assures us that he dutifully 'paid the greatest deference' to the royal physician and showed great solicitation for 'Mother' who was herself ill at the time. And 'though what he suffered in the latter apart of his existence was severe indeed' his mind 'remained perfectly clear and calm to the last' (265–66):

On the Thursday before his death, walking across the room, he looked at himself in the glass (his face being then much swelled and disfigured); he shook his head, turned away, as if disgusted at his own appearance, and told Mr. SHARP, that *his father and mother much grieve, for they knew he was very sick*; this he repeated several times. – At night, growing worse, he appeared to think himself in danger; he took Mr. SHARP by the hand, and, fixing his eyes steadfastly on him, with earnestness said; *Good friend, when you go to Pelew, tell Abba Thule that Lee Boo take much drink to make small-pox go away, but he die; – that the Captain and Mother (meaning Mrs WILSON) very kind – all English very good men; – was much sorry he could not speak to the King the number of fine things the English had got.* – Then he reckoned what had been given him as presents, which he wished Mr. SHARP would distribute, when he came back among the chiefs . . .

Poor TOM ROSE, [interpreter on the Antelope] who stood at the foot of his young master's bed, was shedding tears at hearing all this, which Lee Boo observing, rebuked him for his weakness, asking, Why should he be crying so because Lee Boo die? (266)

These fetching deathbed exchanges, confirming Lebuu's sustained gratitude towards his English mentors, were aimed at reinforcing Keate's overarching emphasis upon the irony that an eager youth who had not only bravely left his family, but journeyed so far to encounter a supposedly advanced culture and had been entrusted into Wilson's care by a philanthropic people who had themselves offered every hospitality to their British visitors, did not live long enough fully to experience all England's wonders and carry his new-found knowledge of the English language, English military might and English cultural sophistication back to his native islands.

Keate's recent editors note how the story of Lebuu's ready domestication and tragic death was designed to provide liberals, abolitionists and primitivist romantics with a suitable counter-example with which to obliterate any lingering negative memories of an earlier much-publicised native visitor from the South Sea Islands, the famous Omai, whose reputation had been clouded by rumours of shallow greed and sexual intrigue.[53] In contrast, after attending Lebuu on his deathbed, Carmichael Smyth had reportedly remarked that 'in living and dying he has given me a lesson which I shall never forget' for in 'patience and fortitude, he was an example worthy the imitation of a Stoic!'[54] Given this exemplary character and the context of British efforts to consolidate colonial expansion, the story of Lebuu's tragic fate raised the vexed problem of native vulnerability to disease, particularly the now preventable disease smallpox, as it impacted upon potentially beneficial encounters. Presented as an embarrassing tale of colonial ingratitude, for the hard-headed imperialist Lebuu's death from smallpox was at the very least a lesson in how colonial and medical mismanagement could thwart the forging of an economically useful alliance, while ameliorist campaigners were able to exploit the pathos of his thwarted enthusiasm for English culture in their calls for a more caring imperialism. As such this story rapidly entered the popular imagination regarding the Pacific. Keate's pathetic narrative was to be recycled well into the nineteenth century in various reprints, redactions, magazine extracts, chap-books and other adaptations, including a school-boy primer and a stage-play.[55] (Illustration 6) As addressed in my final chapter, Lebuu's story

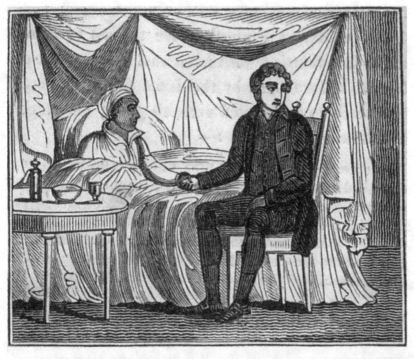

6. Deathbed of 'Prince Lee Boo', illustration from *The History of Lee Boo* (Edinburgh, 1828). One of many popular, sentimental depictions of Lebuu's death as a tale of failed colonial relations.

was later invoked by the poet Robert Bloomfield in his patriotic efforts to promote Jennerian vaccination. More broadly, it illustrates how death from smallpox could be accommodated within sentimentalist discourse for specific political ends. While the polite Georgian literary gaze often sought to draw a veil over the more gruesome aspects of death from smallpox, in the age of inoculation and vaccination philanthropic writers nevertheless exploited the potential for empathy and melodrama in the reactions of the grief-stricken survivors in order to promote a reformist, ameliorative medical agenda.

PART III

Disfigurement

CHAPTER 5

'Beauty's enemy' and the disfigured woman

Sir Novelty: I take more pains to preserve a Publick reputation, then
ever any Lady took after the Small-Pox, to recover her complexion . . .
Colley Cibber, Love's Last Shift (1696).

The threat of permanent disfigurement was both a practical concern of
medical commentators and a dominant motif in imaginative representations of smallpox.[1] Physicians eagerly sought to categorise the marks of
smallpox according to their pet theories: some identified a 'Master Pock',
others colour-coded them according to the dominant humour, while the
late-Georgians meticulously mapped their progressive sizes, shades and
textures in order to compare the severe eruptions of the natural disease with
the milder, less disfiguring effects of the inoculated form.[2] (Illustration 7)
A burgeoning Georgian medical marketplace was also keen to cash-in on
the perennial fear of 'losing face' to smallpox.[3] Flavia, the newly scarred
'Beauty' in Lady Mary Wortley Montagu's famous poem 'After the
Smallpox' (1715), curses the 'cruel Chymists' who hold out false-hopes of
a cosmetic cure: 'Could no Pomatums save a trembling Maid? / How false
and triffling is that art ye boast; / No Art can give me back my Beauty lost'.[4]
Advertisements for patent preparations claiming to prevent scarring
appeared in the pages of *The Tatler, The Spectator* and other periodicals
alongside the many poems and fictional narratives addressing the social
consequences of disfigurement to be discussed below.[5]

Medical writers often cite traditional recipes or surgical interventions
aimed at preventing, reducing, or repairing permanent pitting of the face
merely to dismiss their efficacy.[6] Diemerbroeck's long list includes 'a great
secret amongst the Court's Lady's' of laying 'the caul of a boar-pig twice-
daily' over the affected areas, but he is dismissive of 'the Custom of
Courtiers . . . who more solicitous to preserve their Beauty then others,
use to open the Wheals with a Golden Bodkin to let out the matter before it
corrode, as they pretend, more deep into the Skin'.[7] Fuller is equally
sceptical when recalling how the gullible Sir Kenelm Digby 'commended

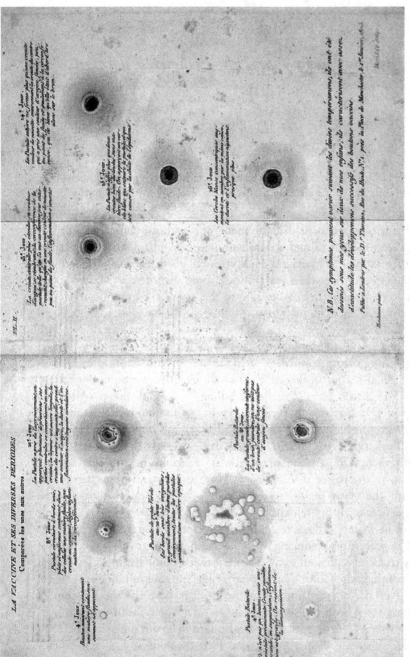

7. Comparison between natural and inoculated smallpox from Robert John Thornton, *Preuves de l'efficacité de la vaccine, suivies d'une réponse aux objections formées contre la vaccination*, Paris, 1808. One of many similar 'pustule charts' through which eighteenth-century physicians sought to give a sense of order to the external symptoms of smallpox.

anointing the face with Oil of Almonds, and then covering it all over with leaf of Gold', claiming that a young maid in whom 'that half her face where the Gold lay, was clear from any Pocks at all, and that other half, where they laid no Gold, was deform'd with Scars'.[8] Though the threat of scarring was not an exclusive concern of the super-rich, the use of such expensive ingredients and implements is indicative of the interests of a courtier class.[9] Diemerbroeck certainly found these special interventions much more popular amongst 'the richer sort and great people'.[10] Faith in laying gold-leaf on a woman's skin undoubtedly had its roots in an ancient notion of talismanic healing by sympathetic magic, but pointedly it also betrays an assumed correspondence between fair female flesh and material wealth.

There was indeed a blatant gender asymmetry in the narrative attention accorded to the social impact of smallpox scarring, with by far the bulk of the material addressing the loss of beauty being directed specifically at the figure of the young, marriageable woman. As Grundy succinctly observes, 'smallpox discourse was gendered: referring to men, it spoke of the danger to life; referring to women, of the danger to beauty'.[11] This bias is evident from a plethora of texts ranging from poems, plays and novelistic episodes to moral essays and conduct books all concerning themselves with the figure of the scarred woman. As Nussbaum observes, this literature reiterates a 'familiar theme that the disfiguring tragedy of smallpox is somehow intrinsic to being female'.[12] In a gendered economy of heterosexual desire, patriarchal power and property-relations, as revealed throughout this chapter, the woman scarred by smallpox functioned as a dreaded but ubiquitous sign of subjective and social disruption.

DISFIGURING DESIRES

'Bellmour: ... thou art as unmmanerly and as unwelcome to a Woman, as a Looking-glass after the Small-pox'. (William Congreve, *The Old Batchelour* (1693))

Appearances obviously mattered to members and would-be members of the late-Stuart and Hanoverian English courts, not least for physically attractive young women who, through choice or coercion, found themselves participants in power games when preferment and the consolidation of potentially profitable dynastic, economic, or political ties might be gained or cemented through arranged marriages, through expeditious extra-marital liaisons or simply by drawing the interested attention of the monarch. The noted beauty Montagu lost her looks to smallpox in 1715 just as she was starting to gain the attentions of George I. Her ambitious husband was reportedly left 'inconsolable for ye disappointment this gives him in ye [career] he had chalkt out of his fortunes'.[13] Discussing the contemporary culture of flattering portraiture, Marcia Pointon observes how, in 'political terms, seeing and being seen was crucially important, whether this meant appearing at the right occasion at court or the circulation of an engraved image'.[14] A woman courtier left badly scarred felt obliged to permanently remove herself from court or at the very least resort to wearing a mask: Ben Jonson, for example, told William Drummond of Hawthornden that Sir Philip Sidney's mother 'after she had ye litle pox never shew her self in Court yafter bot Masked'.[15]

On an individual level disfigurement was no doubt distressful across the social spectrum, but in imaginative literature the threat of scarring from smallpox is presented as predominantly the concern of the young, aspiring, upper-class heiress. Didactic texts advising an affluent readership on matters of health present the preservation of a girl's beauty as a wise investment.[16] While companionate marriage was not unknown, attractive daughters were more marketable daughters; with less likelihood of the financial burden of adult female dependency, they might also prove an additional economic cachet by serving as trafficable commodities through which a propertied patriarchy sought to cement economically and politically advantageous dynastic ties.[17]

Contemporary diaries and letters attest to the gossip-mongering concern in court circles with the fate of 'Beauties' in the smallpox.[18] The young Swift, for example, observing from the fringes of Queen Anne's court often displays a cynical interest in the impending threat of disfigurement. In 1711 he notes waspishly in a letter to Stella that 'one of the Maids of Honor has the Small-pox, but the best is, she can lose no Beauty, & we have one new handsom M[ai]d of Hon[o]r'.[19] In the imaginative and didactic literature generated within and for this upper-class milieu this mercenary tone is invariably projected exclusively onto other women who are portrayed as gloating over the fate of their sexual rivals. Thus in Mary Pix's stage-comedy *The Different Widows* (1703) 'Lady Gaylove' pompously quizzes a woman friend over 'what Proud beauty lies sick of the Small-Pox . . .? I have been so busy with Amours, I haven't had leisure to enquire of the World these two Days'.[20] This is a Hobbesian world where, for every 'Beauty' cast down from her throne, there is another one standing by eagerly waiting to take her place and, in passing, mock at her rival's disgrace. Once scarred, Richard Steele's fictional Parthenissa finds that 'My Lovers are at the Feet of my Rivals [and] my Rivals are every day bewailing me'.[21] In *The Rambler*, the disfigured beauty Victoria remarks that although 'the negligence of men was not very pleasing when compared with vows and adoration, yet it was far more supportable than the insolence of my own sex'. A queen whose 'reign was at an end' she is either ostracised or treated as an object of pity whose 'understanding was impaired as well as my face'. This mercenary context is encapsulated in Victoria's complaints at being shunned, mocked or condescended to by other women using 'all the stratagems of well-bred malignity'.[22]

The most anthologised poem on the 'loss of beauty' theme, Montagu's 'Satturday, The Small Pox', has often been read as a dramatic act of self-exposure, but it can also be approached as a highly contrived response to an established sub-genre of gallant poems addressing the loss of a woman's beauty which emerge in the previous century, and for which Ben Jonson's 'An Epigram, To the Smallpox', first published in 1640 provided an influential early model (it is sometimes associated with the illness of Lucy, Countess of Bedford).[23] Jonson upbraids the 'Envious and foule Disease' as the scourge of an undeserving woman, but his chivalrous defence relies upon a familiar male critique of female cosmetic artifice: 'Were there not store / Of those that set by their false faces more / Then this did by her true?'[24] Jonson angrily demands to know the disease's motivation in attacking a woman of such exceptional integrity who has never 'drawne to practise other hue, then that Her owne bloud gave her': 'Thought'st thou in disgrace Of beautie, so to nullifie a face / That heaven should make no more'?[25] Casting the punishing disease as an envious romantic rival, Jonson surmises that the smallpox's real target was the poet himself. The female victim serves as the passive, desecrated third-term in a triangulation of desire in which the primary relationship is one of male homosocial rivalry between the poet and the disease. In the final couplet Jonson avenges his mistress by asserting that his affections are not diminished and his rival has failed.

Thomas Philipot puts forward similar rhetorical questions in his lines 'On a Gentlewoman much deformed with the small pox' of 1687, insisting that heaven has made a mistake 'And buried all her beautie in her face', but as in many of these later Jonsonian imitations, blame quickly comes to rest with the disfigured woman: 'Each hole may be a Sepulcher, / Now fitly to inter / Those, whom her coy disdaine, / And nice contempt, has immaturely slaine'.[26] Only her black eyes are left 'To mourne at her owne Beauties Obsequies' as disfigurement is cast as just revenge for a beautiful woman's powers of seduction. The charge of slayer-slain was to be repeated in numerous verses in which the pitting of skin is portrayed as a justified wounding of a man-killer.[27] As Anselment notes, being crudely derived from the world of Petrarchan sonnets, many of these verses make grotesque play with images of pock-marked flesh as 'the love-slain who fall to Cupid's bow are buried in the graves and wrinkles of their beloved'.[28] Translating Quillet's *Callipædia* Samuel Cobb typically asks us to consider Aminta's many graces before she fell 'a Sacrifice': 'What Hecatombs of Lovers would she Slay, / Till she became this Tyrant's mournful Prey!' for now 'Her dented Cheeks, where Roses grew before, / And dropping Eyes, distribute Death no more'.[29] Forced comparisons between redness and the cheeks of Aurora or unconvincing reassurances that each 'Pock-Hole' merely Shews (at a Distance) but like *Venus* Mole' typify this tradition and despite occasional reassurances that smallpox can only despoil the transitory body, the underlying message is frequently punitive.[30]

Proverbial claims that smallpox serves as a moral corrective were reinforced by traditional physiological explanations which popularly clung onto some vestigial version of humoral pathology to posit distinctive constitutional preconditions for a given illness. The facial redness symptomatic of smallpox invited visual associations with blushing, signifying a lack of innocence or the hectic warmth of strong passions. Writing on smallpox in 1714 Walter Lynn, one of many practitioners anxious to offer treatments that serve to draw the disease away from the victim's face, suggests that

... there is a greater conflux both of Blood and Spirits to the face of most persons, as appears not only by the Fire in the eyes, especially upon any Passion, but by the more florid or sanguine Colour impress'd upon the face always than upon any other part of the Body. And 'tis generally observ'd, that the higher and fresher this colour is in the face of any one, the more dangerous this Distemper of the Smallpox proves to such a Person.[31]

Such traditional beliefs in temperamental vulnerability made it easy to equate smallpox with the corrupting effects of sexual excess. For example, in the long homiletic letter sent by Matthew Hales, the Lord Chief Justice to one of his sons 'After his recovery from the Small-Pox' in the 1680s, the father attributes the severity of his son's case to youthful intemperance. When urging him in future to avoid 'sinful Lusts' which 'corrupt the Blood, decay and distemper the Spirit, disorder and putrefie the humours, and make the body a very bag full of putrefaction', Hales was implicitly equating smallpox with 'The Great Pox', syphilis.[32]

Smallpox rarely carries the same moral burden as syphilis but, as noted in my introduction, there is ample evidence for the two being related as similar signs of moral corruption. In William Wagstaffe's satirical verse 'translation' of Richard Mead's medical writings, smallpox '... stands next in Blood, the POX'.[33] The verbal, if not visual affinity between the two 'poxy' diseases provided reason enough for this venereal comparison becoming proverbial. In *The Country Wife*, Wycherley exploits this potential for verbal elision when his naive eponymous heroine, Margery Pinchwife is quickly corrected for remarking that her jealous husband 'won't let me go abroad, for fear of catching the pox'. 'Fie' retorts the polite Alithea, ' "The Smallpox" you should say'.[34] At the other end of our period, in 1819 we catch a medical student, the poet John Keats including the following 'Pun' in a letter to his brother George:

> Between the two P-x's I've lost every Lover,
> But a difference I found twixt the great and the small:
> For by the Small Pox I gott pitted all over
> By the other I did not get pitted at all.[35]

This was to be sung to the tune of 'The Harlot's Lament'. Given such persistent colloquial associations between the 'small' and 'great' pox it is perhaps unsurprising to find that one of the earliest, most lurid novelistic representations of smallpox specifically connects disfigurement with female corruption.[36]

The London Jilt or Politick Whore (1683) is anonymous but was probably written by a man for, like many post-Restoration pornographers, the voyeuristic author promises to present 'the Jilt displayed in her true Colours' ostensibly as a warning to dissuade young men from the 'Roving, Libertine, lascivious Course of Life' which ensues when they succumb to 'Female Debauchery', for a whore 'is but a Close-stool to Man . . .'.[37] This denunciation of deceptive creatures with 'stinking Carcasses' is typical of many late-seventeenth century, ostensibly reformist diatribes which place the blame for prostitution firmly with women who all have the potential to be sexually insatiable Syrens.[38] In this fictitious memoir, the Jilt relates 'the Narrative of my Life' as a 'series of . . . Artifices for the ensnaring of Men' (1–2). An only child brought up 'wanton', the Jilt is still in her early teens when her widowed mother, who lives off male admirers, is taken ill with smallpox, 'a Disease which renders people ugly, as well the young as the old'.

[Mother, who was] . . . void of all Comfort upon this Accident . . . wished a thousand times rather to have had the Covent-Garden Gout [i.e. Gonorrhoea]: For she fancied she should be sooner freed from it than these Villainous swellings. Nevertheless they began to break out in such abundance upon her face, that one could have hardly placed a Pins head without touching those Devilish things, which cast the poor woman into such a despair, that Night and day she did nothing else then groan and complain. However, after nine days the Pox began to aposthumate, which render'd her face so dreadful and hideous, that she, who had before resembled a *Venus* in beauty, had then the Figure of a *Medusa*. (22)

Through this metamorphosis from love goddess to monstrous Medusa, seductive femininity is exposed as 'two-faced'. A brutal emphasis upon grotesque physical detail underscores the implicit message that perhaps even more than gonorrhoea, the petrifying face of smallpox represents the truth behind the purportedly deceptive, artful face of female beauty.

The mother's plight is ridiculed through absurd comparison: 'her Nose' is now 'of a prodigious length and Breadth, by reason of the scabs where-with it was so covered all over, that one would have rather taken it for a Steeple'. In keeping with the usual practice of protecting the recovering smallpox patient against shock, daughter and servant keep the mother away from mirrors but when she eventually sneaks her way to a looking-glass she 'saw her face, and Observing that it was so thick, and so ugly, she gave so terrible a Shriek, that all the House rang with it'(22). Such pivotal scenes of traumatic self-recognition are a central feature in fictional smallpox narra-tives. In this particularly violent example the shock of seeing her trans-formed image throws the mother into so 'desperate a Condition, that with both her Hands she scratched her Face, insomuch that the Blood ran down her Cheeks' so that 'that every pit resembled a Cautery' and she 'might justly pass for a Remedy to love' (23). She vainly tries 'all manner of artifices' to repair her looks only to find herself being 'Laughed at by those who before valued her so highly' while 'the most part of our Customers forsook the House' (23). Those who do come are young blades only interested in the daughter. When the disfigured mother eventually gains the attentions of a handsome young 'Surrey Gentleman', her daugh-ter attributes the compliance of this 'young Joseph' more to his desire 'to remedy his Poverty ... than by a passion of Love; for as I said before, since my mother had had the Small pox, she was become so ugly, that a Man must have been extremely sharp set that could have drawn his Knife for such a Piece of Flesh' (23–4). The mother's ability – despite the ravages of smallpox – to attract a young, but entirely mercenary suitor represents a punitive ironic reversal at the same time as encapsulating this sordid world of vanity, venality and corrupting passions. *The London Jilt* is an early example of many similar narratives presenting smallpox disfigurement as just punishment for over-reaching femininity. When old Mr Birimport in Robert Bage's novel *Man as He Is* (1792), asserts that 'Vanity ... makes such terrible ravage in the female mind, for the cure of which, or the prevention, heaven sent the small-pox' we are invited to take it as evidence of his mean nature, but nevertheless he expresses a view implicit in much post-Restoration literature.[39]

TALES OF THE 'AFTER-LIFE'

For the more polite writers of the eighteenth century, the trauma of smallpox disfigurement provided a perennial motif for didactic narratives and moral reflections. In a period when the behaviour of horrified beaus and shocked husbands prompted endless fascination, scarring raised the question of whether love is only skin-deep. When Richardson's pious heroine Pamela contracts smallpox – after fearing for the life of her baby who nearly dies of the disease – her concerned sister-in-law, Lady Davers, writes in hope to her reformed brother that should his wife be left scarred his 'roving mind' will remain 'constant'. Lady Davers is reassured by Mr B's exemplary declaration that 'if I were capable of slighting a person, whose principles beauties are much deeper than the skin, I should deserve to be thought the most unworthy and superficial of husbands', though she is even more reassured by the news that Pamela's 'charming face' has not received 'any disfigurement by this cruel enemy to beauty'.[40] A disfigured bride or wife tested the limits of male fidelity.[41]

In more frivolous contexts a wife's disfigurement could be portrayed as a useful insurance against her infidelity. Oliver Goldsmith's anti-romantic Swiftian ballad *The Double Transformation: A Tale*, tells the story of the belated marriage of Jack, an unworldly college fellow, to an unsuitably coquettish, prodigal wife who is 'Skilled in no other arts' but 'dressing, patching, repartee'.[42] The narrator asks rhetorically 'Could so much beauty condescend / To be a dull domestic friend?' The answer comes with 'That dire disease, whose ruthless power / Withers the beauty's transient flower'. Being 'condemned' to 'hack' the rest of her days with 'anxious Jack', she now troubles herself to please her husband who in turn is 'dazzled to behold / Her present face surpass the old' (371). With cheeks now 'dyed' with humility rather than pride, 'No more presuming on her sway, / She learns good-nature every day; / Serenely gay and strict in duty, / Jack finds his wife a perfect beauty' (371). The relish with which Goldsmith invites his implied male reader to enjoy the irony that Jack prefers a disfigured, but obedient wife suggests displaced anger on the part of a poet who had himself been left badly scarred by smallpox in his youth; born with a receding chin, pock-marks had simply added to the torments of a boy who was to be taunted as ugly for the rest of his life.[43] But Goldsmith's comedy of domestic containment is also a fair reflection of contemporary attitudes. After Charles Wesley's wife Sarah, who had refused to be inoculated on religious grounds, contracted smallpox in 1753 and was left so disfigured that she was barely recognisable, she remarked that it 'afforded great satisfaction to her dear husband who was glad to see her look so much older and better suited to be his wife'.[44]

Social writers were even more engaged by the trauma of the young 'Beauty' whose marriage prospects are suddenly ruined by smallpox. The fictional letter from the ruined beauty 'Parthenissa' and the associated editorial comments of Richard Steele in *The Spectator* (No. 306, 20 February 1712) provided an influential model for many similar episodes in magazines and novels.[45] Parthenissa bewails how it 'goes to the very Soul of me to speak what I really think of my face; and tho I think I did over-rate my beauty while I had it, it has extremely advanced in its value with me now it is lost'.[46] She writes arrestingly as 'one who has survived her self, and knows not how to Act in a new Being' (101). Pock-marks are an obvious visible marker of the disjunctive impact of a sickness episode which, as Brody notes, 'can make us different persons while we remain the same person', but such a total sense of self-loss as that attributed to Parthenissa implies that there had been nothing more to her than the commodity value attached to her outward 'Beauty':[47]

... I cannot enjoy what I am, by reason of the distracting Reflexion upon what I was. Consider the Woman I was did not dye of old Age, but was taken off in the prime of my Youth, and according to the Course of Nature may have Forty Years After-Life to come. I have nothing of my self left which I like ... (101–102)

Thus, in what Campbell terms 'a condensed, *almost* non-temporal tableau', female disfigurement was portrayed as concentrating the process of ageing into one accelerated experience in which 'the effects of a brief life-threatening disease and the effects of the passage of years are rendered identical' because 'both destroy a woman's socially valued appearance' (224–5). The loss of beauty 'that defined a young woman's essential identity constitutes such a sharp break in her life course that her earlier self might as well be declared dead, while her new self is ghostly because it has no place in the material social world'. There is no room here, Campbell concludes, for conceiving any accommodation to time – 'a young woman *is* in the common parlance, "a Beauty" ' – until the attack of disease propels her into an equally undifferentiated state of old age or deformity, an 'Afterlife' that might, as Steele's Parthenissa fears, in reality last decades.[48]

Smallpox and ageing are invariably presented as commensurate fates for the giddy young woman who relies for social power wholly upon her looks. Thus in Pope's *Rape of the Lock*, the advisor figure Clarissa rhetorically reminds the coquette Belinda that 'if to dance all Night, and dress all Day, / Charm'd the Small-Pox, or chas'd old Age away; / Who wou'd not scorn what Huswife's cares produce, / Or who would learn one earthly thing of use?'[49] Traditionally critics have read Clarissa's speech as an ethically normative, humanitarian voice which wisely seeks to remind Belinda of the priority of the spirit over the body, but recent feminist criticism invites us to see Clarissa as simply a cipher, a dramatic mouthpiece for the chauvinistic views of the male poet. Her demand for accommodation within the sexual status quo is merely the internalised acceptance of patriarchal values.[50] Pope the ventriloquist certainly uses the speech to reinforce a false, if culturally pervasive link between smallpox (a disease to which men and women were equally vulnerable), the effects of ageing (which are universal and inevitable) and thwarted female power. With the figure of faded female beauty serving a universal role as a sobering example of the transience of *all* mortal, worldly beauty, the figure of the disfigured, hence disgraced and discarded woman served as a fearful reminder of such impermanence. The bereaved Parthenissa does not simply mourn the loss of her beauty as if this had been a distinct part of her being in which all her self-esteem and social power was invested; rather it was as if her beauty was her entire being, rendering social death commensurate with physical death.

This frequent elision between a threat to beauty and a threat to life invariably rests upon male proprietary assumptions concerning the value of a woman's body. In his 'Supplication for Miss Carteret in the Small-Pox' (1725), for example, Ambrose Philips gallantly intercedes with 'the arbiter of life and death' to preserve the innocent, virtuous life of one who is still 'in the Small-Pox', but when he appeals to the supreme power 'who giv'st angelick grace / To the blooming virgin face' to 'Let the fell disease not blight / What thou mad'st for man's delight', he makes overt the often implicit assumption that female beauty is a gift from the gods designed, as if by pact, for the benefit of male onlookers. The virginal Carteret is to be spared not for her intrinsic, human value, but more as a fetish object of masculine aesthetic pleasure.[51]

Adopting similar chivalrous language, Steele does not take issue with Parthenissa's sense of bereavement, but rather advises her to resign her old 'conquests' and begin her 'new life' by burning all her old love-letters or returning them to her admirers under 'this honest Inscription, *Articles of Marriage Treaty broken off by the Small Pox*' (102). He also prints a reassuring letter from 'Corrina' who finds herself in similar circumstances. Though she has urged a previous flatterer to keep away 'for I am not the same', he is so impressed by her honesty that he now likes her 'above all your Sex' and is eager to ask for her hand in marriage (102). Steele's narrative voice insists that if '*Parthenissa* can now possess her own Mind, and think as little of her beauty as she ought to have done, when she had it, there will be no great Diminution of her Charms' (103). It is not the most beautiful women who 'take possession of Men's hearts' but those who are least self-conscious of their charms. 'Beauties', he argues, are often hated by their husbands because it makes them vain and conceited, while the women best 'formed for making men happy' are those plain, but 'good-humoured creatures' who 'can dance a Jigg, raise a paste, write good hand, keep an Accompt, give a reasonable Answer, and do as she is bid'. Rather than 'offering to administer Consolation to Parthenissa, I should congratulate her Metamorphosis': 'Good-Nature will always supply the Absence of beauty, but beauty cannot long supply the Absence of Good-Nature' (103–104). For Steele and his many imitators smallpox not only provides moral protection against the shallow world of preening and flirtation, it forces its female victims to attend to the development of a dutiful, domesticated character.

Samuel Johnson's very similar account of 'The Miseries of Beauty Disgraced' in *The Rambler* (Nos. 130 and 133, June 1751), is even more concerned with social maladjustment, with blame directed at the educational failings of an irresponsible, shallow-minded mother 'whose face had luckily advanced her to a condition above her birth' and so 'thought no evil so great as deformity'.[52] Obsessed exclusively with cultivating her daughter Victoria's physical appearance the mother had reduced her daughter to a mere 'assemblage of all that could raise envy or desire' (326–7; 330) When Victoria is left scarred at nineteen, it is her mother who 'grieved that I had not lost my life together with my beauty' (330). Such cruel materialism contributes to Victoria's psychological trauma as she struggles to adjust to her new 'self' with her mother 'incessantly ringing the knell of departed beauty' (341). Victoria's consequent self-pity provides an opening for Johnson to intrude his characteristic message that enforced idleness encourages melancholia. Victoria turns in despair to 'Euphemia' who, acting as Johnson's mouthpiece, sententiously urges her to bow to divine providence, reminding her that she has only lost what few possess and 'for the most part possess in vain' and only 'what the laws of nature forbid you to keep long' (345). Once again the disfigured young woman is encouraged to embrace her loss as an opportunity for the development of more lasting accomplishments.[53]

In a useful formulation Nussbaum remarks on the many such narratives in which, 'unsightlyness becomes a legible rendering of a highly valued interior state and a virtuous femininity'.[54] A succinct use of this trope, as later amplified by the eighteenth-century moralists, is found in Thomas Shipman's 'Beauty's Enemy' prompted by the death of Princess Mary in 1660:

> This fatal Mask, that thus beclouds her Eyes,
> Is no Deformity, but a disguise.
> 'Tis but an Angels' Veil she now has on;
> For veil'd they are, when they approach the Throne.[55]

Forging an equation between the rituals of earthly and heavenly courts, Shipman seeks to turn a compliment by playing upon the social pressures placed upon disfigured women to employ costuming to conceal their marked faces from public gaze. But in other hands an already well-worn angelic trope often bears a double-edge.

Jonathan Smedley's consolatory lines 'To Jacynta, lamenting at Cloe's Small-Pox', designed to outwit Jacynta in her cruel triumphalism over Cloe's disfigurement, gallantly insist that Cloe remains 'divinely Fair': 'Were she an Angel heretofore, / As you'd be understood; / Yet, I'm contented, I'll be swore, / With this same Flesh and Blood'. Smedley seeks to relocate value away from sullied flesh towards the transcendent spirit, but the pun on 'an Angel' – meaning both a divine attribute and a coin – keeps the monetary stakes firmly in view.[56] Moreover the reassuring argument for seeing disfigurement as the profitable exchange of evanescent physical features for more lasting mental or spiritual attributes is often achieved at the expense of presenting the disfigured woman's abjection as of itself an aesthetic spectacle. Such voyeurism controls William Pattison's lines 'TO Mrs. MARY FREWEN, Upon Her having the Small-Pox' (1728):[57]

> Let Others pensive o'er their Mirrors trace,
> The beauteous Ruins of a former Face;
> Nor for thy Beauties, lovely Maid repine,
> Thy Beauties mingled in a Mould Divine,
> Can but endure a momentary Pain,
> And like all Heavenly Substance heal again.
>
> And see thy Dangers, and our Fears are o'er,
> Hearts pant, Sighs heave, and Sorrow streams no more!
> As Gold by purging Flame still clearer glows,
> As Virtue from Affliction brighter grows,

> Sweet e'en in Griefs, and e'en in Pangs serene,
> Dawn the dear Glories of Euphrenia's Mien.

Pattison's compliments rely upon a Christian apologetics which insists that physical suffering leads to moral redemption and metaphysical transcendence, but Frewen's experience of a disfiguring illness is defined within the terms of a male gaze which cannot distinguish between the fate of her 'Beauties' from that of her suffering self. Though his muse sings in vain when 'Beauty's in Affliction', yet he anticipates a time

> When every Charm a thousand Charms resumes,
> And fair as Eden, from Confusion blooms,
> Raptur'd He stands, and boldly dares Divine,
> How to an Angel Thou must once Refine.[58]

A reminder of the Fall once again invites us to interpret smallpox as expiation for Eve's original sin but the earlier reference to refining gold means that the punning promise of the transformation of Euphrenia's resistant beauty back into the purity of an 'Angel' once again keeps the argument tied to the exchange values of the marketplace.

An impoverished Pattison was himself to die of smallpox in 1727, his twentieth year, while lodging at the house of the bookseller Edmund Curll. It is probably no coincidence that his defiant invocation of the image of a mirror in the opening stanza of his lines to Frewen betrays the influence of the opening lines of Montagu's now canonical poem 'Satturday, The Small Pox', to which they might even constitute a direct response. Though not available in print during Pattison's lifetime, Montagu's poem is known to have been in circulation in manuscript from 1716 onwards, forming part of a series of six 'Town Eclogues', three of which were eventually published without authorial consent by Pattison's associate Curll in 1718.[59] Of the many poems on this theme it has been by far the most frequently anthologised and discussed.

MONTAGU'S 'THE SMALLPOX'

Initial interest in 'Satturday, The Smallpox' was fuelled by curiosity over Montagu's fate as a one-time court beauty. It continued as a legacy of her pioneering role in introducing variolation (inoculation) into English court circles upon her return from a residency in Turkey in 1719 as the wife of the English ambassador. When Montagu contracted smallpox in December 1715 she was a young, rich, well-connected Whig aristocrat. Despite having eloped and married in defiance of her father's wishes, by this date she had established herself as both a beauty and a 'female wit' at the politically conducive court of the new English monarch, George I. No medical case-notes pertaining to Montagu's severe illness appear to have survived, but in her recent biography Grundy traces the ripples of court gossip, as Lady Mary's contemporaries speculated on the likelihood of permanent dis-figurement.[60] The precise extent of that disfigurement is difficult to establish; anecdotal reports show little consensus beyond the assumption that her court career was over. At the time the most noted damage was the loss of her 'very fine' eyelashes which never grew back, though her own letters reveal that she subsequently suffered from recurrent eye inflammations.[61]

'Satturday, The Small Pox, Flavia' opens with a dramatic stage direction as 'the wretched Flavia' reclines on her couch about to express 'the Anguish of a wounded mind'; like a sulking Venus, 'A Glass revers'd in her right hand she bore; / For now she shunn'd the Face she sought before'.[62] In a valedictory speech, the once beautiful Flavia, now suddenly transformed, raves at her own reflected image in her 'faithless glass'. With the 'bloom' on which she was to rely for 'years to come' ruined, she finds herself alienated from her former self: 'How am I chang'd! Alas! how am I grown / A frightful Spectre, to my selfe unknown!' (lines 5–6). 'Now Beautie's fled, and Presents are no more', Flavia recollects her so recent triumphs when she had full command of the men of the town who showered her with attention at the expense of work, wives and creditors. Wistful nostalgia turns to anger as she notices her own portrait:

> Far from my Sight that killing Picture bear,
> The Face disfigure, or the Canvas tear!
> That Picture, which to Pride I us'd to show,
> The lost resemblance but upbraids me now. (lines 43–6).

In *The London Jilt* the disfigured widow attacks her own face, but here the scarred woman's anger is displaced as she calls for the destruction of her pictorial, public image which, in the commonplace pun on 'killing' beauty, has turned upon itself. In a passage reminiscent of Pope's mock-heroic description of Belinda arming herself for the battle of the sexes in *The Rape of the Lock*, Flavia, is likened to a wounded warrior forced to retreat from the battlefield. She contemplates her now redundant toilette before passing on her weaponry of cosmetics and 'useless Jewells' to 'Fairer Heads': 'No borrow'd Lustre can my Charms restore, / Beauty is Fled, and Dress is now no more' (lines 53–4). In this mock-heroic act of relinquishing her author-ity, Flavia graciously permits 'meaner beauties' to take charge of the battle

over men's hearts, but they should remember that their triumphs are only
made possible by her ruin:

> But oh, how vain, how wretched is the boast,
> Of Beauty faded, and of Empire lost!
> What now is left, but weeping to Deplore
> My Beauty fled, and Empire now no more! (lines 61–4)

The evidence of Montagu's letters suggest that she knew that her lost beauty
was not everything, but traditional approaches have insisted on reading this
poem as an act of personal expression resulting from immediate experience.

At least one of Montagu's contemporaries was aware of a discrepancy
between autobiography and an albeit justified dramatic, poetic license;
Frances Seymour, Lady Hertford, writing to her friend, the Countess of
Pomfret in 1740, considers that nothing,

> ... can be more natural than her [Wortley's] complaint for the loss of her beauty:
> but as that was only one of her various powers to charm, I should have imagined
> she would have only felt a very small part of the regret that many other people have
> suffered on a like misfortune; who have had nothing but the loveliness of their
> persons to claim admiration; and, consequently, by the loss of that, have found all
> their hopes of it vanish much earlier in life than Lady Mary; – for, if I do not
> mistake, she was near thirty before she had to deplore the loss of beauty greater
> than ever I saw in any face beside her own.[63]

Modern readings of the poem as pure autobiography have invariably drawn
attention to the later testimony of Montagu's own granddaughter:

> ... small-pox was a disorder which she had sufficient reason to dread: it carried off
> her only brother, and had visited her so severely that she always said she meant the
> Flavia of her sixth Town-Eclogue for herself, having expressed in that poem what
> her own sensations were while slowly recovering under the apprehension of being
> totally disfigured.[64]

Discussing the frequent supportive use of this passage in autobiographical
readings of the poem, Campbell responds directly to the granddaughter's
claim by arguing that if this be the case then, notwithstanding, Montagu
' "expresses" her own "sensations" in this poem in a distanced and patently
conventional, even satirical, style'.[65] Although much of the poem takes the
form of a long monologue spoken by Flavia, Campbell also observes that 'the
opening lines present her in the third person as part of a dramatic tableaux,
and the monologue that follows emphasises her vanity and histrionic self-
pity in a way reminiscent of the poems of Pope or Gay (indeed Montagu's
eclogues were initiated in collaboration with those very poets)'.[66] We may
never know if it was Montagu herself who, in arranging these eclogues for

publication, placed that on smallpox immediately after 'Friday' in which Lydia laments her 'old age' at thirty-five, but certainly this sequential positioning encourages the reader to link Flavia's trauma to the more general trope of the ageing beauty who suddenly realises that she has become, in Campbell's formulation, 'that despised Other – an old woman'.[67]

Grundy also gives attention to the sequential ordering, noting that in so far as the poem corresponds to the positioning of, for example, 'Winter' in Pope's *Pastorals* or 'Friday' in Gay's *Shepherd's Week* as the closing eclogue in a pastoral cycle, it clearly should refer to death; but while Flavia is attended by sympathetic friends, 'death itself is not the theme, but rather the social death or "loss of face" resulting from the destruction of the beauty which had ensured her conquests and cash presents'.[68] When reading the poem as rooted in autobiography we must therefore bear in mind the degree to which Montagu has consciously (possibly collaboratively) re-shaped personal experience in accordance with the inherited protocols of mock-pastoral elegy or mock-heroic satire. As Campbell observes, these generic considerations 'raise questions about Montagu's placement "inside" or "outside" the scarred woman's suffering, [since] the poem turns out to pose Flavia's problem precisely in terms of the troubled placement of her sense of self'.[69] Putting the problems of a crudely autobiographical reading to one side, this formal complexity of dramatic viewpoint certainly makes Montagu's poem one of the most sophisticated poems on this theme, but where does it stand as a riposte to the usual chauvinistic assumptions concerning the disfigured woman?

Nussbaum claims that Montagu's eclogue 'cleverly documents the way that smallpox exposes the commodification of beauty', but surely as an act of proto-feminist defiance the poem is deeply compromised in the way its speaking subject 'Flavia' can imagine no other fate for herself but social retirement?[70] To read the poem as an example of feminocentric counter-discourse we need to be alert to the possibility of an element of distancing irony in the presentation of Flavia's dilemma. The closing passage of the poem seems crucial, as Flavia's upbraiding of 'the Great Machaon' (probably her family physician, Samuel Garth) for his false reassurances is silenced by an unidentified speaker:

> Cease hapless Maid, no more thy Tale persue,
> Forsake Mankind, and bid the World Adieu.
> Monarchs, and Beauties rule with equal sway,
> All strive to serve, and Glory to obey,
> Alike unpity'd when depos'd they grow,
> Men mock the Idol of their Former vow. (lines 83–8)

Whose voice is this brusquely ordering Flavia to stop whingeing and accept her lot as one of the socially dead?[71] Is this Montagu's actual voice (and opinion), or a ventriloquised version of the sneering, triumphalist voices she was herself exposed to after finding herself in Flavia's position? In this key controlling passage the pun on 'unpity'd' suggests a direct verbal echo of a joke that is known to have been going the social rounds at the very time of composition during the period of Montagu's immediate recovery.

On 26 January 1715, Bridges, (later Lord Chandos) wrote to a Colonel Bladen that 'Montagu is almost recover'd & her sickness has given oceassion for a Pun amongst the Ladies. They say, she was very full and yet not pitted, but She'l live to be reveng'd on some more of her Sex' (the implication is that although her face was 'very full' of pustules she is not pitted / pitied).[72] As it seems very likely that Montagu would have heard about this punning jibe, what now reads like her own deliberate play upon the possibilities of the pun towards the close of 'Satturday' might be taken as an attempt to distance herself from a courtly chorus which cannot imagine any life for a female subject after the 'death' of her beauty. In this context, Flavia's self-dramatising closing speech bidding farewell to society and culminating in her final declaration that she is to retreat from the public gaze to seek nature's solace in 'some deserted place' where she can 'hide in shades this lost Inglorious Face', can indeed be read ironically as a subtle parody of what court society might be expecting of her.

For a far more overt critique of the commodification of beauty we can turn to one of Montagu's imitators, Mary Jones and her provocative occasional poem 'After the Smallpox' (1750).[73] Writing from the position of a middle-ranking social outsider, who gained access into court circles through the patronage of her friend Martha Lovelace the daughter of a baron, Jones approaches the disfigurement theme from a far more distanced perspective than that adopted by Montagu. Jones's opening observation – 'When skilful traders first set up, / To draw the people to their shop, / They strait hang out some gaudy sign, / Expressive of the goods within' – establishes her primary aim of exposing the crude economics underpinning the institution of marriage and the consequent reification of female beauty:

> So fares it with the nymph divine;
> For what is beauty but a Sign?
> A face hung out, thro' which is seen
> The nature of the goods within. (79)

Jones contrasts the coquette who ensnares her beau through 'study'd smiles' with the prude who 'hangs out a frown / To strike the audacious gazer down', observing that it is only the latter who, being 'adorn'd with every grace ... wears a sample in her face' (80). Echoing Clarissa's warning in *The Rape of the Lock*, Jones observes that this is a commodity market in which she who only invests in her physical attributes risks finding that 'all her stock of beauty's gone, / And ev'n the very sign took down'. The sensible Jones might well be addressing Montagu's despondent, self-dramatising 'Flavia':

> Yet grieve not at the fatal blow;
> For if you break a while, we know,
> 'Tis bankrupt like, more rich to grow.
> A fairer sign you'll soon hang up,
> And with fresh credit open shop:
> For nature's pencil soon shall trace.
> And once more finish off your face,
> Which all your neighbours shall out-shine,
> And of your Mind remain the Sign. (80)

A likely source for Jones's shop-trade imagery is Aphra Behn's popular play *The Rover* (1677), in which the high-class courtesan Angellica Bianca advertises herself through the use of a portrait sign-board hung outside her lodgings. Certainly, like Angellica in her defiant exchanges with the play's eponymous rake-hero Willmore, Jones implies that upper-class marriage is nothing more nor less than a sanctioned form of prostitution. Though she does not suggest any way of escaping the marketplace beyond repeating the consolatory commonplace that beauty is fragile and can be replaced by more lasting accomplishments, the cynical exposure of the economic basis of marriage gives this poem a critical edge absent in Montagu's model.

DISFIGURING THE WOMAN WRITER

Disfigurement as both a biographical fact and fictional construct takes on particular resonances amongst post-Restoration woman writers who often found themselves being judged as much upon their physical appearance as their literary merits; women like Delarivier Manley, whose career as novel-ist and journalist has only recently been rescued from two centuries of accumulated moral censure.[74] At the opening of Manley's disguised auto-biography *The Adventures of Rivella* (1714), Sir Charles Lovemore, describes

Rivella's character and appearance: 'I have heard her friends lament the disaster of her having had the small-pox in such an injurious manner, being a beautiful child before the distemper; but as that disease had now left her face, she has scarce any pretence to it'.[75] Lovemore is in conversation with a Chevalier d'Aumont over the requirements of a woman writer to combine intelligence with beauty and a knowledge of love. Despite her unprepossessing appearance the Chevalier is reassured that Rivella's 'eyes love as well as her pen'.[76]

Manley's contemporary Eliza Hayward deliberately appropriates the trope of disfigurement to excuse, if not wholly legitimate her own adoption of a public voice. The young Hayward had found herself the target of one of Pope's cruel attacks in *The Dunciad* where she is portrayed as a monstrous mother 'with cow-like udders', her novels imagined as bastard progeny clinging to this bovine body.[77] At the opening of the first issue of Hayward's journal *The Young Lady* (1756), her eidolon 'Euphrosine', launching herself 'forth on the wide ocean of public criticism', is fearful 'it will be said, that a Young Lady ... is a vain, giddy, senseless thing, totally ignorant of what she ought to know ... incapable of reflection, or of thinking farther than the embellishments of her person ...; – very unfit qualifications indeed for to set up as an Author'. Hayward's fictional persona reassures her prospective readers that

... nature has provided for me a pretty sure defence from vanity, by casting my form in one of her coarsest moulds; she gave no regularity to my features, – no delicacy to my complexion, and render'd both still worse, by letting loose upon me, when I was scarce seven years old, that cruel enemy to beauty, – the small-pox.[78]

Constantly upstaged throughout her childhood by a beautiful older sister, her mother's favourite, Euphrosine took to reading which has proven to be 'the greatest blessing of my life, as it has kept me free from the follies and impertinencies of the age'.[79]

Looking beyond the conventional reassurances, Nussbaum suggests that in some actual cases the scarred woman's transformed condition may have brought some genuine compensations; disfigurement 'ruined women's prospects while offering escape from traditional femininities ... enabling compensatory expression in their lives and work'.[80] Not least such 'compensatory expression' included professional writing.[81] Manley and Hayward head a long line of scarred women, actual and fictitious, for whom literary study and practice is claimed as providing compensation for loss of beauty. In Frances Burney's novel *Camilla* (1796), when Eugenia is left crippled after falling from a teeter-totter (see-saw) and then severely disfigured after catching smallpox when her over-indulgent uncle allows her to wander amongst the infected crowd at a fairground, she develops a love of book learning. This prompts a sympathetic acquaintance to declare that 'Eugenia joins so much innocence with information, that the mind must itself be deformed that would could dwell upon her personal defects, after conversing with her'.[82] Louisa Tunstall, in Sarah Scott's *The History of Sir George Ellison* (1766) – whose 'vivacity was so unbounded as frequently inclined her mother to think that the ravages a very severe small-pox had made in her face was no small blessing' – is one of several similar female smallpox survivors portrayed in Scott's fiction who also find compensatory solace in intellectual pursuits, in this instance by studying geography, astronomy, geometry, history and philosophy as well as acquiring Latin, Greek, French, and Italian.[83] Burney never contracted smallpox herself, but Scott's pronounced concern with these positive psychological adjustments was motivated by her own experience of being left marked by a severe bout of smallpox contracted in April 1741 when she was eighteen; a trauma which had played a key role in redirecting her away from emulating the social success of her equally beautiful sister Elizabeth, towards a life dedicated to writing, domestic female friendship and Christian philanthropy.[84] Addressing how this trauma informed the fiction, Nussbaum remarks that, notwithstanding Scott's acquiescence to 'a culture's idealization of white and smooth skin', she implies that 'the woman who loses her beauty finds her soul'.[85]

Set against this insistence that devotional, educational and philanthropic pursuits represent the exemplary response to disfigurement, the invariably futile attempt at cosmetic repair is targeted for ridicule as an act of deceptive affectation. Johnson's Victoria tries to nurse her wounds in the countryside, but dragged back to town by her mercenary mother she finds herself 'imprisoned . . . as a criminal, whose appearance would disgrace my friends' before being 'tortured into new beauty':

Every experiment which the officiousness of folly could communicate . . . was tried upon me. I was covered with emollients, by which it was expected that all the scars would be filled, and my cheeks plumped up to their former smoothness; and sometimes I was punished with artificial excoriations, in hopes of gaining new graces with a new skin. (341–2)

This carries verbal echoes of Swift's voyeuristic portrait of Celia, the decrepit prostitute in 'The Ladies Dressing Room', who we witness struggling to reassemble the decrepit prosthetic parts of her disease-raddled body. Through

Victoria's sad reflections on how the 'cosmetick science was exhausted upon me; but who can repair the ruins of nature?' (342), we are being given a Johnsonian lesson in the need to know when to bow to divine will.

In Charlotte Smith's novel *The Old Manor House* (1793), the reader is invited to condemn the mature authoress Mrs Manby, when she is described as 'a little, ill-made woman, with a pale complexion, pitted with the small-pox; two defects which her attachment to literature did not prevent her from taking all possible pains to conceal'.[86] In this complex caricature smallpox scars signify moral inadequacies and typically reinforce other physical defects accrued through age. The name Manby can be taken as a pun on her social strategy, for although self-confident with women, she affects a 'tender languor' with men. Her cosmetic attempt to conceal a pock-marked face serves as a metaphor for such hypocrisy as well as being symbolic of her literary deceptions as a plagiarist who simply cons foolish men with recycled plots from 'grotesque' old plays. But while Smith seems to imply that a woman writer should not care so much about her appearance, Manby is mocked not because she is a woman who dares to write (Smith herself was a fully professional novelist), but because she exploits her damaged, fading physical charms to gain the only attention she values, that of men. This caricature resembles the typically snide reports on the elderly Lady Montagu, as brought back by English visitors to Italy where she lived in exile. As Campbell notes, cast as a monstrous or deformed grotesque, for male viewers in particular Montagu came to epitomise 'the horrific persistence of the female body after it has been declared socially dead at the end of its reign of beauty'.[87] Smith's caricature relies upon the same rhetoric through which social transgression translates into physical disfigurement.[88]

The woman scarred by smallpox is a significant concern of post-Restoration writers, often as the subject of a judgemental discourse which casts the disease as a moral agent acting to expose inherent female corruption or curb and domesticate a supposed propensity towards vanity and promiscuity. A dominant didactic narrative implies that to be left disfigured meant being accelerated into a socially meaningless old age, if not a spectral form of premature death, while cosmetic efforts invite mockery. More positively, with a sentimentalised Christian dualism allowing for consolatory gestures foregrounding the eternal nature of the unsullied soul temporarily trapped in corruptible flesh, disfigurement placed young women outside the marriage market, legitimating their pursuit of literary and charitable interests.

CHAPTER 6

'Enamel'd, not deform'd': manly disfigurements

> View what a Ghastly Visage now he wears,
> All crusted o'er! and marr'd beyond our Fears;
> Of ev'ry Sweet dispoil'd, and ev'ry Grace,
> That wore but now such Magick on his Face![1]

The plain-speaking Robert Gould displays typical rage when he invites smallpox to contemplate its own dreadful handiwork in disfiguring the body of young James Margetts. Such angry responses to the destruction of beauty form an essential element in the elegiac tradition, but what could be said to those men who survived and were left scarred by smallpox? For all the abundance of material concerned with scarred women, the relatively few sustained commentaries on the disfigurement of male survivors have been wholly ignored. As a complement to my analysis of the figure of the scarred woman, this chapter examines the significantly different range of aesthetic and moral responses accruing around the figure of the scarred man; a discussion which returns to the testamentary value of autopathography as we consider the psychological impact of scarring as revealed in some notable instances of male writers self-consciously addressing the loss of their own looks.

It has already been noted that in advisory literature addressing how to protect against or reconcile oneself to smallpox scarring was usually addressed to girls. One exception is *Callipaedia*, the popular poetic treatise on child-rearing which warns of how syphilis and other disfiguring illnesses can ruin the romantic prospects of the young. Cobb's 1712 English version isolates the 'peculiar Effect which the Small-Pox has in spoiling a Comly Face' for discussion by including the tale of the unfortunate lad Daphnis alongside that of the nymphs 'Aminta' and 'Galatea':

> Daphnis was once the Beauty of the Plain,
> Till this Contagion seiz'd the lovely Swain.
> How was He Courted! How the Idol grown,

> Of the Fair Sex; and darling of his own!
> Daphnis the Breast of each Beholder fir'd,
> Daphnis alone the longing Nymphs desir'd;
> But now they Pity, whom they once Admir'd.[2]

Like his Virgilian namesake, Daphnis occupies an ideal world of polymorphous love in which he is an idol to 'the Fair Sex, and darling to his own'. Instead of the more usual scene of female homosocial rivalry and the cruel disdain for a fallen 'Beauty', the romantic conventions of literary pastoral encourage Cobb to present a male victim who becomes the object of universal sympathy. As revealed below, pastoral idealism was just one in a range of literary, aesthetic and religious conventions within which male disfigurement might be configured.

'. . . OUT OF FASHION GROWN'

Gould regrets that Margetts's ruined corpse had to be buried at sea, but the poet finds some consolation in the consideration that the family did not have to look on such 'horror'. The image of sullied male beauty was a mainstay of the smallpox elegy, as exemplified in Dryden's lines on Lord Hastings in which the poetic voice seems to vie with the rapacious disease over possession of the bejewelled body of a 'Ganymede'.[3] Related, if less gushingly eroticised homophile sentiments inform other tributes to schoolfriends lost to smallpox. John Oldham's substantial lines 'To the Memory of My Dear Friend, Mr. Charles Morwent' (1684), mourn how 'All the staid Glories of thy Face, / Where sprightly Youth lay checkt with manly Grace, / Are now impair'd, / And quite by the rude hand of Sickness mar'd'. Killed as youthful foppishness was just giving way to the maturity of manliness, Morwent's once well-proportioned body 'Now hardly could be known, / Its very Figure out of Fashion grown'. Forcing a compliment Oldham insists that his friend never looked so fine as on his deathbed:

> And here thy Sickness does new matter raise
> Both for thy Vertue and our Praise;
> 'Twas here thy Picture look'd most neat,
> When deep'st in Shades 'twas set,
> Thy Virtues only thus could fairer be
> Advantag'd by the Foil of Misery. (lines 586–91)

Smallpox forces Morwent to 'wear' a 'ghastly visage' obscuring his 'real' face, but the poet takes on the role of the portrait artist in restoring that face to an admiring world. Out of darkened, swollen features arises a new picture of manly beauty enhanced by suffering. But this is merely an imaginary reconstruction as the actual face of his dying friend was left 'impair'd'.

What consolation could be offered to those young men who, having survived smallpox, were left marked for life? An attempt is made to do so in 'Verses sent to Mr. Bevil Higgons, On his sickness and recovery from the Small-pox, in the Year 1693', from the juvenilia of the dramatist and philosophical writer, Catherine Cockburn (née Trotter) (1679–1749). This critically important poem provides a perhaps unique re-configuration of the consolatory theme usually being offered to women by male poets, for here a girl reassures a young man over the loss of *his* beauty. Written when Trotter was fourteen, the poem's addressee – a minor poet and active Jacobite later known as a pro-Stuart historian – was twenty-three at the time of his illness. Nothing is known of their relationship beyond what is revealed in Trotter's verses which adopt a familiar stance in reprimanding the 'Cruel disease!':

> . . . can there for beauty be
> Against thy malice no security?
> Must thou pursue her to this choice retreat?
> Enough thy triumphs in her wonted seat,
> The softer sex, whose epithet is fair,
> How couldst thou follow or suspect her here?
> But beauty does, like light, itself reveal;
> No place can either's glorious beams conceal.[4]

Assuming that smallpox is primarily the enemy of female beauty, Trotter accuses the disease of straying beyond its normal bounds; it has become what we would now term 'a stalker' who, in picking on a male target, exploits the weakness in beauty's universal power of self-exposure. Comparing his beauty to a fatally 'destructive flame' which 'left no peace in either sex's mind', the second stanza is specifically addressed to Higgons:

> The men with envy burn'd, and ev'n the fair,
> When with their own, thy matchless charms compare,
> Doubt, if they should or love, or envy, most,
> A finer form than they themselves can boast:
> Repine not, lovely youth, if that be lost!
> What hearts it gain'd thee! 'Twas no pride to please,
> To whom that part was lost, which no disease,
> Nor time, nor age, nor death itself can seize.
> That part, which thou for ever wilt retain,
> Fewer, but nobler victories will gain.
> And what all felt, when you in danger were,
> Shews us how needful to our peace you are.[5]

By seeking to rescue an eternal self that will outlast a now disfigured body, Trotter's moral reassurances closely parallel the sentiments conventionally addressed to female victims, but there is no mention here of a catastrophic social death nor any associated need for a retreat from public visibility. On the contrary the young Trotter – writing, one suspects, out of an adolescent infatuation – encouragingly urges 'Go on brave youth, in all the noblest arts, / And every virtue; exercise thy parts'. As the rest of the poem emphasises, the disfigured young Higgons, once the envy of men and women alike, does not find himself being shunned; on the contrary, he has become the focus for stronger and more genuine affections. The threat to his survival has merely exposed how those 'Who feign'd to love you, now no longer would' while those 'who had hid their love no longer could'. Indeed in the conclusion Higgons is cast as being especially blessed: at a time of epidemic he is the only 'one return'd' to his friends among 'ten diseas'd, who heav'nly medicine gain'd'.[6] In contrast to the assumptions of social ostracism and necessary retreat imposed upon his many female counterparts, for the scarred young man recovery brings with it the anticipated expansion and deepening of affective social bonds.

Alexander Brome's poetic epistle 'To a Gentleman that fell sick of the small Pox, when he should be married' (1661), adopts a very different tone to offer similar reassurances. Discussing this poem Anselment describes how 'moments of banter and flights of satire combine with intricate imagery and evident compassion in a deliberately unsettling compendium'.[7] For example, Brome jokingly suggests how his friend's scarring might be put to practical use:

> Were it your Butler's face, a Man would think,
> They had but been new boylings of the drink;
> Or had his nose been such, one would have sowre,
> 'Twere red with anger, 'cause he'd drink no more.
> Or had your keeper such, he'ld sell it all
> For harts-horn to make halfts of knives withal.
> Or if your Cooks were such, how it would fit,
> To grate your ginger, or your nutmegs with it?[8]

Anselment's observation that in wishing to avoid sentimentalism Brome courts the grotesque invites closer scrutiny, specifically in the light of Bakhtin's theoretical concern with the affirmative function of the grotesque in carnival culture. With his unswerving, comic attention to the body's physicality, Brome's Rabelaisian suggestion that the coruscated skin of the smallpox victim might be usefully employed in making knife-handles or serve as a spice-grater superficially partakes of the 'degradation' Bakhtin identifies as the essential principle of 'grotesque-realism'.[9] But Bakhtin also associates such 'reminders that we are all creatures of flesh, and thus of food' (and faeces) with the life-affirmative ability to transform 'cosmic terror into a gay carnival monster'. This function accords with Brome's perceived attempt to bring about an acceptance of 'the unacceptable'.[10]

In fact Brome's closing image of the poet stumbling through 'the vallies of your face' is the very same topographical metaphor employed in Bakhtin's own account of the process through which the traditionally expansive open body of carnival was to be displaced by a more modern, bounded, bourgeois body in which the 'opaque surface and body's vallies acquire an essential meaning as the border of a closed individuality that does not merge with other bodies or in the world'.[11] In this context, Brome's genial comparison between the damaged face of the bridegroom and the red faces of his drunken butler, alongside his ludicrous suggestions as to how his scars might be put to practical use by his gamekeeper and cook, represent an imaginative attempt to 'merge' this 'gentleman' smallpox victim with the wider, revitalising world of the lower orders, a world associated with the affirmative life of the brew-house, kitchen, pantry and marketplace; the life of the family servants whose membership of Bakhtin's realm of festive consumption is eventually confirmed by Brome's insistence upon staging the delayed, yet recoverable marriage feast. As we have noted, poems addressed to female victims can be clumsily grotesque or deliberately cruel, but Brome's bantering style of male-male consolation serves a different purpose to that offered to disfigured women. Instead of the emphasis being upon the inevitability of social death, often encouraged by gloating females, his raillery aims at bringing the scarred gentleman back within a male homosocial circle of hunting, eating and drinking. The gentleman is not allowed to forget that he is scarred, but for a man this does not have to preclude marriage.

A 'SPECTACLE FULL OF DEFORMITY'

Not all responses to male scarring were so consolatory or good-humoured. In the seventeenth century, when smallpox was considered a purging disease of childhood, the disfigurement of young men was occasionally presented as just punishment for overweening pride and vanity. This is illustrated near the opening of James Shirley's 1653 masque *Cupid and Death* where the host of an inn and his chamberlain discuss the impending arrival of two guests, 'Cupid' and 'Death'; the former to be accompanied

by two gentlemen attendants, 'Folly' and 'Madness'. When the chamberlain enquires 'what was the mad-man' before he lost his reason, the host
describes a 'Thing' born 'to a very fair *per* annum' but who 'spent it all in
Looking-glasses':

> For Nature having given him a good face,
> The man grew wild with his own admirations,
> And spent his full means upon flatterers.
> That represented him next to an angel.
> Thus blown up, he took confidence at Court
> A lady of noble blood, and swelling fortune;
> Within three days fell sick of the small pox,
> And on the fourth run mad, with the conceit
> His face, when recover'd, would be like
> A country cake, from which some children had
> New pick'd the plums.[12]

Smallpox is poetic punishment for narcissism and presumptuous social
ambition. We still talk of being 'swollen with pride'. Shirley uses the same
somatic analogy to forge ironic connections between different forms of
bloating: 'blowne up' with vanity, the youth assumes the attentions of a
woman of 'swelling fortune' before an eruption of smallpox has him fearing
that he will be left resembling a richly laden, but greedily plundered fruit
cake. By implying that it was the vain conceit of the fearful outcome of the
disease which caused his madness, Shirley's text relies upon the traditional
psychosomatic theory of a triggered seed discussed in my opening chapter.
In men, such symptomatic, unregulated passion is figured as a sign of
effeminate excess.

The charge of effeminacy is also being levelled in possibly the most
sustained homiletic work prompted by the disease, the *Letter from Sir
Matthew Hale, Kt, sometime Lord Chief Justice of England, To one of his
Sons; After his recovery from the Small-Pox* (1684). Attention has already been
drawn to how Hales associates smallpox with syphilis, but in the present
context this sustained example of patriarchal moral guidance from the pen of
a learned man who wielded considerable authority at a national level
demands further scrutiny. The *Letter* opens with reassurances that although
the 'contagiousness' of his son's disease had required that his father kept his
distance, he now wishes to offer some seasonable advice 'at your coming
abroad' after this 'sore Visitation' because you will be 'subject to
Temptations' amongst 'young and inconsiderate company'.[13] Through his
providential use of his 'Rod and his Staff', God has taken his son 'to the very
Gates of death, and shewed you the Terrour, and danger of it; and after that

he had shewn you this spectacle of your own Mortality' before delivering him from danger 'so that you are as a man new Born into the World' (3). With smallpox 'now become ordinarily very Mortal, especially to those of your Age', his son could easily have become one of the two thousand or so who died of it last year, but God has been merciful and his survival offers the chance of spiritual and moral reformation (6–7).

Hales eagerly reminds his son how the smallpox struck 'when you seemed to be in your full strength' and how it 'rendered you Noysom to your self, and all that were about you, and a spectacle full of deformity, by the excess of your Disease beyond most that are sick thereof'; it was 'a fierce and violent sickness' which 'did not only take away the common supplies of nature, as digestion, sleep, strength, but it took away your memory, your understand-ing, and the very sense of your own Condition, or of what might be conducible to your good' (7). All his son was capable of doing for himself had merely served 'to make your own Condition more desperate, in Case they that were about you, had not prevented it, and taken Care for you'. The symptoms 'and the violence of your distemper, were without Example; and you were in the very next degree to absolute Rottenness, Putrefaction, and Death it self'. His son is urged to 'Look upon the foregoing Description and remember that ... you were as sad a Picture of Mortality, and Corruption, as any thing but Death it self could make' (7).

As if all this were not enough, Hales presents his son with twenty-one points of guidance ranging from reading the scriptures regularly and taking communion once a week, to recommending frugality and honesty and avoiding, whores, gambling and debts. Smallpox, he urges, 'undeceives' vain young men of their arrogant assumptions that religion does not matter by reminding them of the mortality of the flesh and the need to remain temperate and avoid sin and debauchery:

... how pitiful an inconsiderable thing the Body of man is; how soon is the strength of it turned to faintness, and weakness, the beauty of it to ugliness and deformity, the consistency of it to putrefaction and rottenness; and then remem-ber how foolish a thing it is, to be proud of such a Carcass. To spend all, or the greatest part of our time in trimming and adorning it, in studying new Fashions, and new Postures, and new Devices to set it out: In spending our time and provisions in pampering it, in pleasing the Appetite; and yet this is the chief business of most young men of this Age: Learn therefore ... to furnish thy Noble and Immortal part, thy Soul, with religion, Grace, Knowledge, Virtue, goodness, for that will retain it to eternity: How miserable is that mans Condition, that whiles sickness hath made his Body a deformed, weak, loathsome thing, sin hath made his Soul as ugly, and deformed; The Grave will heal or cover the deformity of the former, but the Soul will carry its Ulcers and Deformity (without

Repentance) into the next World: Learn and remember therefore, to have thy greatest care for thy Noblest part ... and as for thy Body, use it decently, Soberly and Comely, that it may be a fair Instrument for thy Soul to use in this Life ... (15–17).

This diatribe against corruptible flesh accords with traditional religious commentaries on the redemptive value of sickness, but it includes the specific and arresting suggestion that smallpox has carved a permanent *aide memoir* on the young man's face: '... let [these lessons] never be forgotten by you, as often as those Spots and Marks in your Face are reflected to your view from the Glass ..., nay as you open your Eyes from sleep, which were once closed, and likely never to be open again; so often and often remember your sickness, and your recovery, and the admonitions that this paper lends you from the Consideration of both' (5). Indelible scars are a form of stigmata, inscribed reminders of mortality and the wages of sin; a somatic sermon permanently etched into the young man's wayward flesh.

Harris, one of the physicians attending Queen Mary in 1694, was to write of her 'pestilential stigmata'.[14] In his *Book of Skin*, Connor remarks on how 'the sign of the cross always implicates the body in writing; it marks the inflicting of the law of absolute identity between Christ and man in the phenomena of the stigmata'.[15] Hales's instinctive approval of his son's pock-marks as redemptive signs was reflected in the folk-practices of the Eastern church for, as Montagu records in one of her Turkish letters discussing preferred methods of making cuts preparatory to inoculation, the 'Greacians have commonly the superstition of opening one in the middle of the forehead, in each arm, and on the breast to mark the signs of the cross, but this has a very ill effect, all these wounds leaving little scars, and is not done by those that are not superstitious, who choose to have them in the legs or that part of the arm that is concealed'.[16] The adoption of inoculation in Europe meant the rejection of this superstitious method, but the secularisation of the skin was to be a slow process as the scarred face of the smallpox victim was only gradually cleansed of the traces of sin.

JOHN DUNTON AND THE DISFIGUREMENT OF 'EVANDER'

The punitive tone of Hales's *Letter* is exceptional, but to point up any relative disparities of tone or representative social attitudes adopted towards male victims when contrasted with those levelled at scarred women is not to underestimate the psychological impact of disfigurement upon the former. Men did undertake cosmetic measures to cover-up the damage: even the Quaker leader George Fox defended his associate William Penn against charges of aristocratic frippery when the latter was attacked for continuing to wear the wig he had adopted to disguise the severe disfigurement he had suffered after contracting smallpox in his youth.[17] Few men can be caught reflecting upon their own experience of disfigurement, but we gain some insight into how the trauma might be absorbed from the autobiographical writings of John Dunton who contracted smallpox in 1674 at the age of fifteen shortly after commencing apprentice with a London bookseller.

Writing some thirty years later Dunton recalled being 'visited with the Small Pox, which were so severe upon me that 'my Eyes were clos'd Seven days': ' 'twas almost a Miracle I surviv'd . . . 'tho' I shall carry the *Pitts*, and the *Signatures* of that Distemper to my Grave'.[18] In a far more facetious literary mood, the adult Dunton also revisits this event when writing his *Voyage Round the World* (1691) where he recounts his early life-story in the third person, calling himself 'Evander'. Here he tells of how smallpox, 'that inveterate Enemy of good Faces, maul'd *poor Evander* at such an unmerciful rate, that you wou'dn't know one snip of him agen, so unlike did he soon grow to what he was before'.[19] Dunton dramatically bemoans his lost looks in a cry far more frequently ascribed to female victims:

But O my *Face*! my Face – Had my *Brains* been only turn'd topsy-turvy, or my Wits lost by this Disease – had my *Eyes* only been weaken'd, obliging me on some occasions to *wink* ever after – why all this might have been born by a Man that had read *Seneca* (as a Fellow said in *Cheapside*, when another took him a kick in the Br –) but to lose a *good Face* – ay – and such a Face as I lost – 'tis *intolerable* – and I cou'd have found in my heart not to have *liv'd afterward.* (43)

Though he admits that he contemplated suicide, the bathetic allusion to Stoicism undermines the ultimate seriousness of the confession. This defensive, self-mocking manner is partly attributable to the fact that the adult Dunton was self-consciously writing with an awareness of a literary tradition which, as we have just witnessed, largely presented smallpox as the enemy of beautiful women: 'O that I had but *Cowley's* Verses on *Madam Philips* by me! I remember he laments her hard Fate, and the cruel ravage that *scurvy lustful Disease* made in her *beauteous Frame*, that I can hardly forbear thinking 'twas writ for *Evander*; and were I little less a man, shou'd think he had mistaken the Names, and writ *Orinda* instead of me' (44–5). For Dunton to identify fully with Philips's fate as memorialised by Cowley would mean a diminishment of his masculine pride, but he proceeds to 'lace' his personal account with some of his own 'biting iambicks against this foul Disease . . . which has so transmogrophy'd *Evander from Evander*' (45). For all their obvious crudity, these verses are noteworthy for their blunt, cavalier portrayal of smallpox as a weapon in a battle-of-the-sexes. Evander's disfigurement is presented as an essentially female insult to a young man's body:

> *Pandora's* Box
> Let loose the [Small] Pox
> To mawl us,
> And with foul scratches,
> Poor ugly wretches,
> Bescrawl us:
> An Envious Jade,
> Thus to invade
> Fair Bodies,
> And make 'em look
> Like Crow, or Rook . . . (44)

In the same sexually suggestive recourse to myth employed by Dryden, Dunton relentlessly portrays the power of smallpox to disfigure as an assault by a woman upon a man who is transformed into an ugly, carrion bird.[20] An original footnote provides the missing epithet 'Small', purportedly dropped from the main text for metrical reasons, but the elision conveniently serves Dunton's purpose in wishing to equate the disease with syphilis, whoredom and 'envious' womankind.

In the second stanza Evander's angry desire for revenge against this attack upon his own 'fair' body targets 'Fortune', who is also cast as a vindictive woman:

> So fair a Face,
> So sweet a Grace
> To lose thus,
> Makes me my self,
> Unhappy Elf,
> Abuse thus.
> With Tooth and Nail,
> And Tongue I rail,
> At Fortune;
> Revenge from Jove,
> For Peace or Love,
> Importune.
> To make her dote,
> Or cut her Throat

Like Dido:
To make the Jade
Wear Masquerade,
As I do. (45)

As in Thompson's images of being possessed by 'Variola', Dunton writes of having his blood invaded by a debilitating feminine force ('Jade', originally the term for a sorry or worthless horse and often applied to untrustworthy women, was also employed as a verb meaning to weary, dull, cloy or cause to flag through excess). It is an image of male bodily integrity being penetrated by an invasive femininity which comes close to implying a reversed form of heterosexual rape. Having asked Jove to take revenge – in a final snipe at deceptive femininity – Evander's fate is likened to being permanently trapped in a masquerade costume.

Dunton follows up this angry doggerel with some self-reassuring, rhetorical reflections upon the fragile, short-lived nature of beauty which is 'but *skin-deep*, and may be all scratch'd away in a moment'. He asks why anyone should '*admire* their own Fine Faces' or be 'tormented at the loss of 'em' when beauty is so superficial?

Were the men all *Evanders*, the Women all *Iris's*, time must come when they'd look as ugly as *Mother Shipton*, or a half-skinn'd *Chapfaln* Scull in a Charnel-house. 'Tis but a few days perhaps, at least years sooner, that this alteration must be made if Sickness had not done it before, and *saved Death the labour*. (45)

As in responses to female disfigurement, smallpox simply accelerates the inevitable process of ageing, but by sarcastically arguing that if '*Proportion and Harmony* be a part of Beauty' then it is 'better have all the parts of the Face agree and be like one another than otherwise', Dunton pushes the argument that beauty rests in the eye of the beholder:

If 'tis a Beauty to have some part of the Face black, why not yet more to have it patch'd all over? Truth is, that *Beauty is Fancy*, at least the most part on't; and as a person may well be angry, and full as justly, that they have lost a *Lap-full of Guineas they dreamt of*, and imagin'd they were telling over, or hugging the *dear Bags* that held 'em, as to have lost that which is little more real than the other. (46)

Dunton concedes the common equation between beauty and riches only to suggest that both are largely imaginary; what some might deem a defect can also be seen as beautiful. But his defensive equation between his own disfigurement and the presence of moles on women which were thought to enhance their appearance (so-called beauty-spots, often artificially rendered using cosmetic patches) betrays his underlying anger.

The racial implications in the allusion to a 'Black' face become more explicit when Dunton, pursuing his relativist argument that the 'most *celebrated Beauties suit* not all', proffers the provocative example of Prester John who 'thinks himself as happy with his black arm-ful of Joy, as the greatest Prince of the *white World* in the Embraces of the most snowy Ladies' (46). As the mythical priestly ruler of an isolated Oriental kingdom – often located in India, but sometimes in Abyssinia – Prester John symbolised the endurance of Christian civilization amidst pagan otherness.[21] By drawing a rhetorical equivalence between the marks of smallpox and skin-colour as the marker of racial difference, Dunton's relativism might have brought him close to a recognition of the untenable aesthetic basis for racial prejudices. But he never gets beyond the assumption that beauty is to be exclusively equated with whiteness as a sign of civility and, by implication, that his own deformity equates to blackness as the sign of a repudiated racial otherness.[22] Based upon this arrested argument Dunton finds no reason why Evander should attach any further value to beauty:

> If it does not like its *old Habitation*, let it find a better, and e'en stroll off about its business like a *Gypsy Quean* as 'tis: (O that thou wer't but as well rid of others as now of thy own) while thou marchest about thine, being well recover'd by the exquisite, and never-sufficiently acknowledg'd kindness of the *best of Masters*, and after *tallowing* thy Face, and *licking* thy Lips, *scrubbing* thy Thighs, and *clawing* thy Haunches, as is usual in those Cases, art return'd *behind the Counter agen* as brisk as old *Æson* when he had cast his Skin, and grew as fresh as a Chrysom Child, tho' past fourscore and seventeen last Midsummer. (46)

In this bravura gesture Dunton keeps the racial analogy subtly in play by casting off 'beauty' as if she were merely a fly-by-night ('Gypsy') prostitute ('Quean'). With 'beauty' sent packing like a cast-off mistress, Dunton boasts of how he scrubbed himself down and returned to his career as an apprentice bookseller, optimistically comparing this resilient young self with Jason's father Aeson who, according to Ovid's *Metamorphoses* (Book VII), has his youth restored by the workings of Medea's magic. Here an Ovidian reference to bodily transformation reinforces a masculine rhetoric keen to assert the achievement of physical restoration and rebirth (also encapsulated in Dunton's image of a 'Chrisom-child', an innocent baby wrapped in a white Christening cloth).

Dunton offers no overt moral reflections upon Evander's illness, but as an episode in his *Life and Errors*, a spiritual autobiography, the survival experience is narrated alongside sexual alliances and political hell-raising as one of many youthful follies. Nevertheless, male disfigurement does not lead to social death nor, as in Thompson's *Sickness*, immediate spiritual revelation. Upon his recovery Evander 'came into a *new World*' but this is not one of either pastoral retirement nor moral and spiritual reformation; on the contrary, '*When I once came abroad agen* ... [I] was employ'd about Town in my *Masters business* more frequently than formerly, being now *Head-prentice*, and ... I fell into acquaintance ...' (45–7). Disfigurement proves no check on Evander's ambitions for social advancement and mobility, nor does it preclude him from erotic courtship for the very next chapter of this fictionalized autobiography is entirely taken up with recollecting Evander's subsequent romantic exploits as he embarks upon his 'voyage around the world'. Dunton even allows his old self to quip that 'Love is a natural Distemper, a kind of small Pox most have either had it, or is to expect it, and the sooner the better ...' (84).[23]

'THE AUTHOR'S PICTURE'

Dunton's disfigurement informed his responses to issues of authorial presentation. In his *Life and Errors* he mocks the fashion for writers placing engraved portraits at the front of their books. Refusing to indulge in such vanity, he substitutes his own verses entitled 'The Author's Speaking Picture, Drawn by Himself', for 'Fain wou'd the Graver here my Picture place, / But I, my Self, have drawn my truer Face'. A 'pretty Phiz', Dunton argues, does not necessarily reveal 'the Inside of a Man'. The engraver's art could only bequeath a 'Dead Face'; but 'Look on the following Leaves and see me Breath' and 'thus does my Speaking Picture conquer Death'.[24]

Dunton's claim here for there being no match between his true character – what he jokingly terms his 'inward Phiz' – and his outward appearance was a deliberate challenge to the claims of the supposedly ancient 'art' of physiognomy, as popularised in such works as Le Brun's *Conférences ... sur l'expression générale et particuliére* (Paris, 1698). Dunton's suggestion that smallpox confounds physiognomic legibility chimes with the remarks of other sceptical commentators who specifically cite the effacement accidentally enacted by the disease as evidence that one's face is not necessarily an accurate 'Index of the Mind'.[25] In his fashionable writings on physiognomy of the 1770s, Johan Casper Lavater sought to lend renewed scientific and ethical authority to the determinist claim that there is a 'sensible harmony between moral and physical beauty, between moral turpitude and corporal deformity', which are innate and inherited.[26] Lavater looks forward to how a 'Medical Physiognomy would employ itself in studying the signs of sickness', but in the meantime has to admit 'to what a pitch may the small-pox disfigure a face, and imprint on it traces never to be erased! How are the most delicate and distinctive features deranged and confounded by this distemper, and every mark by which we know them effaced!' (I, 100) Amongst the many famous plates depicting the faces of the bovine, the melancholy and the aged in Lavater's *magnum opus*, none depict smallpox scarring. Such images would no doubt have posed an insult to the aesthetic sensibilities of the dedicated physiognomist for, as Lavater reminds his readers, just as in 'other times, persons labouring under any bodily defects or blemish ... were all forbidden to approach the altar of the lord' so too 'the entrance of the sanctuary of Physiognomy must, in like manner, be shut against all who appear before it with a perverse heart, squinting eyes, a misshapen forehead, a distorted mouth.' (I, 117). Besides 'the deformity that is the effect of disease and infirmity must gradually disappear, because the virtues ... contribute to the preservation of health'.[27] Virtue will eventually heal scars.

Such problematic assumptions came to concern a renowned victim of smallpox, the Scottish poet, tutor, journalist, translator and musicologist Thomas Blacklock (1721–1791), who had not only been left scarred, but totally blind after contracting the disease when only five months old.[28] Loss of sight was a very common outcome of smallpox – it is estimated to have been responsible for a large percentage of non-congenital cases of blindness – but Blacklock's story is remarkable, not least because in an effort to implement practical measures for the education of the blind, including the use of raised type, he also attacked oppressive social attitudes towards disfigurement and disability.

Blacklock was born into a supportive, labouring-class family in rural south-west Scotland and showed an early aptitude for learning. Following the premature death of his father in a work accident a philanthropic surgeon supported Blacklock's education at Edinburgh University. After his first volume of poems appeared in 1746, Blacklock found that being hailed as 'Caledonia's Blind Bard' left him vulnerable to being treated as a merely curious prodigy. His ability to compose meaningful, visually descriptive verse when he had no recoverable visual memories presented an intriguing epistemological conundrum. His friend the young David Hume saw in Blacklock an opportunity to test John Locke's claims that all ideas derive from the senses.[29] The poet took an informed interest in the philosophical conjectures arising from his own case, but as a scholar of firm Christian faith who briefly entered the ministry, he sided with his more orthodox literary champion, Joseph Spence, who encouraged the idea that the blind poet was blessed with the compensatory spiritual gift of inner vision. Spence goes so far as to claim that his protégé can 'feel colours';

a gift Blacklock later takes the opportunity to deny in his anonymous essay under the heading 'Blind' in *The Encyclopaedia Britannica*.[30]

In the same article Blacklock considers how the blind find themselves caught between thwarting assumptions of limited professional prospects or the inflated expectations imposed upon supposed prodigies. Discussing his own 'case' in the third-person, he talks of being physically abused by an ignorant mob in the street and being treated as a 'raree show' by the *literati*. Numerous anecdotes concern themselves with Blacklock's physical appearance and 'nervous' mannerisms (his blindness militated against his deportment conforming to social conventions). These waver in tone between pity and cruel mockery but collectively attest to the voyeuristic fascination with his corporeal otherness.[31] Amongst the poet's more sensitive visitors was Samuel Johnson – himself visibly marked by the scrofula and smallpox he had suffered in childhood – who breakfasted with Blacklock at Edinburgh in 1773 and 'looked on him with reverence'.[32]

Blacklock's most openly autobiographical reflection upon his physical appearance is the early poem 'The Author's Picture'. First published in 1754 when Blacklock was twenty-three but probably penned earlier, this is a disarmingly candid composition in which he resorts to self-mockery in addressing his own marriage prospects.[33] Blacklock was to bemoan the fact that his blindness deprived him of direct access to books and the visible wonders of nature, but in this poem he expresses far greater anxiety over the apparent disgust prompted by his physical appearance. In a less crude version of what Dunton called a 'Speaking Picture', Blacklock adopts the stance of a self-portraitist standing before a mirror:

> While in my matchless graces wrapt I stand,
> And touch each feature with a trembling hand;
> Deign, lovely Self! with art and nature's pride,
> To mix the colours, and the pencil guide.[34]

Adopting this ironic pose of sightless self-portraitist, the reflected image is provided by the touch of the blind poet-painter's own fingers. Blacklock plays with the figurative meanings attached to the term 'blind'; he may be blind, but 'How vast a crowd by Self, like me, are blind!' With mocking irony he seeks inspiration for the same 'Self' which paints the fop 'in magic colours' and, echoing Pope's Clarissa, he observes that 'When age and wrinkles seize the conqu'ring maid, / Self, not the glass, reflects the flatt'ring shade' (191). Blacklock presents us with his own portrait:

> Straight is my person, but of little size;
> Lean are my cheeks, and hollow are my eyes:

My youthful down is, like my talents, rare;
Politely distant stands each single hair.
My voice too rough to charm a lady's ear;
So smooth, a child may listen without fear;
Not form'd in cadence soft and warbling lays,
To sooth the fair thro' pleasure's wanton ways.
My form so fine, so regular, so new;
My port so manly, and so fresh my hue;
Oft, as I meet the crowd, they laughing say,
"See, see Memento mori cross the way."
The ravish'd Proserpine at last, we know,
Grew fondly jealous of her sable beau;
But thanks to nature! none from me need fly;
One heart the Devil could wound – so cannot I.
Yet, tho' my person fearless may be seen,
There is some danger in my graceful mien:
For, as some vessel, toss'd by wind and tide,
Bounds o'er the waves, and rocks from side to side;
In just vibration thus I always move:
This who can view, and not be forc'd to love? (191–2)

The obvious model for Blacklock's strategy of ironic self-deprecation was
Pope's 'Epistle to Arbuthnot', in which, as Dennis Todd observes, the
satirist confronts 'his enemies by using the conventional images and stereo-
types of monstrosity' while he 'simultaneously defines himself outside of the
imputations of monstrosity'.[35] Like Pope, the blind poet was obliged to
counter the traditional association between bodily defects and deformations
of character, as exemplified in Shakespeare's portrayal of Richard III and
morally endorsed in such works as Francis Bacon's essay 'Of Deformity';
conventional associations between physical deformity, servility, and deception traceable back to the Romans and still active in the eighteenth-century
burlesque theatre and popular novels.[36]

Announcing mid-way through his 'Picture' that now his 'form in all its
glory stands display'd', Blacklock seeks the inspiration to 'paint the mind'
as he adopts the virtuous stance of the retiring, amateur poet: 'Harmless
I live, unknowing and unknown' (193) But behind this Horatian posturing
we detect genuine anxiety over his marriage prospects as Blacklock closes
with a mock-challenge to the ladies:

These careless lines if any virgin hears,
Perhaps, in pity to my joyless years,
She may consent a gen'rous flame to own;
And I no longer sigh the nights alone.

But, should the fair, affected, vain, or nice,
Scream with the fears inspir'd by frogs or mice;
Cry, "Save us, heav'n! a spectre, not a man!"
Her hartshorn snatch, or interpose her fan:
If I my tender overture repeat;
O! may my vows her kind reception meet!
May she new graces on my form bestow,
And, with tall honours, dignify my brow! (193–4)

Blacklock did eventually marry, but for all this comic self-mockery 'The Author's Picture' now reads like a painfully defensive response to the intrusive curiosity over the poet's physical 'otherness' which on occasion did indeed extend to a prurient fascination with his erotic life.[37]

Three extant portraits of Blacklock all portray him in partial profile with closed eyelids.[38] (Illustration 8) The artists may have been simply following the convention for depicting a blind poet as traditionally employed in images of Homer and Milton, but given Blacklock's poetic allusion to his 'hollow' eyes, it might be taken as indication that they had actually been destroyed by the infection. This was the fate of another blind prodigy, Nicholas Saunderson (1682–1739) who, as Lucasian Professor of Mathematics at Cambridge, famously lectured on Newtonian optics and with whom Blacklock was often compared.[39] Saunderson had been left blind at twelve months old by smallpox which 'not only deprived him of his Sight, but his Eyes also, for they came away in Abcess'.[40] (Illustration 9) Anecdotal evidence certainly suggests that smallpox had left Blacklock with some permanent, organic nerve-damage. Spence's anecdotes record how the poet finds it particularly painful 'to dine with a large company' because he has 'a tremor' that 'seizes him all over', which is 'like the *frémir* of the French, which he opposed to the pleasing *frissoner*'.[41] Blacklock's first biographer, the novelist Henry Mackenzie confirms that 'Dr. Blacklock had from nature a constitution delicate and nervous, and his mind, as is almost always the case, was in a great degree subject to the indispositions of his body'.[42] But he was also at pains to insist that the poet's external appearance belied his essential virtue. Mackenzie describes 'The Author's Picture' as the 'ludicrous picture' the blind-poet 'has drawn of himself' in which 'the outline is true' but the 'general effect is overcharged' for although the poet's 'features were hurt by the disease which deprived him of sight . . . yet even with those disadvantages, there was a certain placid expression in his physiognomy which marked the benevolence of his mind, and was extremely calculated to procure him attachment and regard'.[43] In Mackenzie's sentimentalist formulation, despite a febrile, emasculating

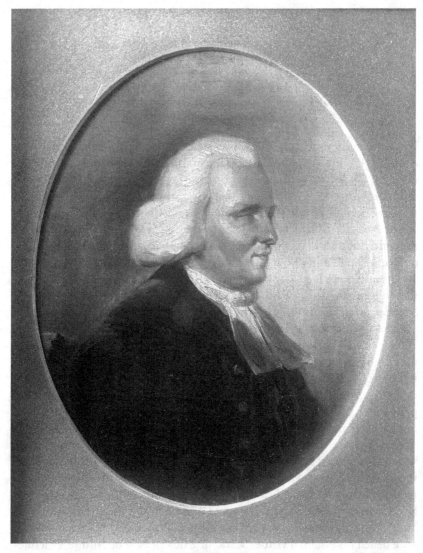

8. Portrait of Thomas Blacklock by William Bonnar, painted in colour on millboard. Having lost his sight to smallpox when only five months old, Blacklock's ability to write convincing visually descriptive poetry intrigued many contemporaries, including his patron David Hume.

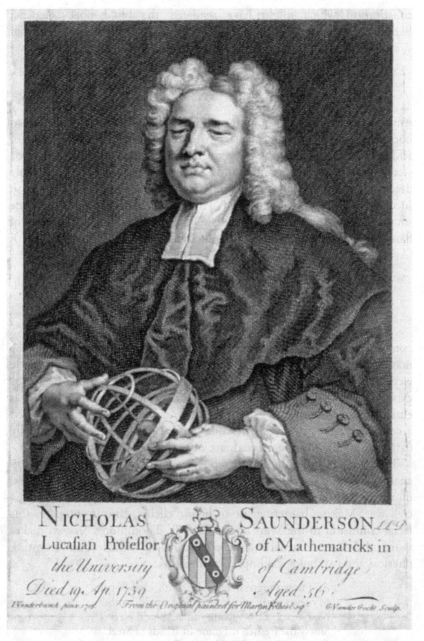

NICHOLAS SAUNDERSON
Lucasian Professor of Mathematicks in
the University of Cambridge
Died 19. Ap. 1739 Aged 56

9. Portrait of Nicholas Saunderson from the frontispiece to his *Elements of Algebra* (Cambridge, 1749), engraved by G. Vandergucht, after an oil original by J. Vanderbanck. The Cambridge mathematician whose eyes were destroyed by smallpox in early infancy. Sauderson's contemporaries were impressed by his lectures on Newtonian optics.

constitution which might have rendered the blind poet splenetic, Blacklock's essentially virtuous, benevolent, balanced and sociable disposition managed to shine through a deceptively unprepossessing exterior.

'ENAMEL'D, NOT DEFORM'D'

Any writer wishing to counter traditional assumptions that deformed bodies house deformed characters had to confront a classical ideal of athletic masculinity against which the damaged physique of the smallpox victim was inevitably found wanting.[44] Male commentators invariably describe smallpox as an emasculating force; an idea rarely expressed so succinctly as in the lines addressed 'To Thomas Stanley Recovered of the small Pox', by the cavalier poet William Hammond, who concludes a list of flattering reasons why 'Nature' has spared his uncle (another royalist poet), from death by suggesting that

> Yet one inducement more thy stay may plead,
> That nature hath so clean thy prison made;
> What though she pit thy skin? She onely can
> Deface the woman in thee, not the Man.[45]

Some obvious Freudian castration anxieties surely inform this, and the many other instances where illness and the threat of disfigurement to male victims is imagined as an encroaching feminisation. But an heroic aristocratic tradition, in which the scars from battle or duelling served as ennobling signs of martial experience and manly fortitude, also provided a comparable, positive aesthetic code within which to frame potentially flattering readings of the marked face of the male smallpox victim.[46]

This is exemplified in Brome's poetic epistle, which exploits a witty analogy between the newly pitted face of the bridegroom and a battlefield on which the red of Mars and the white of Venus are imagined fighting a civil war. Making bantering use of heroic clichés, Brome compares this facial confusion to the Wars of the Roses.[47] Thompson's *Sickness* makes more subtle use of martial and imperialist imagery to reflect on the lasting physical and psychological impact of smallpox:

> And now progressive Health, with kind Repair,
> My fever-weaken'd Joints and languid Limbs
> New-brace. Live Vigour and auxiliar'd Nerves
> Sinew the freshen'd Frame in Bands of Steel.
> As in the Trial of the furnace Ore,
> From baser Dregs refin'd, and drossy Scum,

> Flames more refulgent, and admits the Stamp
> Of Majesty to dignify the Gold,
> Cæsar or George! the human Body, thus,
> Enamel'd, not deform'd, from Sickness' Rage
> More manly Features borrows, and a Grace
> Severe, yet worthier of its Sovereign Form.[48]

A body marked by sickness is like molten metal refined in the furnace of fever. Thompson pursues this image through an extended simile in which the implicitly male smallpox victim is compared with a gold medal or coin stamped with an imperial or royal portrait of a kind typically modelled in imitation of prized antique Roman examples commemorating military victories or dynastic accessions.[49] Thompson's use of 'enamelled' was an apt choice as a recuperative term for the sheet scarring we know he was left with; according to contemporary usages, as a verb it referred to the ceramic process of giving something a hard, glass-like surface but adjectivally it also carried a related, aesthetic idea of decorative embellishment. By insisting upon substituting this positive term in the place of 'deform'd', Thompson portrays smallpox scars in terms of enhancement rather than loss. His simile ultimately implies that by serving to polish, if not ornament a man's features smallpox has merely ennobled his character by rendering it more 'sovereign' (imperialist, economic and numismatic meanings are all being carried in this term). Thus a man's toughened, cicatrised skin produces what Connor – discussing the modern fetishist cult of body-building – describes as 'a reassuring condition of impermeability'. Drawing upon Klaus Theweleit's analyses of the fantasies of early twentieth-century German soldiers, Connor writes of a 'hardness that would enclose, canalize or otherwise discipline the threatening fluidity attributable to the female body, or the feminised interior of the male body'. In the present context, his own description of such shiny skin as a 'visible immune system' is particularly apt.[50]

Writing in 1730, Dr Thomas Dale described the case of a young man with confluent smallpox whose 'whole face was nothing but one continuous Crust, resembling a kind of Parchment, or rather a white Wall'. Formerly a 'Lovely Youth', the disease had erased the young man's features, rendering his face a characterless, blank surface.[51] As discussed in this and in Chapter 5 a disease which could enact such fearful transformations invited questions concerning the continuity of the self and the relationship between one's outward appearance and inner character. The trauma of sudden disfigurement was often made meaningful within a Christian moral context which not only emphasised the impermanence of the flesh

and the spiritual value of personal forbearance, but also invited an interpretation of such loss as a retributive punishment for narcissistic vanity.
Acting as a timely reminder of the ultimate corruption of all mortal flesh,
scarring provided a providential opportunity in redirecting attention to a
higher, transcendental reality. By way of reassurance, such apologists drew
attention to the relative, limited value of social power vested in transient
physical beauty when set against everlasting, spiritual rewards.

But responses were also shaped by both romantic and mercenary conceptions of female beauty or by an heroic, ennobling model of masculinity
as an impregnable, fortress under attack from invasion by a feminised
disease. A disfigured young man could express feelings of anger and despair
and was not immune to judicial moralising, but unless the disease had left
him so deformed that it propelled him into the ranks of the monstrous or
racialised 'other' he could brave it by invoking established models of
military heroism. Unlike the prevalent narrative of the scarred woman
condemned to social death, a degree of facial scarring on a man could be
represented as conferring character, sustaining if not increasing his social
stature. When we are introduced to the gymnastic Godfrey Gauntlet, 'a
soldier from infancy' in Smollett's novel *The Adventures of Peregrine Pickle*
(1751), we are told that he is '. . . remarkably well shaped, and the scars of
the small pox, of which he bore a good number, added a peculiar manliness
to the air of his countenance'.[52] The heroine in Frances Brooke's epistolary
novel *The History of Emily Montagu* (1769), happily falls for an Irish
Captain whose face is 'marked with the smallpox, which in men gives a
sensible look; very manly, and looks extremely like a gentleman'.[53] While
the scarred woman was condemned to a desexualised 'after life' of premature old age, her male counterpart not only expected to remain socially
active, but his pock-marks might even be seen to enhance his sexual
allure.[54]

PART IV

Prevention

Frontispiece

CHAPTER 7

'Beauty's triumph': inoculation

The story of Lady Mary Wortley Montagu's pioneering promotion of variolation amongst influential inner-court circles after her return from Turkey in the early 1720s has often been told.[1] Finding their authority being opposed by an amateur 'female wit', some physicians had initially cast doubt on the efficacy of what they dismissed as an unproven technique practised by ignorant Eastern peasant women, while some members of the clergy had denounced the use of diseased matter to counter disease as blasphemous. Montagu's personal, if largely private efforts towards promoting what came to be termed inoculation in defiance of this medical and clerical opposition has never been in doubt, but her entitlement to be seen as the first European to recognise and adopt the practice has long been a matter of dispute amongst traditional medical historians.[2] But as Grundy observes, recent attention has moved away from the somewhat pedantic matter of a priority claim towards examining Montagu's importance as a creative writer and the import of her reputation as 'female wit' and icon of spoiled beauty; a reorientation exemplified in Grundy's own reappraisals addressing the gendered and racialised discursive contexts within which inoculation was promoted and contested.[3]

We have already seen how Restoration elegists personified 'Variola' as a predatory barbarian attacking an angelic, female Christian beauty. The discovery of the effective use of variolation both in the Orient and (in the New England context), amongst slaves of West-African origin, simply reinforced these xenophobic fears.[4] Writing in 1723 the physician Sir Richard Blackmore was typical of many early sceptics who saw inoculation as just another sign of the English propensity to chase after every fashionable foreign novelty. Blackmore doubted inoculation's efficacy on the grounds that it would have already been adopted by the Christian neighbours of the Ottoman Empire.[5] From the very outset inoculation was associated in the European imagination with the mercenary protection of an economic investment in the commodified beauty of trafficable girls. Blackmore was one of many commentators who propagated the early reports of travellers, notably that of Emanuel Timoni (Timonius) published by the Royal Society in 1713, which claimed that the prophylactic technique originated in the Caspian region amongst Circassian mothers who employed it to protect the faces of their daughters and increase their value as harem slaves.[6] In the British context the value of inoculation as a preservative of female beauty translated into the domestic context of marriage. For example, when Samuel Whyte writes 'On the marriage of Lord Kingsborough' (1772), the assurance of lasting nuptial bliss is credited to the safer inoculation techniques recently adopted by the surgeon Daniel Sutton: 'Oft does *Pandora* blight the blooming Toast / Too oft deforms the envy'd, lovely Wife; / But *Sutton's* saving Art, permit the Boast, / Thy winning Sweetness hath secure'd for Life'.[7] Later Georgian medical opinion often put forward the view that even if 'it proved that inoculation does not lessen the number of deaths' it should still be recommended to protect beauty.[8]

The first half of this chapter addresses how such gendered and racialised rhetoric informed imaginative texts engaged with the inoculation debate as it continued into the later eighteenth century. I begin by considering several poetic tributes to Montagu as medical innovator. All were written by men, but they adopt differing strategies in order to accommodate a female-instigated, dubiously foreign medical innovation into a patriotic enlightenment narrative of Britain's progressive scientific and imperial superiority. The second half concerns itself with how writers sought to articulate the ethical dilemma of a counter-intuitive new medical procedure by which, as one poetic supporter phrased it, 'mortal Venom, Source of Pain and Death, / By Chemistry divine, is chang'd to Balm'.[9] More sceptically, the satirist Nicholas Amhurst refers to the 'inoculating scheme' as that 'strange inverted Science, rash and blind / Which plants diseases, and infects mankind'.[10] The seemingly perverse act of grafting contagious matter into a healthy body not only went against intuitive attitudes towards physical integrity and disease, but posed a practical challenge to traditional relations of trust between the patient and their physician or surgeon; an ethical dilemma for any practitioner who, as a licensed member of the established medical faculties, had sworn adherence to a Hippocratic oath which expressly required him to do nothing to harm the patient. As revealed below, literary texts also provide a subjective insight into the emotional dynamics of this new, uncertain relationship and the wider ethical concerns of inoculees.

'RESERVED FOR FEMALE HANDS': CELEBRATING
LADY MONTAGU

One of the earliest commendations of Montagu as a pioneer of inoculation appeared in *The Plain Dealer* (no. 30: 3 July 1724) in the form of an essay and some accompanying verses 'On Lady Mary Wortley Montagu's bringing with her out of Turkey, the Art of Inoculating the Small-Pox'.[11] Although published anonymously and presented as being ostensibly by different pens, both have been confidently attributed to its proprietor, the dramatist, poet, and journalist Aaron Hill.[12] Reading this prose peroration and poem *in situ*, Grundy finds that Hill 'adds racism to sexism' as he struggles to find a suitable ideological position from which to praise a socially defiant woman as medical innovator.[13] This is not an unreasonable verdict, but this early response still merits attention for the way it exposes how these paternalist anxieties over medical innovation, female embodiment and race were interwoven.

The integrity of the English body-politic is uppermost in Hill's concerns as he addresses the initial resistance to inoculation. As if answering Blackmore, he argues against the vulgar error '*that the English are fond of Novelty*', for although '*ten Englishmen* in twelve, are descendents of *Foreigners*' yet anything new or foreign has always been 'distasteful to us' (239). Arguing from an entrepreneurial Whig position, he observes that although 'our very Laws are precedent' and the rights of parliament are based upon what '*has been* rather than upon *what was*', yet 'scandalous opposition' is given to any bill aimed at encouraging innovative practical 'Publick Benefits' such as those seeking to make rivers more navigable or promote untried trades. The opposition to 'the new practice of Inoculating the Small Pox, on Bodies, purposely prepar'd to receive it' is a further case in point. Drawing attention to the favourable comparative statistics on mortality rates compiled by James Jurin, the Secretary of the Royal Society, Hill recommends inoculation to 'every Parent, who has Reason, or who wou'd save a favourite Child, the promis'd Comfort of his Life' (240–1).[14] Contrary to the opposition from public newspapers generated by 'the Zeal of *Reverend Railers*; who in the holy Blindness of their Passion, have shewn us *Job*, upon his Dunghill; *inoculated*, for the *Small-Pox* by the *Devil*, of a Surgeon!' the case, Hill argues, is rather that 'Providence seems to have guided, and enighten'd Art, in this Practice, to assist, and relieve, nature, for the Preservation of the Human Species' (241). But Hill's contempt is particularly levelled at that 'pious, Older Woman' who tut-tuts that 'God's own Time is Best':[1]

... I rather pity, than grow angry with an unmarried Prude or Coquet when I catch 'em railing at Inoculation, with a Thousand *Excuses* for it, in their *Faces*. – As it is a Comfort to the Miserable, to have companions in their Misery, so, it must be a provocation, to these Fair Invalids, to hear of a Preservation, for other's Beauty, when it is too late, to save their own by it.

YET, these good ladies, unmindful that they carry about with them, the cause of their own peevishness, treat an innocent Practice, when they join the *Chorus* of *Railers*, as the *Indian* did the Looking-Glass, which he found on the Sea-Side. – He was frightfully Ugly; threw away the Glass, in a great Rage, with this comfortable Observation: – *I might have guessed thou wert good for nothing: Thou would'st not have been left here else.* (243)

Crudely attributing opposition to inoculation with the purported envy of ageing spinsters Hill makes a doubly offensive comparison: an anecdote designed to reinforce a racist stereotype (which combines assumptions of native stupidity with physical inferiority) is used to demean and dismiss both the disfigured woman and the native who both fail to recognise the supposed benefits of European technology. Culture is implicitly a privilege only available to the white and the beautiful (and marriageable), as Hill mocks those who supposedly fail to recognise the advancement of reason and civility over 'ugliness'.

Notwithstanding, the very next paragraph is devoted to extolling the blessings the English owe to distinguished women like Montagu, an 'Ornament to her Sex, and Country, who ennobles her own Nobility, by her learning, wit, and Vertues' and who, while 'accompanying her Consort in *Turkey* observ'd the Benefit of this practice, with its Frequency, even amongst those *obstinate Predestinarians*, and brought it over for the Safety and service of her Native *England*; where she consecrated its first effects, on the persons of her own fine Children!' (243). It is here, after acknowledging Montagu's recognition by the Royal family, that Hill places his verse encomium.

Hill's poem turns the introduction of inoculation – a divine gift – into a mythic fable; one which rests upon Montagu's reputation as a beauty coupled with an assumption that women, as represented by the nine muses, are typically driven by envy. Catching sight of Montagu's face, the muses immediately succumb to jealousy but eventually, after being 'Charm'd into love of what eclips'd their fame' they awaken Apollo as the god of beauty, wit and healing to beg 'some favour from your throne, / What could you bid her take, that's not her own?' Montagu is already possessed of both beauty and wit, for neither of which she owes anything to Apollo. He is left with only one other gift left to offer her, 'Physic':

> A skill! your godlike pity will endear.
> Form'd, to give wounds, which must no ease procure,

Atone your influ'nce, by new arts, to cure.
Beauty's chief foe, a fear'd and fierce disease!
Bows at my beck; and knows its God's decrees.
Breath'd, in this kiss, take power, to tame its rage,
And, from its rancour, free the rescued age:
High o'er each sex, in double empire, sit:
Protecting beauty, and inspiring wit.[15]

Hill's foundational myth misrepresents inoculation and Montagu's role in its adoption. A medical knowledge initially passed on between women is imagined as the supposedly flattering gift of a gallant male god. As Grundy observes, Hill's fable conveniently disregards the fact that Montagu's famous looks had already been damaged by the disease, as it 'neatly reduces her from agent to object'. Inoculation's primary purpose is presented as the preservation of female beauty, not human *lives*. Nor is it as if Apollo is portrayed as granting inoculation so that other women will not have to suffer what Montagu underwent when she lost her own beauty; rather, the gift is presented to her so that, as one 'Form'd, to give wounds, which must no ease procure' she can 'Atone' for the pain that her beauty has supposedly caused amongst a supposed train of spurned male admirers and envious rival women.

The nationalist emphasis in Hill's positive account of inoculation confirms how Montagu's promotion of inoculation quickly became enmeshed within wider patriotic claims concerning British technological progress and cultural superiority. This imperialist appropriation reaches an apogee in William Lipscombe's popular Oxford prize poem of 1772 on 'The Beneficial Effects of Inoculation', the most ubiquitous, if not the most sophisticated eulogy to Montagu as medical pioneer (it was anthologised in various contexts in 1784, 1792, 1807 and 1810).[16] Lipscombe sets Montagu's achievement within a familiar historical canvas in which smallpox stands as the perennial scourge of the young maidens of Egypt, where it had its supposed origins in the 'monster-teeming slime' of the Nile.[17] Deflecting attention away from inoculation's Oriental origins, smallpox figures as a tyrant against which neither a futile and misguided Islamic worship nor the Mithraic gods of the Persians could offer protection. In this typically slanted historical geography smallpox is a noxious emanation of the effete climate of the Orient from where, once 'Cloy'd with the luscious banquest of the East', it then turns towards Europe in search of a 'nobler feast', until eventually 'he saw Britannia rise, / Her beauteous lustre struck his ravish'd eyes' (3).

Like Hill, Lipscombe celebrates Montagu's achievement in terms of a patriotic chivalry, implying that she employed her own physical charms in the service of the nation to become the champion of a threatened female beauty which in turn inspires masculine 'Valour': 'INOCULATION, heav'n-instructed maid, / She woo'd from Turkey's shores to Britain's aid'. Montagu is not represented as championing an enlightened medical innovation on the basis of reasoned observation; she simply performs an act of sexual seduction, employing her supposedly superior British charms to 'woo' the prize from an Ottoman Empire associated with a weakness for sexual excess. But unlike Hill, Lipscombe does not steal Montagu's thunder by casting inoculation as ultimately a male gift, he does however displace attention onto the figure of Britannia as a more acceptable, idealised symbol of heroic femininity. It is Britannia who describes 'the vaulted dome' of London's smallpox hospital, erected by 'the sons of Albion' and overseen by the welcoming presence of the two sacred, virgin sisters 'meek Benevolence' and 'soft-eyed Pity' (8). And it is Britannia who recalls how Montagu, her 'country's champion', who knew that '... when beauty's charms decay'd, / Britannia's drooping laurels soon must fade' (3–4). The poem ends with Britannia waving her 'ensign o'er the Monster's head', while triumphantly announcing smallpox's defeat: 'Let now no more thy touch profane defile / The sacred beauties of Britannia's Isle ...' (7). Inoculation continues to be equated primarily with the protection of female beauty, but this has now been subsumed within a more blatantly chauvinistic narrative of women's supportive, decorative role in the heroic fight for British imperial dominance.

Lipscombe's trumpeting contrasts with Montagu's own style for she largely shunned open debate and certainly did not go out of her way to seek public recognition (though she had continued to encourage inoculation by offering private advice and by deliberately taking her inoculated daughter along with her when attending inoculations to display her own trust in its efficacy). For a more subtle tribute, we have the conclusion to the popular, six-book poem *Infancy, or the management of children* (1774–1776), by the physician-poet Hugh Downman who in offering a sustained warning of the dangers of neglecting to inoculate denounces the shameful failure to erect a public monument in recognition of Montagu's role as medical pioneer.[18]

Downman prefaces his tribute by rehearsing the usual formulaic story of smallpox as a foul legacy of Islamic attempts at expansionism, offering a series of pathetic poetic cameos adapted from Thucydides, notably the mother bewailing the loss of the babe her own breath has infected (VI: 510–27). As the disease for which neither the Romans, Greeks, nor Rhazes the Arabian could find an 'antidote', smallpox left ancient medicine 'whelm'd with shame' and even 'baffled' all Sydenham's bold efforts to quell 'the rank malignant nature of the pest'(VI: 527):

> The triumph was reserved for female hands;
> Thine was the deed, accomplish'd Montague!
> What physic ne'er conjectured, what described
> By Pylarini, by Timoni sketch'd,
> Seem'd to philosophy an idle tale,
> Or curious only; She, by patriot love
> Inspired, and England rising to her view,
> Proved as a truth, and proved it on her son.
> A manly mind where reason dwelt supreme
> Was her's, the little terrors of her sex
> Despising, by maternal fondness sway'd,
> Yet bold, where confidence had stable grounds.
> How far superior to the turbann'd race
> With whom she sojourn'd, scrupulous, and weak! (VI: 444–557)

Accurately describing Montagu's role in taking seriously a practice that had been presented rather dismissively by such earlier travellers Pylarini and Timoni, and recognising her brave step in arranging for the inoculation of her own son, a woman's achievement is rightly celebrated, but only at the expense of a blatantly absurd slur against the supposedly effeminate Turks.[19] Downman perhaps had more justification in choosing his next target:

> Yet, this is she, whom Pope's illiberal verse
> Hath dared to censure with malicious spleen,
> And meanly-coward soul. Redoubted Bard!
> What hath thy satire [. . .] of profit e'er produced,
> Of high advantage to thy natal land,
> Compared with her bequest? Thy numbers charm
> The listening ear, and with thy polish'd stile
> Taste is enamour'd; she hath been the cause
> Of heart-felt joy to thousands, thousands live,
> And still live thro her. (VI: 558–72)

Acknowledging Montagu's patriotism in promoting a medical innovation which benefits 'the world', this recognises the need to recover her reputation from the damage caused by Pope's notorious slanders (a task recently taken up again by feminist historians), but nonetheless, in what Wendy Frith describes as an 'ideological sleight of hand', Downman attributes Montagu's achievement to her purportedly 'masculine mind'.[20] Frith observes how Downman's claims of racial superiority are left wholly unquestioned, as Montagu is finally presented as a mere 'conduit, whereby the superstitious and unenlightened practices of the Turks were transported to England, where they were transformed into a rational procedure for the benefit of humanity (i.e. the English upper classes)'.[21] Montagu is portrayed as exceptional amongst her sex, otherwise dismissed as weak and timid, while the stress is placed upon motherliness as her prime motivation.

Notwithstanding these typical rhetorical biases, the personal motivations fuelling Downman's sincere concern with promoting the prevention of smallpox deserve recovery. He had begun to write poetry in the 1760s as a medical student at Edinburgh, where he boarded in the house of a smallpox victim, the blind poet and tutor Thomas Blacklock and they later maintained a literary correspondence.[22] At Edinburgh Downman was also taught by Professor William Cullen, the most influential medical theorist of his generation. Of all the Edinburgh medical faculty Cullen is afforded particular praise in *Infancy* as the dedicatee of Book III where he is commended as a figurehead of medical enlightenment. In his published lectures Cullen placed emphasis upon the environmental causes of disease. A keen advocate of inoculation, which he believed proved that smallpox is 'a disease arising from a specific contagion', Cullen even suggested that in time the method might be adapted for other diseases.[23] He also privately supported a group of Downman's fellow medical graduates who sought to eradicate smallpox through a planned, philanthropic programme of *universal* inoculation.[24] Downman's argument at the conclusion to *Infancy*, which accords with Cullen's published advice concerning when and at what age it is safe to inoculate, was integral to this enlightened medical campaign.

Such practical advice is specifically directed towards mothers and female nurses in whom, as care-givers, the primary responsibility for the health of children is firmly invested by the admonitory voice of the professional male physician-poet: 'let every prudent matron be resolved / To obey the call of duty and of love' (VI: 602–603). Downman flatters this imagined reader with a classical model of heroic motherhood, inviting her to compare her own feelings upon viewing the joyful prospect of her children being at last able to 'overcome' the 'plague Variolus' with the similar relief felt 'As Hercules / The spotted snakes defeating, transport flush'd / Alcmena's glowing cheek' (VI: 503–506). They should not yield to 'superstition' but trusting the wisdom of 'experience' they must 'let thy child / Encounter in his native shape the fiend, / And brave his violence' by anticipating his 'threaten'd blow' through the use of inoculation. (VI: 576–9) Countering religious objections, he also lends Old Testament authority to inoculation as divine intervention by making a potent allusion to the sacrificial tale of Abraham and Isaac: 'So when the Patriarch's arm / Was stretched to wound his son, an Angel came / And saved the victim from impending death' (VI: 583–5). Where Lipscombe recalls how 'Blind Superstition' had once stood in the way of medical progress, Downman argues for inoculation as a rational duty in this, our enlightened 'Aera, when mature, / And vigorous reason prospers' over the 'groundless fears' of 'fondness or religion' (VI: 607–608). Refusing to have one's child inoculated is likened to someone who, being afraid to step into 'a shallow frith', is later left having to risk drowning when the tide has risen. He also argues on the basis of statistical probability, insisting that to inoculate is not to tempt providence, because from 'providence flows reason to mankind' and 'reason teaches us to fly from ill' and 'covet good': 'The invention, the success, / Is the true warrant of approving heaven' (VI: 625–30).

Set against these appeals to rational religion and the relatively new science of statistical probability, blame for the failure to inoculate continued to be directed at female timidity. Downman paints a very sorry picture indeed of those 'unhappy beings' who, having once refused inoculation themselves either 'from idle dread' or 'weak maternal love', now refuse to have their own children protected. 'Tho' rare examples now', he presents these faltering few as social outcasts, who 'pine in solitude, oppress'd / By anxious thought' for whom 'the voice of music breathes / Its choral notes unheard; the stage displays / The living manners, and the assembly beams / With sprightliness and elegance, in vain' (VI: 644–8). A mother's failure to inoculate her children is doubly irresponsible; it not only puts them in permanent fear of catching the disease but disables them from social participation which is not only therapeutic for the individual but necessary to the conduct of civilised life. Those who wisely inoculate, the physician-poet urges, will reap the pleasurable benefits of a now medically regulated sociability.[25]

In directing their campaign at women, professional advocates of inoculation had also often appealed to their supposed vanity. Complaining in 1733 at the abysmal failure of the British to adopt inoculation, the popular practitioner Thomas Dover makes no mention of Montagu, but does highlight the example set by Queen Caroline, it being 'unpardonable' not to take 'Notice of her Majesty, as a great Promoter and encourager of this Practice' when all must agree that she 'is as much superior in her Understanding to the generality of her Sex'.[26] In an age when everyone readily runs into 'any Mode of Fashion', he is baffled by the failure of 'the Ladies' to 'imitate the Queen' by adopting inoculation to protect their own beauty:

Is Beauty, that arrives to such Perfection in the *English* climate, or so little Importance, that it is beneath our Care? What miserable Havock, what terrible

Changes has this one Distemper produced in the most lovely and amiable Part of Creation? The Ladies may possibly smile to hear a Man of Seventy use such warm Expressions, but I may venture to say with Mr. Dryden

> Old as I am, for Ladies love unfit,
> The Power of Beauty I remember yet.[27]

Downman is less flirtatious, if equally condescending when addressing his own 'preceptive notes' primarily to neglectful or unreliable 'matrons' who are deemed in need of rational, male professional guidance:

> We write to reason: Hence ye doating train
> Of midwives and of nurses ignorant!
> Old beldames grey, in error positive,
> And stiff in prejudice, whose fatal care
> Oft death attends, or a life worse than death (I: 26–31)

Such demonisation of supposedly ignorant female lay-practitioners and credulous, weak-willed mothers was commonplace enough, but with regard to inoculation it seems particularly patronising. Having been originally championed by a woman amongst other mothers in her own aristocratic circle, anecdotal evidence suggests that the fraught responsibility of electing to inoculate offspring in the face of conflicting advice from family members, friends, physicians and clergyman often fell to mothers, though not without raising questions over which parent has ultimate authority over their offspring.

ELIZABETH GRIFFITHS, INOCULATION AND FEMALE AUTHORITY

Inoculation is at present more in fashion than ever; half of my acquaintance are shut up to nurse their children, grand-children, nephews, or nieces. I could be content, notwithstanding the fine weather, to stay in town upon the same account, if I were happy enough to see my son desire it, but that is not the case; and, at his age, it must either be a voluntary act, or left undone. (Frances Seymour, Countess of Hertford to Lady Pomfret, London, April 1741.)[28]

Hertford's son, George Seymour, Lord Beauchamp, was to die of smallpox on his nineteenth birthday, less than three years after his mother penned this letter. In hindsight, especially for anyone who has also read Thompson's elegiac lines, Hertford's expression of respect for her only child's wish not to be inoculated takes on an air of tragic irony. Montagu, who had originally arranged for her own son's inoculation at Constantinople without even his absent father's approval, would have had little sympathy. Writing in 1723 to inform her daughter of the death of 'our nephew, Lady Gower's son of the smallpox', she remarks that

I think she [Gower] has had a great deal of reason to regret it, in consideration of the offer I made her two year together of taking the child home to my house where I would have inoculated him with the same care and safety I did my own. I know nobody that has hitherto repented the operation though it has been very trouble-some to some fools who had rather be sick by the doctors' prescriptions than in health in rebellion to the college.[29]

Controversy over the moral responsibilities of parents, particularly moth-ers, with respect to uncertain medical procedures has not gone away, as witnessed in recent heated debates in Britain over widespread rejection of the MMR vaccine as a possible cause of autism. In her 1769 novel *The Delicate Distress* Elizabeth Griffiths exploits the intimacy of a fictional exchange of letters between upper-class women to explore the domestic dilemma that smallpox inoculation posed.[30] As illustrated below, the epistolary form enabled Griffiths to offer a minute exploration of how the risks and etiquette of inoculation come to be debated and negotiated within one extended family circle. Dating from the period when inocu-lation was starting to be widely accepted, the debate is not so much over basic safety and efficacy, but more over questions of familial authority and procedural etiquette. In particular Griffiths dramatises how the emotional burden of overseeing a still risky procedure often falls on women over whom more distantly involved men hold decisive power.

At the opening of the novel Lady Straffon reveals her plan to avoid causing her husband, Sir John, unnecessary stress by forgoing accompany-ing him on a trip to Paris in order to oversee the inoculation of their children in his absence. 'I shall not acquaint him with my intention, till it is over' she writes in confidence to her sister, Lady Woodville:

I know he wishes it to done; and I would spare him the anxiety of a fond father, upon such an occasion. I know too, he will be vastly obliged to me, for laying hold of this opportunity; for it is an invariable maxim, that all men hate trouble . . . and choose to be out of the way, when there is any disagreeable operation to be performed.' (9)

Lady Straffon's young sister-in-law Lucy has also 'determined to take her chance, with my children' because 'she could not answer it to her con-science, to marry Sir James Miller, who seems to be enamoured of her face, till she has put her features beyond the common danger of an alteration' (9). Lucy has just informed Miller that she intends being inoculated, but 'he opposed it with the utmost vehemence, and told many stories, upon that subject, to intimidate her' but 'in vain she continued firm to her purpose' (10). Miller entreats Lucy to go ahead with their marriage 'before the operation' and that he will then give his consent for her to undertake it ten days after. When Lucy refuses this offer 'the altercation grew warm on both sides' and being 'chosen umpire' Lady Strafford takes Lucy's side. Miller departs in anger leaving Lucy full of forebodings over the union ever happening. Reconciled to the possibility of losing either her beauty or even her life to 'this experiment', Lucy is inconsolable at the prospect of losing Miller, but the entrance of Sir John, who is to be kept in the dark, 'put an end to the subject of inoculation' (10–11).

Griffiths has rapidly generated a situation of intrigue between two women, one of whom assumes control over the bodies of her children and the other over her own, but Lucy's motive in seeking to preserve her beauty serves to complicate the issue. While these are presented as genuinely rooted in a desire to serve her betrothed's interests, his dramatised opposition opens up the question of it being deemed selfish. Yet Griffiths is surely directing her readers' sympathies through Lady Woodville's reply: 'I feel for you on your children's account, and for Lucy on her own. She has long determined on inoculation and ... I admire her fortitude, but fear I should not be able to imitate it' (11). Lady Straffon subsequently reports that within an hour of her husband's departure, 'Mr Ranby inoculated Lucy and my dear children'. Despite her faith in the goodness of providence 'the mother could not stand it'; 'I was forced to retire to my closet' where 'I repented of not having acquainted Sir John with my design, and thought, that if a misfortune should happen to either of the children, even his grief would seem a constant reproach to me'. She resorts to prayer, and as 'the rectitude of my intentions confirmed my resolution' is left feeling 'perfectly calm and resigned' (15). Although 'the children are in a fine way and have received the infection', Lucy has not and 'insists upon being inoculated again tomorrow'. In the meantime Lucy's fiancé tells them 'that he should not see us again, till this affair is over' and starts to pay court to an 'artful and agreeable' Miss Nelson. The cautious Lady Woodville responds with 'apprehensions for poor Lucy': 'I almost wish she may not receive the infection' since 'there have been numberless instances of persons who have never had the small-pox; and I think it is like forcing nature, to make a second effort' (23). In her next, Lady Straffon can report that 'the mother's fears are lost in the happy certainty of my children's recovery' but 'poor Lucy continues extremely ill, though, thank God ... is pronounced out of danger'. Lucy's poor response is attributed to psychological stress, for although 'the small-pox was as favourable to her, as possible ... the emotions of her mind, on account of that wretch, Sir James Miller, have thrown her into a violent fever'. This accords with contemporary thinking over the need for the subject to be both physically and mentally strong at the time of inoculation. In a parting letter to Lucy, Miller – who has jilted her for Miss Nelson – explains that while he is 'glad that her beauty is out of danger, as there was no doubt it would procure her a better husband, than him' yet 'he should endeavour to look out for a wife who was less anxious about her features' (26). The narrative voice implies that Lucy is well rid of him but she dreads the return of her brother, while the older women are left wondering how to avoid a duel ensuing when Sir John eventually hears of Miller's 'base' behaviour. As this blow-by-blow distillation illustrates, Griffiths deftly exploits concerns over inoculation (including the practical matter of whether it is efficacious to make a second attempt at inoculation when the first fails to 'take'), as the dramatic focus for airing questions regarding the independent authority of both mothers and prospective wives and, along the way, the moral duties of a brother towards his unmarried sister. But one crucial relationship is left unexplored; that between the inoculee and inoculator.

THE POETICS OF INOCULATION

By the 1770s the ritual of choosing to submit oneself to inoculation and hopefully recovering from the mild form of smallpox it triggered had already prompted occasional poems which struggled to articulate the mixed feelings of trepidation and celebration involved.[31] One of the very earliest examples, Richard Savage's 'The Animalcule. A Tale. Occasioned by His Grace the Duke of Rutland's Receiving the Small-Pox by Inoculation' (1726), opens with an anxious invocation in which the poet admits that this is a novel subject resistant to poetic elevation: 'In Animalcules, muse, display / Spirits, of name unknown in song!'[32] In a desire to dramatise the internal, physiological drama of inoculation Savage emphasises how, once the decision to be inoculated has been made, the battle with the disease is beyond the patient's control, taking place as an internal struggle within the most intimate, labyrinthine recesses of the body. But, as Savage's modern editor Clarence Tracy notes, this attempt to make fresh poetic conceits out of a new medical practice founders in a metaphoric muddle for although 'The Animalcule' was prompted by a patron submitting to inoculation in April 1725, Savage 'is less concerned with inoculation than with the spermatic animalcule' and in so doing shows 'little scientific knowledge, his poem being an elaborate conceit, in which he traces the descent of the gene of literary patronage from the Greeks to the Duke of Rutland'.[33] Allusions to microscopic 'mites' probably owe a far greater debt to Swift's mock-scientific imagery than to any actual medical treatise and when Savage imagines a 'subtle spright' entering into Rutland's bloodstream along with the variolated form of smallpox, like a guardian spirit acting to remove the infection from his heart, the source is clearly Pope's mock-Rosicrucian machinery in *The Rape of the Lock*. Savage's poetic analogies rely upon the traditional assumption that smallpox is already present in the body and yet, like many theorists, he is ultimately unable to reconcile this internal seed model with the increasing evidence for external contagion provided by inoculation. But if the poet confuses an animalculist theory of smallpox, particularly as boosted by the discovery of micro-organisms by the microscopist Anton van Leeuwenhoek (1632–1723), with the latter's discovery of spermatozoa, he was doing no more than many medical theorists who, when faced with a lack of accurate empirical evidence, rarely hesitated over imagining what reproductive pathogenic processes might be at work. But while Savage awkwardly appropriates the language of the new reproductive science to serve what is essentially a traditional compliment poem, the notion of animalcules does at least allow him to re-imagine the battle between the individual victim and smallpox as a more complex encounter. This fight is now to be won by knowing when to yield ground to 'the tumour's rage' by counter-intuitively allowing the enemy into the fortress of the body.

Savage's odd poem can be set alongside his mockery of the opposition to useful innovations in 'The Authors of the Town' (1725), a satire on the literary abuses of the age, where he sarcastically observes: 'If next Inoculation's Art spreads wide, / (An Art, that mitigates Infection's Tide) / Loud Pamphleteers 'gainst Innovation cry, / Let *Nature work* – 'Tis natural to die'.[34] The high-profile experiments with inoculation, first tested on condemned Newgate prisoners in 1725 before being given to members of the Royal household had indeed prompted a pamphlet debate which through periods of abatement and intensification was to continue to the end of the century. The publication of an annual sermon, many by leading clerics, in support of the charitable inoculation programme at the London Smallpox Hospital is a measure of the extent to which religious opposition to inoculation was in abeyance by mid-century, but as Downman's poetic championing in the 1770s implies, inoculation continued to pose a unique challenge to the art of professional persuasion. Disrupting the expectations of patients who traditionally do not seek to *receive* disease from their physician or surgeon, this 'inverted' science of inoculation demanded a new relationship of trust. Patient heroism now lay in the counter-intuitive act of allowing oneself to be infected.

Samuel Bowden's occasional verses 'To A Young Lady at Holt, on her Recovery from the Small-Pox, By Inoculation' published in 1754 represent a physician's own attempt to portray the emotional drama surrounding his use of a still controversial medical intervention.[35] Bowden practised at Frome, in Somerset, where he had family connections with the prominent non-conformist circle to which the poetess Elizabeth Rowe had been attached.[36] But 'Sylvia', the inoculee whose 'painful' but 'pleasing flight' back to health prompted Bowden's verses was the younger, more obscure poetess Esther Lewis (later Clark, 1716–1794).[37] Bowden's poem belongs with other poetic and epistolary exchanges printed in his *Poems on Various Subjects; with some Essays in Prose* (Bath: 1754), in which this literary doctor encourages Lewis to publish her own poetry.[38] Bowden played upon his paternalist role as Lewis's physician in an Apollonian friendship in which medical and poetic concerns are closely allied. Exploiting the fact that Lewis resided 'in the midst of rural contemplation' by the mineral springs at Holt in Wiltshire, Bowden teasingly prescribes the waters as the cure for her flagging muse:[39]

When your muse sleeps, she ought to be summon'd to her duty, and rous'd out of such a dangerous slumber. 'Tis a kind of alarm. As in a lethargy the most stimulating applications are best, to quicken the patient, and remove the stupor. As you have been silent for some time, it makes some suspect you are infected with some of those comatose symptoms, which, if not prevented in time, may end in total stagnation . . . I advise therefore, by all means, to exercise genius, and set your facultys to work; and to drink, at proper medical hours, some of your *Castalian* waters, observing a due poetic regimen in the mean time.[40]

In her lively reply Lewis runs with Bowden's medical analogy, politely accepting his diagnosis, for while she 'has not been seiz'd with a rhyming fit this long time' she grows fond of 'indolence'. She thanks him for his 'friendly advice to my muse' but fears 'her case is desperate' and even the 'strongest antihypnotics' would be applied in vain. Promising to attempt a poetic riposte, she warns Bowden to take care that he is 'not infected by the stupefying fog' himself and prescribes a 'drink a cup or two of coffee, as an antidote against morbific effluvia of a muse who sings in her sleep'. Self-consciously reversing the conventional terms of a doctor-patient relationship, Lewis begs Bowden's pardon 'for taking the liberty of advising you; for 'tis certainly somewhat preposterous for the patient to advise the doctor; but women are fond of novel ways'.[41] From the evidence of these witty letters, Lewis had a strong grasp of medical terms and proved herself open to 'novel ways' by submitting, at Bowden's hands, to inoculation.[42]

Like other smallpox poets, Bowden is aware that his subject matter may not be readily adaptable to the aesthetic codes of poetic language: 'Your health restor'd – the muse attempts to write. / Inoculation! unharmonious name! / And dire disease, afford no grateful theme; / Yet thus inspir'd, no dangers shall dismay, / When friendship prompts, and Sylvia smooths the Way' (49). And like other literary champions of inoculation he sets the minimal risks of the practice against the long and tragic sweep of history when, from 'age to age' the 'spotted monster with polluted gore, / Breath'd putrid death at every poison'd pore'. Comparing smallpox contagion to insects in an 'Eastern Breeze', Bowden repeats the story that inoculation was originally employed by Circassian mothers for the purpose of preserving their daughter's beauty in order to retain their retail value for a Turkish market in 'Seraglian-slaves'. But it is with an extraordinary lack of interceding comment that Bowden jumps straight from this picture of sexual enslavement to his own personal injunction that 'Blest be th' invention, and the art ador'd, / Which sav'd mankind, and Sylvia's Health restor'd'. His interrogatory demand – 'Say, Sylvia, how debating passions sway'd, / With pulse alternate, when th' attempt you weigh'd?' gestures towards a concern for the emotional stress surrounding his patient's brave decision to undertake a risky medical procedure, but it is Bowden himself, in his own role of wise doctor, who responds to this purely rhetorical question by launching into a self-defensive counter-argument to the charge of blasphemy:

> To graft distempers, and inflict disease,
> Seem'd a bold challenge on divine decrees.
> Too fast comes sickness, with its solemn train,
> Shall mortals then anticipate their pain?
> Ingenious – nature's artifice to ape,
> And seek diseases which they may escape.
> But preservation turns the dubious scales,
> And reason o'er fantastic fears prevails:
> Obvious the choice, let prejudice depart,
> To die by Nature – or to live by Art (52).

Passing concern for Sylvia's fears serves to highlight male medical heroics. Even when he returns to her feelings by asking her to 'Say, with what thoughts your beating breast was fill'd, / When in your veins the poison first distil'd?', a complimentary comparison between her 'sedate' bravery and the stoic virtue displayed by Socrates when he drank the 'mortal mixture of the poison'd cup' is somewhat undercut by the subsequent borrowing of Pope's playful use of mock-epic machinery in *The Rape of the Lock*, which lends an incongruous flirtatious tone to Bowden's address:

> More anxious far attentive Sylphs stood round,
> And conscious Muses hover'd o'er the wound:
> For all the light militia of the sky
> Still round their favourite fair patroling fly.
> From the Pandoran box, with heavenly art,
> And balm divine, some chace the destin'd dart;
> While some with poppy fans soft sleep infuse,
> And o'er your pillow pour pacific dews.
> Protected thus – what dangers cou'd you dread,
> While tutelary Saints watch'd round your bed? (53)

The Pandora allusion complicates Bowden's gallant tribute to the role of female attendance on the sick poetess leaving his closing insistence that Sylvia should mark her recovery by offering up 'Some grateful Hymn to that Protecting Power / Who thus preserv'd you in the dangerous hour' open to mixed interpretation: is this 'Protecting Power' the spirit of inoculation, Sylvia's sylph-like nursing attendants, or Bowden the heroic physician? Bowden does at least acknowledge Sylvia's powers as a poet when he concludes with the flattering charge, 'Let others their own way the Powers address, / Sylvia's must be a Hecatomb of Verse' (54).

Lewis's own verses 'On Recovery from the Small-Pox by Inoculation' must have been composed in direct response to Bowden's injunction since they conclude with her thanking him for having 'Prescrib'd the way to make the dire disease / With soften'd symptoms gently seize'.[43] The overall religiosity of Lewis's poem and her choice of Pindarics suggests a literary model in Elizabeth Rowe (who wrote a 'Hymn of Thanks. On my recovery from the Small-Pox').[44] Lewis's presents her own prayer

> To HIM, who blest those means, which reason's voice
> Bade human prudence makes its choice
> To free the mind from anxious fears,
> And easier make my future years.[45]

Without underplaying her trepidation, Lewis portrays her submission to inoculation as an example of how we should put our trust in a merciful God who, by acting through 'Nature' to direct 'human skill',

> Points out a way by which Mankind,
> With safety o'er that dreadful gulph may steer,
> Where myriads perish each revolving year.

> Then since thy Maker smooth the wave,
> Don't thou refuse thyself to save
> But wisely trust him with the life he gave.[46]

Conscious that submitting to inoculation might be considered a defiance of divine will, Lewis contrives to argue that although she fully accepts that her death is entirely in the hands of her maker, nonetheless 'He' has provided inoculation as a means of assuaging some of the anxiety aroused by the constant fear of smallpox.

This accommodating argument follows that endorsed by the leading dissenting theologian, Phillip Dodderidge through his publication of *The Case of Receiving the Small-Pox by Inoculation; impartially considered and especially from a religious point of view* (from a manuscript by David Some dating from 1725). It is regrettable, though far from unusual, that in buttressing this rationalist argument for the safety and sanctity of inoculation with her own personal testimony, Lewis punctuates her sincere, experiential response by compounding the usual assumptions concerning female vanity. Her formulaic litany of the historical horrors of smallpox concludes with the predictable observation that as well as killing thousands, smallpox has often 'kill'd the peace of man' by ruining 'Beauty's fair field': 'For O! few females can despise / Those charms which catch a gazer's eyes'.

Casting inoculation as beauty's protector proved a lasting rhetorical trope. From later in the century we have Anna Seward's 'Verses, Sent with some ornaments for the hair of Miss Margaret Knowles, on Her Recovery from Inoculation for the Small Pox, in her 17th Year', in which the poet offers a 'Nymph' 'praise, for having dared disarm / The dread contagion of its power to harm, / Furrow the cheeks, and blast their rising bloom'. Seward presents a young woman's recovery from inoculated smallpox as a necessary, female rite-of-passage, assuring Knowles that she can now step 'fearless tho' beauty's demon cross thy way'.[47]

This enduring cultural linkage between inoculation and the investment of female power in the ability to capture a male gaze is most fully encapsulated in *Inoculation; or Beauty's Triumph; a Poem* (Bath: 1768), in which the dramatist Henry Jones announces that 'No more shall fell deformity arrest / The radiant Angel, in her bright Career'.[48] Although Jones, like Hill and Lipscomb, celebrates inoculation as a national achievement, he never mentions Montagu but rather devotes the first half of *Beauty's Triumph* to a sustained tribute to 'SUTTON'. This could possibly allude to the surgeon-apothecary Robert Sutton (1708–1788), but by this date it more likely refers to his enterprising son Daniel Sutton (1708–1788) who in 1766 had personally inoculated 7,816 patients.[49] In the wake of the severe smallpox epidemic of 1752, this family of Suffolk surgeons were responsible for successfully promoting a safer and cheaper inoculation technique, marking the start of a second, popularising phase in the history of smallpox prevention.[50]

Until the 1750s inoculation was often a private, domestic affair requiring elaborate and expensive preparatory regimens and aftercare which, despite many local charitable efforts, kept it largely a preserve of the urban rich.[51] This situation was to be transformed with the emergence of new sites of medically managed sociability. By 1757 Robert Sutton was advertising in the *Ipswich Journal* that he had 'hired a large commodious House' where 'gentleman and ladies will be prepared, inoculated, boarded and nursed, and allowed tea, Wine, Fish and Fowl, at seven Guineas each, for one Month', with suitably reduced provisions and rates for farmers, and 'the meaner sort' (there was also a free service to the poor).[52] The Suttons went on to open a range of 'Inoculation Houses' throughout Suffolk and the adjacent counties, designed to cater to different social classes. The publication at Bath in 1768 of Jones's poetic eulogy to 'Sutton' probably coincided with a working visit to the spa by Daniel Sutton who, by this date, had taken to touring the country undertaking mass inoculations in response to local outbreaks. Sceptics like George Saville Carey in his theatrical apprentice-piece *The Inoculator, a Comedy* (1766) bawdily mocked this new class of medical entrepreneur as exploitative, Volpone-like quacks, but celebrating the Suttonian breakthrough, the first half of *Inoculation; or Beauty's Triumph* presents their endeavours as a national achievement.

Jones's poem opens with a melodramatic image of Sutton the medical hero, with the surgeon imagined stopping the arm of 'tyrant' death despite opposition from 'Superstition' who, in a resemblance to earlier personifications of the fury smallpox, stands 'With magnifying Mirror, broad revers'd / That teems with spectred and fantastic Forms / With ideot Terrors and distorted Shapes, / The ghastly Brood of credulous Conceit'. Sutton's method, Jones declares, outshines the achievements of all the learned physicians; if the whole medical pantheon from Hippocrates to Boerhaave were to come back to life they would think that 'Nature, since their Time, had chang'd her laws'. Sutton's far 'nobler and unmatch'd discovery' even tops that of Columbus in finding America whose 'vast Domain' of gold and diamonds bears no comparison with rescuing millions of human lives from the threat of smallpox.

We are witnessing the emergence of the heroic rhetoric that eventually came to inspire efforts towards global eradication. Jones even anticipates

the conquest of death itself, but for all this vision of the universal adoption
of the Suttonian technique, the hyperbole is haunted by anxieties over the
prevalence of moral as much as physical corruption; an innate degeneration
which is once again traced back to female sexual transgression. Women are
cast as the key beneficiaries of inoculation, but they are also the primary
source of the first falling away from the original divine order of creation
which lies at the root of disease and deformity:

> Oh! Hadst thou Power to purge the darker Passions
> From the human breast, with moral Medicine,
> And inoculate the Soul; couldst thou, SUTTON,
> Quick kill the Seeds of each Distemper there,
> Of each irruptive Fever, that deforms
> The Maker's Image, in the outward Frame
> With marking, deep degrading Spots, those Banners
> Of frail Defect, those Legacies of EVE,
> That give th'angelic human face the Lye,
> And bring that fatal Apple to our View.

Set against this pointed reminder of the burden of original sin, Jones
invokes three exemplary aristocratic women, all court beauties exceptional
for their piety, virtue and learning. The first is Mary (Panton), Duchess of
Ancaster and Mistress of the Robes to Queen Charlotte since 1761, whose
portrait by Reynolds was often reproduced in print. Jones wishes that
Sutton was able to 'ingraft' her fine qualities into the 'lovely Daughters
of Britannia' other women:

> Oh! could thy Art her pure, her polish'd
> Humane Accomplishments, serene, ingraft
> With Wonder-working hand on all her class,
> Her envy'd and exalted Class: Oh! could thy Hand
> Her mental Medicine blend through each distemper'd
> Intellectual Mass, and mix her Virtues,
> With the British fair . . .

Jones also compliments the political hostess Elizabeth Percy, Duchess of
Northumberland – another Lady to the Bedchamber of Queen Charlotte
and another sitter for Reynolds – wishing that Sutton 'Couldst thou
NORTHUMBERLAND's Contagion spread / the pure Infection of her
generous Soul, / Through Courts and palaces, where Monarchs reign'.[53]
Jones wishes that Sutton could 'mix the private, with the public Weal, /
And make all Hearts, all princely Hearts like hers' (9). Jones ignores
Montagu's historic role in introducing inoculation, giving all the credit
to a male surgeon, but he does exploit a metaphoric conception of

inoculation as the benign transmission of wisdom to promote a call for female moral example from above. While exalting and flattering these exemplary women of the courtier class Jones acknowledges that corruption dwells in palaces, but in his insistence upon the need to seek out a 'moral medicine' with which to cure a perceived degeneracy amongst 'the British fair', he reinforces a persistent association between smallpox and female weakness.

CHAPTER 8

'Cow mania': vaccination, poetry and politics

Edward Jenner's *Inquiry into the Causes and Effects of the Variolae Vaccinae, a disease discovered in some of the western Counties of England . . . and known by the name of The Cow Pox* (1798), a thin quarto volume of seventy-five pages printed at the expense of its author, a Gloucestershire surgeon, has rightly been described as a 'revolutionary work'.[1] It carries a modest dedication in which Jenner remarks how 'in this age of scientific investigation, it is remarkable that a disease of so peculiar a nature as Cow pox, which has appeared in this and some of the neighbouring counties for such a series of years, should have so long escaped particular attention'. In an effort to test local folk-wisdom that farm labourers who were commonly infected by cow-pox became resistant to smallpox, Jenner's initial experiment had involved taking the infected matter of the relatively harmless cow-pox from the milking hand of the dairymaid Sarah Nelmes and inserting it into the arm of a healthy eight-year-old boy who subsequently showed few symptoms and was rendered immune to smallpox. As Tim Fulford and Debbie Lee have recently observed, appearing at a moment of national crisis when Britain – beset by naval mutinies and unrest amongst the labouring-classes fuelled by pro-French radicalism – was preparing for a threatened invasion, Jenner's discovery was notable for not being 'derived from medical authorities, but from the oral tradition of Gloucestershire villagers'. The *Inquiry* simply offered 'a series of stories about dairy maids, farm hands, paupers, and man servants whose daily, pastoral activities brought them in touch with cows and cowpox, and thus made them immune to smallpox'. Jenner's major medical discovery was not 'rooted in visions of national and international conquest but in the bodies of those who worked in the English countryside'. Like Wordsworth and Coleridge's *Lyrical Ballads*, first published in the same year, the humble story of 'the dairymaid with a sore hand' was a tale of such 'rural simplicity' that initially at least it barely registered 'in a metropolis alarmed by the threat of revolution and invasion' (140).

It was Jenner's friend and biographer, John Baron who first reflected on how the leading physicians occupying 'prominent stations in the metropolis could not so readily admit the claims of a provincial physician, who held no place in either of the great corporations which preside over medicine and surgery in this country'.[2] Jenner did gradually find professional allies, but as another supporter, the poet Charles Frognall Dibdin was to recall, 'What a fight he had to encounter for the establishment of his beloved VACCINATION!'. Unlike Montagu, who had preferred to use her private connections to work behind-the-scenes at court, Jenner, who had a 'passion for *poetising*', made deliberate efforts to gain the support of imaginative writers in an often highly personal campaign to gain professional approval and governmental support.[3] As Fulford and Lee observe, with Jenner seeking 'the services of romantic poets, who lent their verse to his efforts to create the taste by which his discovery might be enjoyed by the people' this was a campaign 'that from the start, presented science through the medium of poetry' (139). Indeed Dr Benjamin Moseley, in his eagerly adopted role as Jenner's chief professional opponent, was to make the characteristically alarmist claim that in 'the year 1798 the Cow Pox Inoculation Mania seized the people of England *en masse*' as 'the English language expired under the load of Cow Pox Pæns'.[4] This closing chapter explores this propagandist use of pastoral poetry in the promotion of a ground-breaking medical procedure which finally made it possible to imagine the global eradication of smallpox.

'COW MANIA'

The Jennerian adoption of a pastoral idiom needs to be set against the markedly anti-pastoral rhetoric of an energetic anti-vaccination movement. Cow-pox was a familiar, relatively benign, locally sporadic disease which produced sores on the hands of milkers, but as early as 1799 the haughty Moseley, anxious to defend his own vested interest in inoculation, starts to attack its use against smallpox as the product of parochial gullibility, disparaging this 'new star in the Æsculapian system . . . first observed in the Provinces'.[5] Moseley claims that vaccinated patients were developing a scrofulous bestial disease. He conjures up salacious images of women chasing after bulls and mockingly wonders whether 'the human character may undergo strange mutations from *quadrupedan* sympathy; and that some modern Pasipaë may rival the fables of old' (Pasipaë gave birth to the monstrous Minotaur) (183). No-one, he argues, can possibly know 'what may be the consequence of introducing the *Lues Bovilla*, a bestial humour – into the human frame . . .?' Moseley's neologism is an etymological adaptation of *Lues Venerea* (i.e. syphilis) deliberately designed to counter Jenner's term *Variolae Vaccinae* and foster the implication that cow-pox implants a bestial form of syphilis. It was inevitable that a technique which involved the injection of matter derived from domestic beasts would raise concerns over the potential dangers of eroding a species boundary, but medical and lay opposition to the prophylactic use of cow-pox crudely exploited intensified post-revolution fears of constitutional degeneracy at both an individual and national level.

Moseley found an ally in William Rowley, a successful man-midwife, whose polemical *Cow-Pox Inoculation no Security Against Small-Pox Infection, to which is added the Modes of Treating the Beastly New Diseases Produced from Cow-Pox* (1805), includes two hand-coloured engraved plates depicting 'the COW-POXED OX-FACED BOY, and the GIRL, [afflicted] with that dreadful disease, the Cow-pox mange, evil, abscess, and other similar proofs of Cow-pox impurities, or beastly *ulcers*'.[6] (Illustration 10) When Rowley exhibited these cases at a public lecture, Moseley observed 'that the boy's face seemed to be in a state of transforming, and assuming the visage of a cow' (viii). Reinforcing Moseley's analogy between 'the Cow-pox mange' and syphilis, Rowley asks 'Who would marry into a family, at the risk of their offspring having filthy beastly diseases?' (vi). He also backs up this anti-vaccination argument by drawing upon Levitican taboos against defilement from contact with beasts, and he makes much of a comparison with the failed, blasphemous experiments of seventeenth-century virtuosi who tried to transfuse 'the blood of beasts into the veins of human beings to . . . prolong life to eternity' which ended in death or madness (8). Vaccination, Rowley insists, is another example of how 'Visionary conceits, irrational projects, and an obstinate perseverance in error, united to uncontrolled arrogance, are frequently the causes of great evils in the political, moral and physical world' (1–2). Ranting against 'Cow Mania' as the triumph of passion over reason, Rowley's rhetoric echoes that in Burke and other pro-government accounts of how the French mob were too easily carried away by misguided demagogues (5). 'Cow-pox infatuation' is represented as part of the same revolutionary political fervour that overthrew the French *ancien regime* and now poses a direct military threat to Britain.

Such insinuations were to be bandied on both sides; Baron later wrote that the 'British Forum' established in 1808 to oppose Jenner and who published a 'Cow-Pox Chronicle, a newspaper with mock-advertisements . . . seems to have been a place somewhat akin to that in which the Jacobins

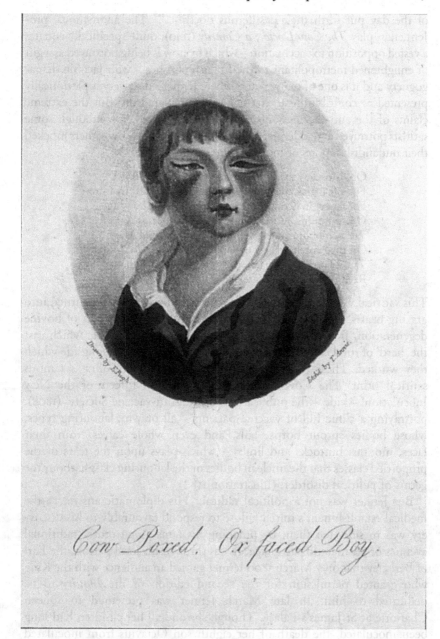

10. 'The Cow-Poxed Ox-Faced Boy' from William Rowley, *Cow-Pox Inoculation No Security Against Small-Pox Infection* (London, 1805.) As part of the anti-vaccination campaign, this purported victim of 'cow-mania' had been exhibited as a warning at Rowley's London lectures.

of the day put forth their pestiferous doctrines'.[7] The anonymous, pro-Jennerian play *The Cow Doctor; a Comedy* (1810), quite specifically equates a vested opposition to vaccination – which by now is being portrayed as a gift of enlightened metropolitans to the English parishes – with Jacobin demagoguery and it is one of many places where Jenner's discovery is patriotically presented as contributing to the fight against Napoleon. But the extreme claims of the anti-vaccinationist may have back-fired, for although some satirists portrayed a mad Jenner riding his hobbyhorsical cow, others mocked their outlandish reports of mooing mutants:

> Oh, Moseley! thy book nightly phantasies rousing,
> Full oft makes me quake for my heart's dearest treasure;
> For fancy, in dreams, oft presents them all brousing
> On commons, just like little Nebuchadnezzar.
> *There*, nibbling at thistle, stand Jem, Joe, and Mary,
> On their foreheads, O horrible! crumpled horns bud;
> *There* Tom with his tail, and poor William all hairy,
> Reclined in a corner, are chewing the cud.[8]

This satirical vision of a countryside in which the swains have turned into grazing beasts works by offering a deliberately comic prospect of bovine degeneration. It also implicitly mocks a conservative rhetoric which cast the 'herd' of rural labourers as being little above the beasts alongside which they worked. These fears are mockingly visualised in Gillray's famous satirical print 'The Cow-Pock, or the wonderful Effects of the New Inoculation! – vide – the publications of the Anti-vaccine Society' (1808), portraying a clinic full of vaccine patients – all brawny labouring types, whose bodies sprout horns, tails, and even whole calves from their faces, mouths, buttocks and limbs – which plays upon the fears of the propertied classes that the unclean bodies of the labouring class harbour the germs of political disorder. (Illustration 11)

But Jenner was not a political radical.[9] His diplomatic answer to the medical establishment's initial failure to respond favourably to his discovery was to side-step them by pursuing his aims along more traditional avenues of aristocratic patronage. It was through his local patron, the Earl of Berkeley that on 7 March 1800 Jenner gained an audience with the King who granted permission for the second edition of the *Inquiry* to be dedicated to him. In late March Jenner was presented to Queen Charlotte at St James's Palace. Though she and all her children had long been inoculated, the death of her eighth son Octavius from inoculated smallpox meant that she took a genuine interest in the discovery of a potentially safer method. The same month, Jenner was also received by

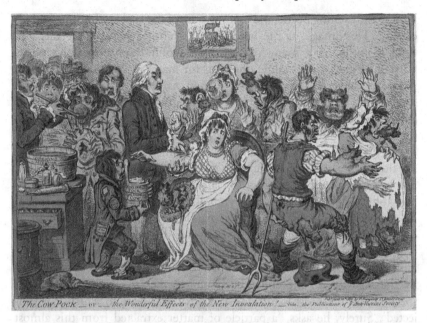

The Cow Pock — or — the Wonderful Effects of the New Inoculation! — vide — *the Publication of ye Anti Vaccine Society*

11. James Gillray, 'The Cow-Pock, or the wonderful Effects of the New Inoculations! – vide – the publications of the Anti-vaccine Society', 1808. Gillray's politically suggestive caricature of a vaccination clinic, prompted by contemporary medical propaganda that the use of a bovine serum will trigger 'Cow-Mania'.

the Prince of Wales at his rival court at Carlton House, thus assuring that his project was also authorised by the heir who would stand regent should the king's madness return.[10] Though it was some years before Jenner was required to vaccinate any royal children, this rush of royal assent immediately rendered vaccination an approved topic for drawing-room discussion: in November 1800, Jane Austen attended a house-party where her hosts 'alternately read Dr. Jenner's pamphlet on the cow pox'.[11]

To counter charges that cow-pox vaccination represents a blasphemous erosion of the firm category division between humanity and the beasts, Jenner deliberately cultivated a romantic rhetoric in which his pastoral medicine figured as a benign symbol of the natural powers of healing.[12] He fostered a public image of himself as a philanthropic country surgeon (later doctor), who only spent time in dirty, expensive London long enough to seek official recognition for his discovery. Upholding this myth, Dibdin later recalled how 'no man hated pomp and display more thoroughly' and 'having had his system established to his satisfaction' he 'retired to his native village – the enjoyment of his garden, his roses and honeysuckles, the hum of the evening beetle, the echoing note of the cuckoo, his flute and his cigar'.[13] This image of the vaccinator as retiring romanticist was also fostered in Jenner's many portraits.[14] In John Raphael Smith's pastel portrait of 1800, for example, the basis for many variant engraved prints, Jenner is depicted with his own natural hair, leaning informally with hat-in-hand against a tree, before a middle-ground pastoral scene of cows and a milk-maid. The country seat of his neighbour and patron Lord Berkeley is visible on the wooded horizon.

Even when portrayed at study indoors Jenner's accoutrements emphasise the pastoral message by including the image of a sacred cow.[15] This had first been adopted by Jenner's associate, the philanthropic Quaker physician John Coakley Lettsom, for symbolic inclusion on the frontispiece to his *Observations on the Cow-Pock* (1801). (Illustration 12) Countering fears of 'Cow-Mania', Lettsom waxes lyrical over the cleanliness and domestic benefits of the cow, marvelling at how an 'animal whose lactarious fountains afford in our infancy a substitute for that of the parent . . . is destined by the sagacity of one enlightened philosopher to protect the human species from the most loathsome and noxious disease to which it is subjected'. Surely, he asks, 'a particle of matter extracted from this almost sacred animal, can excite no disgust?'[16] The Jennerian Society officially adopted the holy cow as the icon for their benign revolution in pastoral medicine, including it on their commemorative medals.

Jenner, whose extant poetry reflects his early interest in the close observation of nature that ultimately led him to investigate cow-pox, shared the popular taste for pastoral verse.[17] Although he encouraged others to exploit this literary fashion to further the vaccination cause, this posed a challenge at a time when critics were often observing how previous efforts to eulogise inoculation had resulted in some dismal compositions.[18] In his *Biographia Literaria* Coleridge recalls a line from 'an Oxford copy of verses on the two SUTTONS, commencing with "INOCULATION, heavenly maid! descend!"' as a prime example of 'the madness' of hysterically weak 'Pseudo-poesy' which 'bursts upon the reader in sundry odes and apostrophes to abstract terms'.[19] But in half-remembering Lipscombe's prize-winning ode, it should be emphasised that Coleridge was targeting the over-use of trite personifications, *not* the smallpox theme *per se*. In the autumn of 1811, the poet was writing to Jenner to request where he might find 'the best and fullest history of the vaccine matter as preventive of smallpox' since he had long 'planned a poem on this theme, which after long deliberation, I have convinced myself is capable in the highest degree of being poetically treated, according to our divine bard's own definition of poetry, as '*simple,*

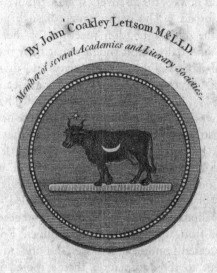

Observations

on the

COW-POCK;

By John Coakley Lettsom M&L.L.D.

Member of several Academies and Literary Societies

Printed by Nichols & Son Red Lion Passage Fleet Street

for Joseph Mawman, Poultry.

1801.

12. Frontispiece of John Coakley Lettsom, *Observations on the Cow-Pock* (1801). Countering fears of 'Cow-Mania', Jenner's followers adopted the healthy, domestic icon of a sacred cow.

sensuous . . . and impassioned'.[20] In tandem with his plans for this poem he had been approached by *The Courier*, the leading evening newspaper to which Coleridge had contributed for a dozen years, to contribute a series of essays on vaccination (though the poet considered it a sorry situation that it

should be necessary 'in this the native country of the discoverer' to still have
to promote the method). In the same letter Coleridge places Jenner in this
personal pantheon of progressive scientists and flatteringly acknowledges
the vaccinationist's contribution to human welfare.[21] Like many of
Coleridge's literary plans neither *The Courier* articles nor his vaccination
poem ever materialised but Jenner considered his interest 'very important'
at a time when many other, often less gifted poets had already been
forthcoming.[22]

By 1800 Jenner was being addressed in numerous odes, operas and other
verse eulogies and as news of his discovery spread, tributes to 'Vaccinia' also
poured in from abroad.[23] The performance of such poetry formed an
essential part of the annual London meetings of the Royal Jennerian
Society; a literary bias reflected in the fact that their resident inoculator
between 1806 and 1808 was the aspiring actor and dramatist Dr James
Sheridan Knowles.[24] Much of this verse is insubstantial and of little artistic
merit. For his own *Vaccination; a Dramatic Poem* (1810) Knowles borrowed
Hecate and the three witches from *Macbeth* to conjure up a Shakespearian
vision of the monstrous birth of 'Variola' so 'rank, that e'en the mother
loath'd to touch', but of more interest are his heartfelt, documentary
footnotes in which he bears witness to how opposition to vaccination by
mercenary practitioners with a vested interest in inoculation simply pro-
longs the miseries of London's wretched, overcrowded migrant workers,
amongst whom smallpox remains rife.[25] Jenner's most accomplished poetic
champion emerged from this displaced urban milieu; Robert Bloomfield,
the largely self-educated London shoemaker and one-time farm-labourer,
had a commitment to the vaccination theme rooted in his first-hand
experience of the devastating impact of smallpox amongst labouring-class
families.

Bloomfield's rapid emergence as a popular poet rested upon his claim
to rustic authenticity in his autobiographical poem *The Farmer's Boy*
(1800). The critic Nathan Drake was one of many to praise it as the work
of a 'genuine and original poet'. Castigating the numerous pastoral
poems displaying 'a servile adherence to classical imagery and custom'
which cannot achieve that 'fecundity in painting the economy of rural
life, which this poem, drawn from actual experience, so richly
displays', Drake found *The Farmer's Boy* to be 'literally the composition of
the character it describes'.[26] This shared astonishment at how many
'curious and striking circumstances peculiar to the occupations of the
British Farmer' had 'escaped our poets previous to the publication of
Mr. Bloomfield's work' had opened up an ideal critical window through

which to promote Jenner's discovery of a medical marvel in the same humble walk of life.[27] Bloomfield's pro-vaccination poem, *Good Tidings; or News from The Farm*, eventually appeared in May 1804. A reconstruction of its pre-publication history will reveal how the composition of a populist poem of medical reform was being shaped by the forces of politicised patronage.

ROBERT BLOOMFIELD: PROPHYLACTIC POETRY
AND PATRONAGE

The earliest evidence of any personal contact between Bloomfield and Jenner dates from July 1802, but in the January of that year the poet had already been in close discussions with Nathan Drake, himself a practising physician.[28] In January 1802 Bloomfield asked for Drake's opinion on 'the Vaccine'.[29] Bloomfield had just returned from being a New Year guest at Drake's home at Hadleigh, Surrey where the physician raised a subscription of twelve guineas for the poet from his local literary coterie. The timing makes it very likely that rather than being commissioned by Jenner, as has often been assumed, Bloomfield's pro-vaccination poem had originally been encouraged by the poet's contact with Drake who later supported the project by providing comments on a late draft and by composing a polemical medical essay designed to serve as a preface.

In fact at this date Jenner was already actively engaged with another poet, Thomas Frognall Dibdin, who was being 'urged to attempt a poem in blank verse, entitled VACCINIA'.[30] Raising a problem intrinsic to didactic poetry, Dibdin considered it a 'mediated work' in which 'the notes' were 'preferable to the versification', since the former 'was to be considered merely as a sort of peg to hang notes upon' to which end he had 'set about reading the whole history of smallpox, resolving to make it out (which in reality it has been) the most frightful scourge of humanity'.[31] By October 1803 Dibdin had sent a polished draft of 'Vaccinia' to Jenner who was anxious to keep close control over a text which was to be printed at his expense: 'I hope that *no proof-sheet* has yet gone finally to the press without my inspection'.[32] Unaccountably 'Vaccinia' never appeared and Dibdin later lost the manuscript after lending it out to a friend.

By the early summer of 1802 Jenner appears to have been offering Bloomfield similar support, but in a letter to his brother George dated 21 July, Robert expresses doubts over accepting this patronage: 'I have seen Dr. Jenner, and his kindness almost induced me to show him the little progress I have made in pursuit of his subject, but I suddenly determined to the contrary, and doubted of the propriety of so doing'.[33] As he was writing this letter, another arrived from Jenner inviting him to tea. Fearing that he may be in pursuit of a 'wrong scent', yet reluctant to pass up the opportunity of serving a significant patron, Bloomfield sought his brother's advice:

What shall I do – leave 150 lines of an unfinished subject in his hands? I am bounded to consult Mr. [Capel] Lofft and the Duke [of Grafton], and to submit my pieces to their judgement, and never will do otherwise; and yet it is hard to say no in such cases as this. I wish I could suspend his curiosity six months and take my chance. He is a very amiable man and perhaps rates my abilities too high.[34]

With Bloomfield anxious to keep on the right side of his existing patrons, Jenner continued his approaches on his periodic visits to London. Both Robert and his brother Nathaniel, also a poet, attended the Jennerian Society dinner held on 17 May 1802 to celebrate the doctor's fifty-third birthday.[35] On 2 August Bloomfield reported receiving a 'a letter from Dr. Jenner at Cheltenham enquiring my determination as to the poem "On Vaccination", and expressing great interest in my welfare'.[36]

In the meantime Nathaniel had published his own 'Lyric Address to Dr. Jenner', probably composed for the 1802 birthday event. Capel Lofft's biographical preface to the volume of Nathaniel's verses in which this lyric appears, makes sympathetic mention of the personal circumstances behind this tribute in which the voice of experience warns of the dangers of neglecting to vaccinate. Not only had the Bloomfield brothers lost their father early to 'that dreadful disease the SMALL-POX' (around 1767), but Nathaniel had also lost 'two sweet Boys who both died within a few days of each-other' and even 'while this Preface was in the Press' it has 'been fatal to another promising Child, THOMAS; born Aug. 1799':

The Father, oppress'd with grief, reproaches himself for not having inoculated this Child with the Small-Pox. But when it is consider'd how formidable, after two such Losses, the Small-Pox, in any form must appear to affectionate Parents, I think it will be evident that he is too severe to himself in this reproach. The inoculated Small-Pox is sometimes fatal: had he inoculated the Child he would have reproach'd himself, and still more feeling than justice, for doing so.[37]

After the death of this third child in November 1802, Robert had taken another nephew Tom, into his own home, resolving to have the boy vaccinated because 'I am inexpressably [sic] hurt and confounded at this stroke and it shall operate as a powerful stimulous on my Mind in pursuit of that great Momentus Subject'.[38] He also began to have his own children vaccinated, although in the case of his daughter Mary it took four attempts before the serum would 'take'.[39]

In his equivocal prefatorial comments on Nathaniel's pro-Jenner lyric, Lofft does not feel qualified to offer an opinion on 'the Merits of VACCINE INOCULATION', even though it does now seem to find 'a general reception in the *medical* World'. Eager to distance himself from his protégé openly taking Jenner's side in the controversy, Lofft asks us to consider that 'poetical Merit is comparatively independent on the correctness of a philosophic System or Hypothesis'. It is with considerable condescension that he implies that the uneducated poet's endorsement is simply an emotional, 'knee-jerk' response to domestic tragedy: 'reflecting on his former Losses and present calamities, the Author could not but feel a deep Interest in whatever seem'd likely to obviate such an Evil to others'.[40]

Robert was shortly to subject his own pro-Jennerian poem to Lofft's scrutiny. By July 1803 the poet had been in receipt of Drake's comments on a draft of his own 'Vaccine Poem' along with a draft copy of the physician's prefatory essay, both of which the poet forwarded to Lofft. The latter's responses, contained in a long reply to Bloomfield dated 10 July 1803, reveal the conflicting editorial pressures that shaped the final appearance of *Good Tidings*. Although Lofft largely upheld many of Drake's 'objections to particular lines' and approved in principal to the use of what was clearly a polemical preface, he baulked at a couple of paragraphs in which the physician 'recommends that inoculation for the smallpox be prohibited by authority; and that every minister be enjoined to recommend to his parishioners vaccine inoculation as a moral and religious duty'. He considered such demands 'quite incompatible with liberty, civil and religious, and with good policy'. Inoculation has proven a 'great mitigator' of the evils of smallpox – he has had three out of his own four children inoculated – and therefore does not 'see the right which Government and Legislature have to prohibit this practise entirely', especially when many do not yet trust the new method of vaccination: 'For a century medical reasoning and general benevolence have been exerted to conquer the repugnance to inoculation for the small-pox, and now that repugnance is so very nearly annihilated, how strange it would be to say we forbid you under severe legal restrictions from using this precaution'.[41] A libertarian in medical as in other matters, Lofft objected to coercion at every level, thinking it enough to regulate inoculation and publish rules for keeping it safe.

At this date Bloomfield had only just repaired his relationship with Lofft after a heated dispute over his patron's inclusion of politically explosive editorial annotations in revised editions of *The Farmer's Boy*. Lofft was a wealthy oppositional Whig barrister who had agitated against the American War and the slave trade. A personal friend of Fox and such leading social reformers as Clarkson, Howard, Godwin and Wilberforce, he was considered something of a firebrand. In 1800 his name had been struck off the roll of magistrates because of his 'improper interference' in jumping on the prison-cart to try to save the life of a poor girl condemned to death for a paltry theft. Lofft's promotion of the Bloomfield brothers as labouring-class poets could never be seen as politically neutral. *The Farmer's Boy* itself avoids obvious party-bias, but Lofft's pointed prefatory comments on the suppression of press freedoms and the educational value of the now outlawed debating societies had rendered it a vehicle for oppositional comment.[42] Bloomfield himself politely tried to remind Lofft that his use of an appendix to the third edition of *The Farmer's Boy* to address his own controversial dismissal as magistrate had been widely 'disapproved'.[43]

Tension between the poet and his editor had reached a crisis over the latter's plans to append similar 'political notes' – some containing party-political comments – to individual poems in Robert's projected volume of *Rural Tales*.[44] Bloomfield was 'proud of the approbation of such a man as Mr. Fox and should be glad the public should know' but he wished it could be presented 'in a more unexceptionable shape'. He begged Lofft to agree to have any editorial notes placed at the end, leaving the reader free to form their own initial judgements of the poems (9). Taking offence, Lofft had threatened to have no more to do with Bloomfield, drawing the correct assumption that the poet's real concern was to distance himself from his patron's radicalism.[45] Lofft insisted that what 'I said of Mr Fox I said less for the sake of Mr. Fox than for the sake of my country and posterity' with the hope 'that it may lead . . . the public to learn better to distinguish . . . between those who have plunged us into such a war and so long kept us in it, and those who would have prevented our ever rushing into that direful whirlpool' (10). Faced with further bad press after Lord Grafton gained him a place at the Stamp Office, by 1803 Bloomfield was certainly feeling that he was being drawn into a whirlpool: 'I have been extravagantly applauded; few men have had a severer trial . . . I feel my situation to be novel; the world looks at me in that light; I am extremely anxious on that account' (12). His pro-vaccination poem was completed amidst this increasing sense of personal crisis: 'Extreme publicity begins to be more and more disgusting to my feelings . . . Dr Jenner is in town, and has written to me' (30). Obliged 'to wriggle amongst a quarrelling set of candidates for fame and . . . money' (13), Bloomfield had fought to keep his poetry free of Lofft's attempts at party-political appropriation but in the event the beleaguered poet did choose to support Jenner's controversial

social cause. Smallpox was a theme close to Bloomfield's domestic experience and in the event he was to prove that it could lend itself to the 'simple',
'impassioned' treatment which Coleridge had always felt it warranted.

BLOOMFIELD'S *GOOD TIDINGS*

When *Good Tidings, or News from the Farm* was finally published in
May 1804, it did not bear Drake's polemical preface nor any editorial notes
by Lofft, but it did carry an authorial dedication to Jenner and a brief
'Advertisement' in which Bloomfield confirms the autobiographical basis
for some of the poem's key incidents: the 'account given of my infancy, and
of my father's burial, is not only poetically, but strictly true' and 'I have
witnessed the destruction described in my brother's family'.[46] The poet
also prays for the 'universal adoption' of Jenner's technique and confirms
that he has himself 'insured the lives of four children by vaccine
Inoculation, who, I trust, are destined to look back on Small-pox as the
scourge of days gone by'.[47] The day of publication deliberately coincided
with Jenner's birthday, and extracts were recited at a special meeting of the
Royal Jennerian Society held in London.[48] Suitably flattered, Jenner presented Bloomfield with an engraved inkstand.[49]

The opening of *Good Tidings* presents a vignette of rural innocence
blighted in the figure of a blind boy, a 'child in everything, but sight',
whose participation in youthful, pastoral companionship and whose enjoyment of nature has been hindered by his affliction. As Fulford and Lee
observe, this pathetic scenario represents an arresting manipulation of an
image of 'a simple, innocent child of nature at play' that we are all now very
familiar with from the poems of Wordsworth, Coleridge, and Blake.[50]
Bloomfield's blind child can shout along with his playmates as they cavort
on the village green, but when the 'grove invites' and 'delight thrills every
breast / To leap the ditch and seek the downy nest' he suddenly 'feels his
dreadful loss'. Forced to stay behind, he sings to himself as he 'plucks by
chance the white and yellow flow'r' to bring home to his distraught mother:

> She blest *that* day, which he remembers too,
> When he could gaze on heav'n's ethereal blue,
> See the young spring, so lovely to his eyes,
> And all the colours of the morning rise. – (13)[51]

When the narrator asks the mother 'When was this work of bitterness
begun?' she wipes away her tears before responding to this 'dagger of a
question':

'My boy was healthy, and the rest was sound,
When last year's corn was green upon the ground:
From yonder town infection found its way;
Around me putrid dead and dying lay,
I trembled for his fate; but all my care
Avail'd not, for he breath'd the tainted air;
Sickness ensu'd – in terror and dismay
I nurs'd him in my arms both night and day,
When his soft skin from head to foot became
One swelling purple sore, unfit to name:' (14)

She concludes with a pathetic account of her desperate efforts to nurse her
sickening child, her guilt that she did not do enough, and her thwarted
hopes that he would once again look into her loving eyes: 'GOD keep
small-pox and blindness from your door!' (15) Where the reader of a
pastoral poem expects to be presented with a rural idyll, Bloomfield
confronts them with this emblematic tale of the misery caused by a
contagion which pointedly emanates from the towns and destroys any
hopes of domestic rural happiness.

Fulford and Lee interpret Bloomfield's introduction of a scene of such
harsh social reality into his pastoral vision as part of a strategy to resolve
what they usefully identify as 'a tension that went to the very heart of his
poetic authority'; one also shaping the work of his contemporaries
Wordsworth and Clare, who made claims for the ideals of traditional
pastoral being 'observable in the lives of contemporary rural labourers'
(150). The largely self-educated author of *The Farmer's Boy* had been
advertised as 'literally a Cow-boy', but even by the time Lofft had first
'discovered' him, Bloomfield had already been displaced from his rural
origins having served an unofficial apprenticeship in London as a tailor.
Publication of *The Farmer's Boy* brought further social displacement as he
gained the attentions of aristocratic patrons amongst the metropolitan
cognoscenti. As Fulford and Lee observe, this increasing tension between
his public, poetic image and actual social positioning quickly 'became
threatening to his commercial prospects and to his sense of identity' such
that 'the very continuance of a rural way of life upon which Bloomfield's
poetic authority depends' was at stake in *Good Tidings* (150–1). Having
established his reputation as a poet who 'by virtue of his peasant upbring-
ing ... could uniquely root the personal ideal in the real', the scourge of
smallpox 'threatened Bloomfield's precarious poetic career because it
exposed a fatal gap between the real world of farm labourers, of which he
had personal experience, and the idealized version of it which his

publication as a "pastoral" poet committed him' (151). Bloomfield's own sense that the tale he now chose to tell of rural woe might undermine an established pastoral ideal is evident from his apologetic 'Advertisement' where he pleads that 'if I may escape the appearance of affectation of research, or the scientific treatment of the subject, I think the egotism, so conspicuous in the poem ... ought to be forgiven'. More specifically this reads like an assertive response to Lofft's earlier comments on Nathaniel's unscientific, emotional championing of Jenner. In the face of a largely metropolitan, professional, theoretical 'scientific' medical debate, Robert follows his brother in rooting his personal bid for authority in his own felt experience of harsh rural social conditions for which a ready and natural ameliorative solution is now available.

Like earlier poetic witnesses to the horrors of smallpox Bloomfield was conscious that his subject matter might be thought objectionable, remarking in the same 'Advertisement' that although 'to the few who knew I have employed my thoughts on the importance of Dr. JENNER's discovery' the topic has 'almost unexceptionally appeared a subject of little promise; peculiarly unfit for poetry', but my chosen 'method of treating it has endeared it to myself, for it indulges in domestic anecdote'. This autobiographical dimension dominates the first half of the poem – and the first part to be written – as Bloomfield draws upon his childhood memories of his mother nursing six children through smallpox and the death and rushed burial of their father:

> Midnight beheld the close of all his pain,
> His grave was clos'd when midnight came again;
> No bell was heard to toll, no funeral pray'r,
> No kindred bow'd, no wife, no children there; ...
> Religious reverence forbade to speak:
> The starting Sexton his short sorrow chid
> When the earth murmur'd on the coffin lid,
> And falling bones and sighs of holy dread
> Sounded a requiem to the silent dead! (24)

At this sombre point Bloomfield anticipates the likely response of those readers who admired *The Farmer's Boy*; 'who o'er the pictur'd Seasons glow'd' and have since held 'the lowly minstrel dear'. Pausing to anticipate their likely objections – 'Why tell us tales of woe, thou didst give / Thy soul to rural themes, and bade them live?' (24) – Bloomfield 'Himself appeals' to them, asking directly

> What if that child were He!
> What, if those midnight sighs a farewell gave,

> While hands, all trembling, clos'd the father's grave!
> Though love enjoin'd not infant eyes to weep,
> In manhood's zenith shall his feelings sleep? (25)

Openly defying the convention-bound reader's sentimental expectations, Bloomfield alerts them to his own near-fate as a smallpox victim and asserts his moral right to bear witness on behalf of the innocent dead. He is not prepared to bury the emotional scars of a childhood, youth and adulthood continually blighted by smallpox along with the family dead:

> Sleep not my soul! indulge a nobler flame:
> Still the destroyer persecutes thy name.
>   Seven winters cannot pluck from memory's store
> That mark'd affliction which a brother bore;
> That storm of trouble bursting on his head,
> When the fiend came, and left *two children* dead!
> Yet, still superior to domestic woes,
> The native vigour of his mind arose,
> And, as new summer's teem'd with other views,
> He traced the wand'rings of his darling Muse,
> And all was joy – this instant all is pain,
> The foe implacable returns again,
> And claims a sacrifice; the deed is done –
> Another child has fall'n, another son!
> His young cheek even now is scarcely cold,
> And shall his early doom remain untold? (25–6).

The smallpox is inimical to the rural muse. Wresting editorial control, Bloomfield's inclusion of a personal footnote at this point stating that 'I had proceeded thus far with the Poem, when the above became a powerful stimulus to my feelings, and to the earnestness of my exhortations' reinforces his claim that these harsh domestic realities are a valid stimulus to write and dramatically underscores the continued immediacy of his pressing social theme (26).

Bloomfield makes some conventional apologies for displaying private grief, but all will probably now concur with Fulford and Lee's observation that it is his inclusion of personal recollections that 'constitute the most powerful passage in the poem as smallpox menaces the Bloomfield family's domestic bliss'.[52] Its earliest readers certainly shared this view; in his positive notice in the *Annual Review*, Robert Southey remarks that while many readers 'will recollect the Oxford verses "Inoculation! heavenly maid descend!", the 'Farmer's Boy has too much good sense to deal in these despicable common places of *poetastry*': everyone 'will be interested by the ... account of the poet's own escape from small-pox in infancy, and of his father's death' which is all 'strictly true'.[53] Even Lofft considered that the second half was 'not in general equal in originality and animation and pathetic effect to the beginning'.[54] But as Fulford and Lee suggest, pathos 'is not the poem's final solution to the tensions in Bloomfield's position: Edward Jenner is'. The discovery of cow-pox serum gave the poet a means of recuperating his original pastoral vision since vaccination 'made the pastoral ideal liveable – at least in one poem' by allowing 'it again to appear rooted in actual rural life' (152).

In fact Bloomfield had already employed this counter-move within the coterie context of Jenner's birthday celebrations in May 1803 in a lyric praising the doctor's gift to 'mild Beauty' as the 'Sweet handmaid of Liberty'. This impassioned eulogy concludes, 'From the field, from the farm, comes the glorious treasure, / May its life-saving impulse – all fresh as the morn- / Still spread round the earth without bounds, without measure . . .'[55] In *Good Tidings* the same politically nuanced message is conveyed in a more nostalgic, personal tone:

> Sweet beam'd the star of peace upon those days
> When Virtue watch'd my childhood's quiet ways,
> Whence a warm spark of nature's holy flame
> Gave the farm-yard an honourable name,
> But left one theme unsung: then, who had seen
> In herds that feast upon the vernal green,
> Or dreamt that in the blood of kine there ran
> Blessings beyond the sustenance of man? (16–17)

Here Fulford and Lee usefully observe how, for a brief moment, 'Bloomfield's pastoralism offers to become socially radical' as 'not only is rural life preferred to urban but, as in the *Lyrical Ballads*, rustics seem wiser than gentleman' (151–2). But if Jenner's dependency upon folk-wisdom puts rustic experience before professional theory, Bloomfield immediately goes on to commend Jenner for recognising the therapeutic value of a mistrusted rustic practice and placing it under the acceptable lens of rational science:

> When the plain truth tradition seem'd to know,
> And simply pointed to the harmless Cow,
> Doubt and distrust to reason might appeal
> But when hope triumph'd, what did Jenner feel? (18)

Unable to countenance that the answer to smallpox might literally lie in the humble hands of rural labourers, the opposition to Jenner's discovery had indeed employed an anti-pastoral rhetoric loaded with threats of contamination from below. Rowley in particular latches onto Jenner's (mistaken) belief that cow-pox originates 'from the greasy ulcerous heels of the horse', to deliberately accentuate a chain of contamination implicating 'beasts, filthy in their very nature' with the rural labourers who attend them: 'The milkers of cows, after dressing the greasy heels of horses, carried filthy infection to the teats and udders of cows, and thus communicated the infection to cows. Then the cows, labouring under this infectious disease, communicated it to man. Here appear three personages concerned, the greasy-heeled horse, the horse doctor, the cow-milker ...' (7). Where Jenner's opponents had mocked the idea that a reliable protection against smallpox could be found in the purportedly sub-human world of the farm labourer, Bloomfield incorporates the healing powers of cow-pox into his realistic, yet restorative, optimistic pastoral vision. *Good Tidings* opposes the anti-vaccinationist's accounts of mangy cow-poxed bodies by invoking a floral analogy which, as my study has shown, had been a mainstay of earlier smallpox poets:

> In ev'ry land, on beauty's lily arm,
> On infant softness, like magic charm,
> Appear'd the gift that conquers as it goes;
> The dairy's boast, the simple, saving *Rose*! (19)

'The Vaccine Rose' had been Bloomfield's working-title for the poem.[56] This had surely met with Jenner's approval for, as Dibdin recalled, one of the physician's 'happiest, and very characteristic sayings was, that he considered the genuine vaccine pustule as the section of a pearl on a rose-leaf!'; a comparison first prompted by questioning from Charles Fox whose 'mind had been a good deal poisoned as to the character of cow-pox by his family physician Moseley'.[57] Hazlitt later quipped that 'we have known a Jennerian Professor as much enraptured with a delineation of the different stages of vaccination, as a florist with a bed of tulips'.[58] With such botanical analogies clearly forming a plank in the Jennerian counter-attack against charges that vaccination is unnatural, why did Bloomfield change his title to 'Good News from the Farm'?

This may be a reflection of pressure from Lofft who disapproved of 'Vaccine Rose' finding 'a trifling allusion in it ... founded on a very slight affinity'.[59] More importantly the final wording of the title brings with it a distinctive note of journalistic realism as if to emphasise the underlying political message. When Bloomfield does invoke the botanical metaphor in the body of the poem itself he puts it into service as a recuperative political symbol, serving to 'cleanse' the origins of vaccination by casting the marks of cow-pox as merely a floral attribute of the healthy bodies of rural labourers. In *The Farmer's Boy* Bloomfield had already portrayed milking cows as a clean, democratic, enjoyable pastoral chore:

> Forth comes the Maid, and like the morning smiles;
> The Mistress too, and follow'd close by Giles.
> A friendly tripod forms their humble seat,
> With pails bright scour'd, and delicately sweet. [...]
> And crouching Giles beneath a neighbouring tree
> Tugs o'er his pail, and chants with equal glee;
> Whose hat with tatter'd brim, of nap so bare,
> From the cow's side purloins a coat of hair,
> A mottled ensign of his harmless trade,
> An unambitious, peaceable cockade.
>
> (*Spring*, lines 190–204)[60]

Praising those 'most original parts of' *The Farmer's Boy* 'which paint the various occupations of the Farmer and his household' amongst which 'milking forms a very important office', Drake had drawn particular attention to the originality of this last image of a 'peaceable cockade'.[61] By describing the hairs adhering to a cowman's hat in terms of a symbolic badge of political or military allegiance, Bloomfield was subtly enfranchising the rural labouring-poor, giving due recognition to their deserving place in the polity, while at the same time reassuring his upper-class readers that the peasantry peaceably accept their place in the social order. This was an appropriately unthreatening, quietist pastoral vision to which Jenner could comfortably have his vaccination message attached.

JENNER'S GIFT TO THE WORLD

The second half of *Good Tidings* argues for the recognition of Jenner as a medical hero of global stature, and to that end studiously endeavours to place the value of vaccination within a historic, patriotic and imperialist context. An authorial footnote acknowledges Bloomfield's dependence upon William Woodville's *History of the Inoculation of the Smallpox in Great Britain* (1796), as the source for the poetic rehearsal of an established narrative of how smallpox arose in the languorous bowers of Arabia before sweeping through India, Britain and Peru like a conquering army.[62] But Bloomfield's subsequent efforts to place the potential benefits of vaccination in a global context should be read in the context of the medical opposition to cow-pox vaccination which, from the very outset, had sought to tie it to racist fears of miscegenation.

Moseley's first scare-mongering account of the phantom *Lues Bovilla* had appeared in the context of his *Treatise on Sugar, with Miscellaneous Medical Observations* (London, 1799), offering practical advice to slave-owning plantocrats. Here the physician forges analogies between cow-pox and the contagious, disfiguring tropical disease yaws (also known as framboesia or 'button scurvy') which he had witnessed amongst Jamaica's plantation slaves. The result is to tie the use of cow-pox to his own blatantly racist medical theories associating negritude with a barely suppressed bestiality supposedly revealed by yaws which he claims is a disease endemic to Africans.[63] Noting how the need to quarantine yaws victims by sending them into the hills encouraged their recourse to 'Obi, the "black art" of Africa' and thus fostered slave-revolts, Moseley goes on to describe how

... some of these abandoned exiles lived, in spite of the common law of nature, and survived a general mutation of their muscles, ligaments, and osteology; became also hideously white in their woolly hair and skin; ... and their limbs and bodies twisted and turned, by the force of the distemper, into shocking grotesque figures, resembling woody excrescences ... or old Ægyptian figures, that seem as if they had been made of the ends of the human, and beginnings of the brutal form; which figures are, by some antiquaries, taken for gods, and by others, for devils. (187–8)

The metamorphosis of black slaves into the colour of their masters is presented as a bizarre form of mocking parody but ultimately betrays their proximity to brutes. Moseley's conversations with slaves had taught him that inoculation for smallpox 'was practiced in Africa long before Inoculation was used in Asia, or in Europe', but his denunciations of the Jennerians repeatedly play upon anxieties over miscegenation and associated fears of racial, sexual, and satanic degeneracy. 'The people of England', he claims, are sprouting hideous horns and 'becoming like inhabitants of the wilderness' (90).

In sharp contrast Bloomfield acknowledges that, despite Montagu giving the 'spotted plague one deadly blow', this deadly poison is still being introduced by white adventurers into native populations with disastrous consequences (17). In particular he lingers sympathetically upon the impact of smallpox on native American populations, though it should be noted that in portraying the Cherokee tribal elders approaching the American government 'for information on the subject of Vaccine Inoculation', 'Till forth their chiefs o'er dying thousands trod / To seek the white man and his bounteous God', he eagerly upholds white supremacy. In particular Bloomfield appeals to his reader's patriotism, arguing that while vaccination is a British discovery, and already being exported in a gesture of global philanthropy, due credit is not yet ours.[64] Dramatising Jenner's own private observation that 'From the potentate to the peasant in every country but this, she ['Vaccinia'] is received with grateful and open arms', *Good News* caters to the sentimental tastes of ameliorist readers already accustomed to reading exotic pastorals as exemplified in the popular tale of white betrayal, 'Inkle and Yarico'.[65] When Bloomfield writes of 'Candian treachery and British strife / The Sword of commerce, nations bought and sold', he pointedly refers to recent native rebellions and threat posed to the stability of empire by the over-mercenary behaviour of the East India Company. In this context vaccination offers a means of colonial pacification; a 'good angel with balmy breath' speeding through Ceylon and India who will owe us more than 'mines of gold' as 'England strikes down the nation's bitterest foe' (30).

In support of this argument that the gift of vaccination can further the imperialist project, Bloomfield invokes the popular tragedy of 'Prince Lee Boo' which, as I discussed in Chapter 4, was originally reported in George Keate's *Account of the Pelew Islands* (1788). Bloomfield's own sentimental-ised version draws out the central irony that an eager youth, having bravely left his family and journeyed so far to encounter a supposedly advanced culture, did not live long enough to experience fully its wonders and carry his knowledge of English sophistication back to his native islands:

> A stranger youth, from his meridian sky,
> Buoyant with hopes, came here – but came to *die*!
> O'er his sad fate I've ponder'd hours away,
> It suits the languor of a gloomy day:
> He left his bamboo groves, his pleasant shore,
> He left his friends to hear new oceans roar,
> All confident, ingenuous, and bold,
> He heard the wonders by the white men told; ...
> In manhood's ripening sense and nature's prime.
> Oh! had the fiend been vanquish'd ere he came,
> The gen'rous youth had spread our country's fame;
> Had known that honour dwells among the brave,
> And England had not prov'd the stranger's grave:
> Then, ere his waning sand of life had run,
> Poor ABBA THULE might have seen his son! (33–2)[66]

Bloomfield exploits the pathos of paternal loss to highlight how Jennerian vaccination could now prevent the repetition of this tragic failure to return benevolence with benevolence. Of course it could also be read as the tale of a wasted opportunity to impress the advantages of British culture on a friendly ally whose native islands had obvious potential as a way-station in

the East India's Company's efforts to find a route into the lucrative
Moluccan spice-trade.[67]

Bloomfield's confession of intense personal interest in Lee Boo's story
represents a crucial act of cross-cultural emotional identification between
himself – a rural English parochial labourer who, upon arrival in London,
had been able to improve himself through an eager capacity for learning –
and Keate's portrait of the princely oriental Lee Boo as 'an amiable youth'
with an 'ardent desire for information' tragically 'cut off in the moment
that his character began to blossom'. As a potential emissary of England's
cultural supremacy, 'What hopes might not have been entertained of the
future fruit such a plant would have produced!'[68] Taking this irony to
heart, Bloomfield exploits the pathos of a now preventable tragedy to
present his own positive argument for the morality of contact. His poem
envisages a future in which vaccination removes the risks of physical
contamination and enables such purportedly improving, benevolent
cross-cultural encounters.

As if in fulfilment of Bloomfield's vision, three years after *Good Tidings*
appeared reports reached London of 'The Address of the Five Nations of
Upper-Canada to Jenner after Colonel Francis Gore, Lieutenant-Governor
presented them with Jenner's work on vaccination'. Jenner was sent a belt
and a string of 'Wampum'. Making much of this exchange Baron published
a facsimile print of the tribal leaders' signatures and pointedly emphasised
how 'such tokens and assurances of regard from the unsophisticated children
of the wilderness were highly acceptable to Jenner, more especially when
contrasted with the ingratitude of too many of his own countrymen'.[69]

Bloomfield's moving accounts of the tragic domestic impact of smallpox
amongst rural communities at home and upon indigenous, tribal societies
abroad impressed itself upon his literary champion Southey, the one-time
radical, now poet laureate. Southey had declared *Good Tidings* 'not inferior
to Robert Bloomfield's former productions – no trifling praise' and subsequently gave him practical support.[70] Southey's own paean to Jenner as
saviour of the world's children was to appear some years later in the overtly
oppositional context of his anti-abolition poem *A Tale of Paraguay* (1825) in
which the physician is commended for having taught us how to tame

> ... the lamentable pest
> Which Africa sent forth to scourge the West,
> As if in vengeance for her sable brood
> So many an age remorselessly opprest.
> For that most fearful malady subdued
> Receive a poet's praise a father's gratitude.[71]

Casting smallpox as the vehicle for a retributive counter-attack against the oppressions of the Atlantic slave trade Southey deftly appropriates the received narrative of smallpox's torrid origins to serve his abolitionist agenda. This frames a harrowing account of how the 'hideous malady' almost wiped-out the 'feeble nation of Guarani'; the peaceful remnant of the natives of Paraguay already weakened by 'perpetual wars', who had retreated into upper reaches of the Mondai river.[72] In Southey's mythic tale, the entire tribe is killed off by smallpox – 'Unwept, unshrouded, and unsepulchred' – except one couple, Quiara and Monnema who, like Adam and Eve are left to begin anew, but whose paradise is eventually destroyed by enslaving Spanish colonialists. Southey's inclusion of a substantial footnote quoting Alexander Mackenzie's 'dreadful picture of the effect of small-pox among the North American Indians' lends eye-witness, documentary credence to an enlightened message that vaccination offers an opportunity to make moral reparation for the decimations of colonial oppression. In the twentieth century similar sentiments were to help motivate the efforts of the World Health Organisation in their eventually successful project to effect the global eradication of smallpox.[73]

Epilogue

The bloated body of the smallpox victim incited revulsion, but as this study has illustrated, despite such horrific symptoms this once ubiquitous disease did not wholly overwhelm the salve of words through which many helpless onlookers sought to comprehend and ameliorate its disruptive impact. Medical and literary texts shared a common inheritance of tropes, myths and moral narratives aimed at lending some coherent meaning to the largely inexplicable actions of this contagious, deadly and disfiguring disease. The adoption of inoculation did not bring about an immediate rejection of traditional models which considered smallpox to be the purging of the maternal legacy of an innate germ of corruption. Even as traditional notions of contagion by conceit or maternal imprinting came to be rejected in the light of increasing evidence of external, particulate infection, popular understandings of smallpox as a fear-inducing spectacle continued to bear a psychological dimension. This is most vividly illustrated when we balance the largely 'external' descriptions of clinicians with the neglected narratives of those who survived.

The recovery of autopathographical texts has been the most satisfying aspect of the present study. William Thompson's spiritual journey or John Dunton's facetious recollections of being disfigured are imaginative acts of accommodation and healing which allow us an insight into the religious and literary preconceptions which undoubtedly shaped all responses to smallpox, confirming what Gilman rightly terms the 'complex interaction of social and biological forces that we call "disease" '.[1] More fundamentally the indelible traces of Variola on the body suggested a literary act in themselves. Dunton, for example, writes of smallpox leaving its 'signature' on his face.[2] Elsewhere pock-marks are frequently being equated with the overwriting, over-printing or crude defacement of a page of script. Thomas Philipot ends his verses 'On a Gentlewoman Much deformed with the Smallpox' with the assurance that 'She needs no glosse to veile those scars, / And those Hebrew Characters, / Which (like letters) do display / The stories of her Beauties sad decay'.[3]

Brome's lines 'To a Gentleman that fell sick of the small Pox when he should be married' rely upon a compelling, extended analogy between the materiality of the poem itself as marks on paper and the corrugated face of the gentleman victim: 'When you view these cheker'd lines and see, / How (bate the colour) like your face they be. / You'll think this sheet to be your looking glass, / And all these spots, the Eccoes of your face'.[4] Reassuringly, Brome argues that such a reading will yet reveal 'the alphabet of love': 'These things I guess not by your face, I find / Your front is not the Index of your mind. / Yet by your Physiognomy, thus much is meant, / You are not spotless though you're innocent'. Smallpox is the 'spiteful' enemy of romance, but Brome assures his male friend that in its attempts to 'write Foul' where love has pitched his tent it will be opposed by the triumphant Cupid:

> Then blush no more, but let your Mrs. Know,
> They're but Love-letters written on your brow,
> Etch'd by th'engravers hand, there she may see,
> That beautie's subject to mortality. (107)

The analogy with literary inscription was an obvious, yet compelling recourse for imaginative writers, for as Connor observes 'Behind every myth of the coming of writing lies a myth of the marking of bodies and faces previously dreamed perfect'.[5] Roland Barthes, who 'reads writing itself in terms of a dermatological dynamic of abrasions, tears, lesions in imaginary veils and surfaces', is just the most influential modern theorist to play with the skin-writing analogy.[6] But such tropes, as Connor notes, have a very material basis in parchment and vellum: 'for centuries of manuscript and book production, books were primarily things of skin'.[7]

But if the scarred face of the smallpox survivor presented a living palimpsest, such a disfiguring act of re-inscription posed a hermeneutic problem, challenging established interpretative assumptions of a direct equivalence between aesthetic appearance and moral character. In comic verses answering the question 'PHYSIOGNOMY, If always an Index of the Mind?', Temple Luttrell mocks traditional claims that man 'Doth from the moment of his birth / Bear on the tablet of his face / (As on the outside of a case) / A schedule what the mass contains . . .', adding that 'smallpox may smear the writing / When Nature hath left off inditing'.[8] Recognising this problem, Lavater could imagine how a 'Medical Physiognomy would employ itself in studying the signs of sickness, as manifested upon the human body', but leaving this task to the medically trained, the fashionable physiognomist never fully confronts the challenge of smallpox.[9]

Smallpox may have confounded the determinist doctrines of fashionable physiognomy, but nonetheless it prompted many acts of judgemental interpretation. Anyone might be touched by the accidental tragedy of smallpox but, as we have seen, disfigurement was presented as the particular scourge of marriageable young women. Doomed to an 'After-Life' of social death and protracted old-age, the disfigured 'Beauty' haunts eighteenth-century poetry and fiction, a spectral reminder of the evanescence of the corruptible flesh. A punitive narrative portraying smallpox acting providentially to chasten transgressive women was a persistent fictional device, most blatantly in Amelia Opie's novel *Adeline Mowbray* (1805), in which the eponymous heroine is effectively punished for her youthful transgression into political radicalism by being left scarred after attending the sick child of a morally degraded servant to whom she had previously set a bad moral example. Despite consolatory voices pointing to the spiritual and intellectual benefits of being excluded from the marriage game, the often abject figure of the scarred woman continued to haunt the literary imagination into the Victorian era. The most famous chastening use of female scarring as a novelistic plot device is found in Charles Dicken's *Bleak House* (1853). Esther Summerson's disfigurement after contracting smallpox while dutifully nursing her loyal servant Charley renders her all the more suitable to become the devoted wife of her paternalistic guardian.[10] In creating the dramatic scene in which Esther finally plucks up the courage to look at herself in a mirror Dickens was simply reworking a well-established motif.[11]

If the more potentially heroic figure of the scarred man did not necessarily accrue the same punitive assumptions, it was often difficult to cast aside the inevitable traces of moral taint; smallpox propelled its victims into the realms of the grotesque and the monstrous. Ancient, elitist associations between disfigurement and servility – the mainstay of caricaturists – must have been reinforced by actual social divisions if we consider the evidence that the gentry advertised for nurses and other servants who were visibly marked (it being common knowledge that you cannot have smallpox twice).[12] With the practice of inoculation being gradually adopted by members of an urban propertied class as eager to protect their complexions as much as their lives, severe smallpox scarring became increasingly a sign of lower-class origins. Despite the propagandist efforts of Robert Bloomfield, throughout the nineteenth century, class mistrust compounded by conscription generated strong resistance from within the urban poor to parliamentary moves to impose compulsory vaccination. It was to take over 150 years for the Jennerian dream of global eradication to be fully realised.

The last reported case of naturally acquired smallpox was in 1977, but despite repeated calls for its destruction *Variola Major* is not extinct. The world's last *known* stocks of the virus are held under military protected, laboratory management by the US Centers for Disease Control (CDC) in their facility in Atlanta, and by the Russian State Institute of Virology and Biotechnology ('Vector'), in Siberia.[13] I began my research for this book prior to the violent events that have come to be abbreviated as '9/11', but much of it has been written in a climate of newly intensified fears that smallpox might be appropriated for use as a terrorist weapon. With small-pox once again haunting the popular imagination hopefully we shall find a common language which enables us to continue our hard-won control over the 'spotted monster'.

Appendix: smallpox in Georgian portraiture

Written reports attest to smallpox scars disfiguring the faces of numerous *literati* and other prominent public figures, yet few contemporary portraits depict any traces of the disease. None of the extant portraits of the novelist and 'Living Muse' Charlotte Lennox, for example, bear out contemporary descriptions of her as being plain and 'much pitted with the small-pox'. Similarly Marcia Pointon has observed how none of the portraits of Lady Mary Wortley Montagu give the slightest hint of pitting. In this context Pointon writes of two contrasting, if interdependent and mutually defining bodies: on the one hand 'the mythicized and idealized portrait that has helped to define the historical personality of Montagu' and on the other what we know to have been a scarred 'biological body subject to decay, a body that is apparently "natural" but is equally the site of interpretation and projection' (141). The failure of these two 'bodies' to match is of course a reflection of artistic and social conventions which required portraitists to flatter and idealise their clients.[1] As the vain fop Sparkish insists in Wycherley's *The Country Wife*, 'painters don't draw the smallpox, or pimples, in one's face'.[2] By the time Lady Mary May died of smallpox in 1681, she had followed landed tradition in already having ordered her own tomb for Mid Levant church, Sussex, but when the sculptor John Bushnell added pock marks to her effigy it came to be seen as evidence of his encroaching madness.[3]

We might expect a male artist to idealise a woman client in particular so as to flatter fathers and husbands if not the sitter herself, but as Pointon explains, the formality of eighteenth-century male portraiture is 'formality defined . . . by implicit contrast with that to which it is other, by its hieratic and symbolic separation from the grotesque disorder into which – without the perpetual replication of these ordered and dignified representations of the idea of social man – it would disintegrate'.[4] Thus in numerous examples of male victims where witnesses attest to sometimes severe facial scarring, no such disfigurement is apparent in the canvas portrait. For example, none of the extant likenesses of the poet and historian John

Pinkerton, including an elegant Tassie medallion, betray the face of a man John Nichols described as having 'a very small, sharp yellow face, thickly pitted by the small-pox'.[5] Similarly, anyone who sees Scottish artist David Allan's dapper self-portrait, nor his equally elegant portrait by Domenico Corvi would be surprised to read a contemporary description of his 'long, sharp, lean, white coarse face, much pitted by the small pox'.[6]

The realistic portrayal of pockmarked faces belonged to 'the inverse world of caricature'.[7] Hence Pope, in his deeply ironic mock-treatise on how to achieve 'the Bathetic' in art, facetiously assures any would-be portraitists that 'many Painter's who could never hit a Nose or an Eye, have with Felicity copied a small-pox'.[8] But a few notable exceptions suggest that there was some room for bringing the ideal and the biological into greater proximity, particularly in mature subjects. We know that the Old English scholar Humphrey Wanley suffered smallpox in childhood, but of the four portraits executed in his lifetime by Thomas Hill only the last, now in the Bodleian Library, reveals a countenance 'absolutely peppered with variolous indentations'.[9] Similarly, Josiah Wedgwood's contemporaries report that he was badly scarred by the confluent smallpox he survived before he was twelve, but amongst all the numerous portraits in circulation his modern biographer can only find one, a paste medallion modelled by William Hackwood in 1782, which 'faithfully records the scars of smallpox, commonly seen among all ranks of the population at that period but seldom visible in contemporary portraits'.[10] The fact that these exceptions are all male subjects supports Campbell's observation that in this period the fears of male writers and artists for the loss of self in ageing focus upon impairments in the faculties of perception (she cites two of Reynold's mature self-portraits in which the artist struggles to hear and also his portrait of the older Johnson shown straining to read), while in marked contrast, the loss of self 'definitively lost by women through disease or age depends not on physical faculties of perception but on physical appearance'. For women 'the problem of the self's dependence on a body that may change over time is located on the surface of that body, or (more precisely) in the impression made by that body on the eyes of others'.[11] Thus a nostalgic William Hazlitt was able to recall his earliest attempt at portraiture; 'a picture of my father, who was then in green old age' drawn 'with strong-marked features, and scarred with the small-pox' and 'with a broad light crossing the face, looking down, with spectacles on, reading'.[12] Tom Paulin, who recently tracked this painting down to the reserve collection of Maidstone Museum only to find it badly blistered, writes fondly of the father's 'old, benevolent, bespectacled, craggy, doubly pocked face'.[13] Crucially, in Hazlitt's painterly eyes his father's smallpox scars simply served to supplement other signs of old age in what Paulin reverently reads as a respectful depiction of mature, patriarchal wisdom.

Two particularly notable depictions of men bearing pock marks are the engraved portraits of the poet William Thompson 'Aet 57' (circa 1759), and the essayist and MP, William Hay (in neither case has the original oil been traced).[14] We know nothing of the circumstances surrounding the production of Thompson's portrait. (See illustration 2) The composition of the engraving suggests it may have been designed as a frontispiece. No such use has been traced, but this rare instance of medical realism must have surely been at the behest of the sitter, providing us with a suitably frank record of the author of *Sickness*.

We are more fortunate with William Hay, who recorded his motives for being depicted with smallpox scars in his remarkable *Deformity; an Essay* (1754). This autobiographical polemic addressing contemporary, demonising attitudes towards disfigurement has been under-recognised as a key intervention in the history of disability.[15] Hay had been left badly scarred by a severe case of confluent smallpox contracted in early adulthood. His son recollected that after leaving Oxford in 1715 Hay had pursued law at the Temple ' 'till obliged to relinquish the prosecution of that study, on his sight having been much injured by the small-pox, which he had in so terrible a manner that his life was despaired of, but was favourably saved by Dr. Mead's having ventured on what was then thought a desperate experiment' (Mead made controversial use of purgatives).[16] But Hay's was an exceptional case because the scars of smallpox were overlaid onto a body that had already rendered him vulnerable to being categorised as monstrous for, in his own words, he was 'scare five Feet high' with 'a distorted frame of body' after 'my back was bent in my Mother's Womb'.[17] While candidly exposing the physical, social and psychological consequences of his disabilities, the mature Hay recollected the actions of his doting parents:

When I was a Child I was drawn like a Cupid, with a Bow and Arrow in my hands and a Quiver on my Shoulder: I afterwards thought this an Abuse, which ought to be corrected: when I sate for my Picture some Years ago, I insisted on being drawn as I am, and that the strong marks of the Small pox might appear in my face, for I did not choose to cover over a Lye. The Painter said, he was never allowed such liberty before; and I advised him, if he hoped to be in Vogue, never to assume it again; for flatterers succeed best in the World; and of all Flatterers, painters are the least liable to be detected by those they flatter. Nor are the ladies the only persons concerned for their Looks.[18]

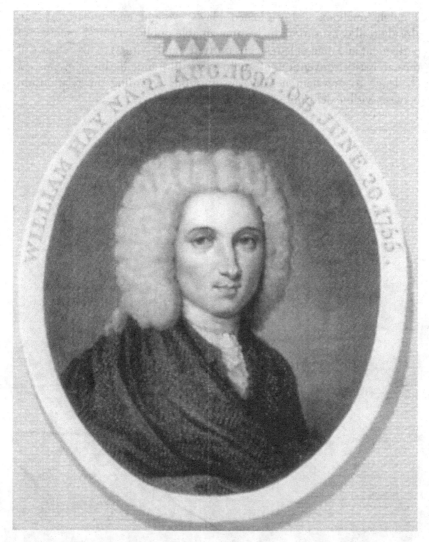

13. Portrait of William Hay MP, detail from the frontispiece to *The Works of William Hay Esq.* (London, 1794). As a champion of the deformed, Hay ordered this unknown portraitist to include his smallpox scars. Cross-hatching indicates that almost half of Hay's face had been left marked by the sheet-scarring found in more severe cases of the disease.

An engraving derived from this defiant adult portrait forms part of the frontispiece to *The Works of William Hay, Esq.* (1794), where an outlined area of hatching serves to delineate a very substantial patch of continuous scar tissue covering about a quarter of the subject's face. (See illustration 13)

Though smallpox had weakened Hay's eyesight and undermined an already frail constitution, he became an able public servant, a member of parliament and man of letters. His portrait stands witness to his defiance of the narcissistic conventions of studio portraiture and, like his *Essay*, posed a challenge to prevalent negative assumptions regarding the relationship between visible deformities and moral character.

Notes

PROLOGUE

1. Samuel Pepys, *Memoirs of Samuel Pepys ... and a selection of his private correspondence*, ed. Lord Braybrooke, 2 vols. (London, 1825), II, Part ii, pp. 197–8.
2. See Steven Connor, *The Book of Skin* (London: Reaktion, 2004), pp. 109–10.
3. *The Collected Works of Samuel Taylor Coleridge: Marginalia, IV*, eds. H. J. Jackson and George Whalley (Princeton, NJ: Princeton University Press, 1998), p. 83.
4. See G. S. Rousseau and David Boyd Haycock 'Framing Samuel Taylor Coleridge's Gut: Genius, Digestion Hypochondria' in G. S. Rousseau, Miranda Gill, David Haycock and Malte Herwig, eds. *Framing and Imagining Disease in Cultural History* (London: Palgrave Macmillan, 2003), pp. 231–65; Neil Vickers, *Coleridge and the Doctors* (Oxford: Clarendon Press, 2004).
5. See Gert H. Brieger, 'The Historiography of Medicine' in *Companion Encyclopaedia of the History of Medicine*, eds. W. F. Bynum and Roy Porter (London: Routledge, 1993), pp. 24–44.
6. Richard Holmes, *Coleridge; Early Visions* (London, Sydney, Auckland and Toronto: Hodder and Stoughton, 1989), p. 62.
7. Molly Lefebure, *Bondage of Love; a Life of Mrs Samuel Taylor Coleridge* (London: Victor Gollancz, 1986), pp. 104–17.

INTRODUCTION

1. James Moore, *The History of the Smallpox* (London, 1815) and Charles Creighton, *A History of Epidemics in Britain*, 2 vols. [1891, 1894] (London: Frank Cass and Co., revised 1963), II, pp. 434–631. The major modern accounts are C. W. Dixon, *Smallpox* (London: J. and A. Churchill, 1962), Donald R. Hopkins, *Princes and Peasants, Smallpox in History* (Chicago and London: The University of Chicago Press, 1983), reissued as *The Greatest Killer: Smallpox in History* in 2002 (all references are to the 2002 edition); J. R. Smith, *The Speckled Monster: Smallpox in England, 1670–1970, with particular reference to Essex* (Chelmsford: Essex Record Office, 1987). For Restoration perceptions of increased virulence see

Genevieve Miller, *Adoption of Inoculation for Smallpox in England and France* (Philadelphia: University of Pennsylvania Press, 1957), chapter 2.

2. Creighton, *History of Epidemics*, II, p. 434.
3. Miller, *Adoption*, p. 26.
4. Brome, Herrick, Denham, Cotton and Marvell also contributed. See H. T. Swedenberg Jr. 'More Tears for Lord Hastings', *Huntingdon Library Quarterly*, 16 (1952–1953), pp. 43–51; Michael Gearin-Tosh, 'Marvell's "Upon the Death of Lord Hastings"', *Essays and Studies*, XXXIV (1981), pp. 105–22; and Ruth Wallerstein, *Studies in Seventeenth-Century Poetic* (Wisconsin: University of Wisconsin Press, 1950), pp. 115–22.
5. Samuel Johnson, 'Life of Dryden' in *Lives of the English Poets*, ed. G. Birkbeck Hill, 3 vols. (Oxford: Oxford University Press, 1905), I, pp. 331–485; 333.
6. Summarised in Aaron Santesso, '*Lachrymae Musarum* and the Metaphysical Dryden', in *The Review of English Studies*, new series vol. 54, no. 217 (2003), pp. 616–17.
7. As cited in Santesso, '*Lachrymae Musarum* and the Metaphysical Dryden', p. 621.
8. *Ibid.*, pp. 620 and 622, footnote 29.
9. For more 'astronomical conceits' see Raymond Anselment, *The Realms of Apollo: Literature and Healing in Seventeenth-Century England* (Newark: University of Delaware Press, 1995), p. 204 and Santesso, '*Lachrymae Musarum*', p. 625.
10. Barbara Maria Stafford, *Body Criticism: Imaging the Unseen in Enlightenment Art and Medicine* (Cambridge MA, 1991), pp. 281–39; Connor, *Book of Skin*, p. 95.
11. For 'imagining disease' in this period see Roy Porter, *Bodies Politic; Disease, Death and Doctors in Britain, 1650–1900* (London: Reaktion, 2001), pp. 89–128. 'Variola' does not feature in his discussion, but Porter usefully emphasises the important role of visible external symptoms in holistic diagnostics, and surveys the ways in which diseases were personified in literature and pictorial art.
12. For the term 'framing' see introductions to *Framing Disease: Studies in Cultural History*, eds. Charles E. Rosenberg and Janet Golden (New Brunswick: Rutgers University Press, 1992) and *Framing and Imagining Disease in Cultural History*, eds. G. S. Rousseau *et al.* (London: Palgrave Macmillan, 2003), pp. 1–38.
13. Representative essays in *Literature and Medicine During the Eighteenth Century*, eds. Marie Mulvey Roberts and Roy Porter (London, 1993). There has been no comprehensive account of smallpox from a literary perspective as we have for other diseases: for plague and syphilis see Margaret Healy, *Fictions of Disease in early Modern England: Bodies, Plagues and Politics* (Basingstoke: Palgrave, 2001); Susan Sontag, *Illness as Metaphor* (New York, 1978), (for cancer, TB); Susan Sontag, *AIDS and its Metaphors* (Harmondsworth: Penguin, 1989); Roy Porter and G. S. Rousseau, *Gout, the Patrician Malady* (New Haven and London: Yale University Press, 1998); Roy Porter, *Mind-Forg'd Manacles: Madness and Psychiatry in England from the Restoration to Regency* (London, 1987; reprinted 1990).

14. See Howard Brody, *Stories of Sickness* (Oxford and New York: Oxford University Press, [1987] revised second edition, 2003); Arthur Kleinman, *The Illness Narratives: Suffering, Healing and the Human Condition* (New York: Basic Books, 1988) and A. W. Frank, *The Wounded Storyteller; Body, Illness and Ethics* (Chicago and London: Chicago University Press, 1995).

15. Anselment, *Realms*.

16. Isobel Grundy, 'Medical Advance and Female Fame: Inoculation and its After-Effects', *Lumen*, XIII (1994), pp. 13–42 and *Lady Mary Wortley Montagu: Comet of the Enlightenment* (Oxford: Oxford University Press, 1999); Jill Campbell, 'Lady Mary Wortley Montagu and the "Glass Revers'd" of Female Old Age' in Helen Deutsch and Felicity Nussbaum, eds. '*Defects': Engendering the Modern Body* (Ann Arbor: University of Michigan Press, 2000), pp. 213–51.

17. Campbell, 'Lady Mary'; Felicity Nussbaum, *The Limits of the Human: Fictions of Anomaly, Race, and Gender in the Long Eighteenth Century* (Cambridge: Cambridge University Press, 2003), ch. 4, 'Scarred Women: Frances Burney and Smallpox', pp. 109–32.

18. Tim Fulford and Debbie Lee, 'The Jenneration of Disease: Vaccination Romanticism and Revolution', in *Studies in Romanticism* (Boston) Volume 39 (Spring 2000), I, pp. 139–63.

19. This occurred in Somalia, but the last recorded death from smallpox was at Birmingham after the virus accidentally escaped from a UK research laboratory and infected a photographer working in the same building.

20. Details in Smith, *Speckled Monster*, Appendix 1, pp. 179–82. Other clinical information drawn from F. Fenner et al., *Smallpox and its Eradication* (Geneva: World Health Organisation, 1988).

21. Robert Bloomfield, *Good Tidings, or News from the Farm* (London, 1804), p. 24. (See Chapter 8 below.)

22. Martin Lleulyn, 'An Elegie on the Death of the Most Illustrious Prince Henry, Duke of Gloucester' (Oxford, 1660) (quoted in Anselment, *Realms*, p. 194).

23. Cited in Anselment, *Realms*, p. 194.

24. Smith, *Speckled Monster*, pp. 179–82.

25. Stephen Taylor, 'Benjamin Hoadly', in *Oxford Dictionary of National Biography* (online) (hereafter *ODNB*).

26. Robin Reilly, *Josiah Wedgwood 1730–1795* (London: Macmillan, 1992), pp. 4, 249.

27. Rebecca Mills, 'Jane Bowdler', *ODNB*.

28. Marcia Pointon, *Hanging the Head: Portraiture and Social Formation* (New Haven and London: Yale University Press, 1988), p. 142.

29. Sara to S.T.C., 1 November 1798 in Molly Lefebure, *Bondage of Love; a Life of Mrs Samuel Taylor Coleridge* (London: Victor Gollancz 3, 1986) pp. 105–107. See also Sara's letter to her husband in *Minnow Among Tritons: Mrs S. T. Coleridge's Letters to Thomas Poole, 1799–1834* edited by Stephen Potter (London, 1934), I, and her letters to Thomas Poole in Mrs Henry Sandford, *Thomas Poole and his Friends*, two vols. (London and New York, 1888) I, pp. 281–2; 284–5; 292–3.

30. Anselment, *Realms*, p. 196, citing Sontag, *Illness as Metaphor* (1978), pp. 58, 73.
31. Sontag, *Illness as Metaphor / AIDS and its Metaphors* (Harmondsworth, 1983), p. 32. Further references are to this combined edition.
32. Brody, *Stories of Sickness*, p. 57.
33. *Ibid.*, pp. 83–4. Brody acknowledges that compared with the plague or even syphilis, cancer and Tuberculosis are seen as highly individualistic so you can ask 'Why me?' They seem to carefully select their victims, encouraging a blame-the-victim attitude which starts looking for a psychological type'.
34. Anne Hunsaker Hawkins, *Reconstructing Illness: Studies in Pathography* (West Lafayette Indiana, 1999), p. xvii (citing Sontag, *Illness*, p. 2) and p. 24.
35. Porter and Rousseau, *Gout*, p. 285.
36. Sander L. Gilman, *Disease and Representation: Images of Illness from Madness to AIDS* (Ithaca and London: Cornell University Press, 1988), p. 7.
37. The earliest use of 'smallpox' cited in *OED* is in a letter dated 1518 amongst the State Papers of Henry VIII. See Anselment, *Realms*, p. 171 (and pp. 131–71 for primary and secondary sources on syphilis).
38. Richard Mead, 'Discourse on the Small-pox and Measles' in *The Medical Works* (Edinburgh, 1775), p. 229. Mead's 'Discourse' first appeared in 1748, but had been written in the 1720s during a fierce controversy over how to treat smallpox.
39. *Ibid.*, pp. 230–35 where Mead offers a standard history. Donald R. Hopkins, *The Greatest Killer: Smallpox in History* (Chicago and London: The University of Chicago Press, 1983), pp. 22–23; Sheldon Watts, *Epidemics and History: Disease, Power and Imperialism* (New Haven and London: Yale University Press, 1997), pp. 84–111.
40. Andrew Tripe MD [William Wagstaffe] *The Small-Pox, a Poem in Five Cantos, Form'd on the Plan of Dr. Mead's prose on that Subject* (London, 1748), p. 13.
41. *Ibid.*, p. 5.
42. First published in a Greek translation in 1548, Rhazes's *Treatise on Smallpox and Measles* later appeared in numerous Latin translations. Mead commissioned the first translation direct from the Arabic into Latin, then English (see his *Works*, p. 227). Early authorities are extracted in Saul Jarcho, *The Concept of Contagion Medicine, Literature and Religion* (Malabar Florida: Krieger Publishing Company, 2000).
43. For smallpox and colonialism see Watts, *Epidemics and History*, pp. 65–115. For the Americas see Hopkins, *Greatest Killer*, pp. 204–94 and R. G. Robertson, *Rotting Face: Smallpox and the American Indian* (Caldwell ID: Caxton Press, 2001).
44. For exclusionary Old Testament laws concerning lepers see Saul Nathaniel Brody, *The Disease of the Soul: Leprosy in Medieval Literature* (Ithaca: Cornell University Press, 1974) and Brian Murdoch, *Adam's Grace: Fall and Redemption in Medieval Literature* (London: D. S. Brewer, 2000).
45. Edmund Massey, *A sermon against the dangerous and sinful practice of inoculation* (London, 1722).

46. Patrick Delany, *An Historical Account of the Life and Reign of David, King of Israel*, 3 vols. (Dublin: third edition, 1743), III, p. 460 and Chapter VII *passim*. Psalm XXXVIII, for example, has 'My wounds stink, and are corrupt'. Commenting on a draft of Delany's retrospective diagnosis, a physician (Dr Richard Helsham?) suggested elephantiasis as described by Araeteus, but Delany carefully rules this out.

47. For earlier uses of Job see Healy, *Fictions of Disease*, p. 44.

48. John Dunton, 'The Weeping Elegy' in *Athenianism; or, the new projects of Mr. Dunton* (London, 1710), p. 58.

49. Paul Hammond, ed. *The Poems of John Dryden* (London and New York: Longman, 1995), I, p. 6. Eric Partridge, *A Dictionary of Slang* (London: Routledge, 2000), Definition 10.

50. Mary Douglas, *Purity and Danger: An Analysis of the Concepts of Pollution and Taboo* [1966] (Harmondsworth, 1970), pp. 114–19 and *passim*.

51. Gilman, *Disease and Representation*, pp. 2–3.

52. My own approach accords with that of Healy, *Fictions of Disease*, pp. 5–7.

53. Gilman, *Disease and Representation*, p. 2.

54. In this context, Gilman invokes some introductory remarks in *Iconography* by W. J. T. Mitchell, who rejects 'a facile relativism' in favour of 'a hard rigorous relativism that regards knowledge as a social product. A matter of dialogue between different versions of the world, including different languages, ideologies and modes of representation' (*Disease and Representation*, p. 20). For other theoretical accounts of the ontology of illness see Bryan S. Turner, *The Body and Society* (London, revised 1996), pp. 197–235.

55. For 'disease as construct' see Healy, *Fictions of Disease*, pp. 5–13. As someone who once undertook mortuary work I also offer no excuses for 'cluttering up the field with real bodies' (p. 11), and endorse Healy's cogent arguments for not ignoring 'extra-textual biology' and for reconstructing diseases within their socio-historical contexts.

56. Porter and Rousseau, *Gout*, p. 284.

57. See Anselment, *Realms*, pp. 23–5; 30–1.

58. G. S. Rousseau, 'Medicine and the muses: an approach to literature and medicine' in Marie Mulvey Roberts and Roy Porter, eds. *Literature and Medicine During the Eighteenth Century* (London: Routledge, 1993), pp. 23–57, and *passim*.

59. Samuel Bowden, *Poetical Essays on Several Occasions*, 2 vols. (London, 1733; 1735), I, pp. 37–8.

60. *Ibid.*, p. 41.

61. Ovid, *Epistolæ Ex Ponto*, III, ii. English translation from Henry T. Riley *The Fasti, Tristia, Pontic Epistles, Ibis, and Halieuticon of Ovid* (London, 1905).

62. See, for example, John Lamport [Lampard] *A Direct Method of ordering and Curing People of that Loathsome Disease, the Small-Pox* (London, 1685), p. 2.

63. For these and other sources see Jarcho, *Concept of Contagion*, pp. 1–20; for Lucretius see Healy, *Fictions of Disease*, pp. 1–2.

64. Thompson, *Sickness; a Poem in Five Books* (London, 1745), p. 246.

65. Thomas Sydenham, *The Whole Works* (London, 1740), vii.
66. Lucan, *Pharsalia*, LIB IX, lines 946–955, as quoted in Richard Mead, 'Discourse on Smallpox and Measles', in *Works*, p. 239.
67. Gilman, *Disease and Representation*, p. xiii.
68. *Ibid.*, p. 10.
69. Smith, *Speckled Monster*, p. 179.

CHAPTER I

1. Henry Fielding, *A Journey to This World and the Next*, ed. Ian A. Bell and Andrew Varney (Oxford: Oxford World's Classics, 1997), p. 7. Further citations provided in brackets.
2. First published 1744; this episode appears in Book VII, Chapter X of 'Volume the Last' issued in 1753. Citations, hereafter in brackets, refer to Sarah Fielding, *The Adventures of David Simple*, ed. Malcolm Kelsall (London: Oxford University Press, 1969).
3. For virology see J. R. Smith, The *Speckled Monster: Smallpox in England, 1670–1970, with particular reference to Essex*, (Chelmsford: Essex Record Office, 1987), pp. 179–82 and F. Fenner et al, *Smallpox and its Eradication*, *passim*.
4. Genevieve Miller, *Adoption of Inoculation for Smallpox in England and France* (Philadelphia, 1957), p. 241.
5. Charles E. Rosenberg, *Explaining Epidemics and other Studies in the History of Medicine* (Cambridge: Cambridge University Press, 1992), p. 295.
6. Ibid., p. 295.
7. Roy Porter, 'The Eighteenth Century' in Lawrence I. Conrad, Michael Neve, Vivian Nutton, Roy Porter and Andrew Wear, *Western Medical Tradition 800BC to AD 1800* (Cambridge: Cambridge University Press, 1995), pp. 407–408.
8. Mead, *Works*, pp. 254–5.
9. Hopkins, *Greatest Killer*, pp. 32–3.
10. Isabelle Pantin, 'Fracastoro's *De Contagione* and Medieval Reflections on "Action at a Distance"' in *Imagining Contagion in Early Modern European Culture*, ed. Claire L. Carlin (London: Palgrave Macmillan, 2005), p. 3–15.
11. Though often attributed to Arabic sources by medieval and Renaissance Europeans, Jarcho can only find the idea in the writings of 'Haly Abbas' (*Concept of Contagion*), p. 23.
12. Miller, *Adoption of Inoculation*, pp. 242–56.
13. Vivian Nutton, 'The Seeds of Disease; an Explanation of Contagion and Infection from the Greeks to the Renaissance', *Medical History* 27 (1983), p. 2.
14. Anon., *A Short Treatise of the Smallpox, shewing the Means how for to govern and cure those which are infected therewith* (London, 1652), pp. 51–2.
15. Ysbrand van Diemerbroeck, *The Anatomy of Human Bodies ... To which is added a particular treatise of the small-pox and measles ... Translated [from original Latin] by William Salmon* (London, 1694), p. 30. Further references given in brackets are to this edition.

16. Thomas Fuller, *Exanthematologia, or an Attempt to Give a Rational Account of eruptive fevers, especially of the measles and smallpox* (London, 1730), p. 189. Further references in brackets.
17. See *Emotional Contagion*, eds. Elaine Hatfield, John Cacioppo and Richard Rapson (Cambridge: Cambridge University Press, 1994).
18. *The Diary of John Evelyn*, ed. E. S. de Beer, 2 vols. (Oxford, 1955), IV, p. 425.
19. Jonathan Swift, *Journal to Stella*, ed. Harold Williams, 2 vols. (Oxford, 1963), II, p. 217.
20. *Horace Walpole's Correspondence with George Montagu*, eds. W. S. Lewis and Ralph S. Brown Jr, 2 vols. (London and New Haven: Oxford University Press and Yale University Press, 1941), II, p. 56.
21. See Thomas Cadogan, *De Animi Pathematum, vi et modo agendi in inucendis vel curandis morbis* (Leiden, 1767). Discussion in Antoine Luyendijk-Elshout, 'Of Masks and Mills: The Enlightenment Doctor and his Frightened Patient' in *The Languages of Psyche: Mind and Body in Enlightenment Thought*, ed. G. S. Rousseau (Berkeley and Oxford: University of California Press, 1990).
22. John Woodward, *The State of Physick and of Diseases; with an inquiry into the causes of the late increase of them, but more particularly of the small-pox* (London, 1718), p. 69.
23. See *Galen on the Passions and Errors of the Soul*, trans. Paul W. Harkins. Introduction by Walter Riese (Columbia, 1963) and for the concept in eighteenth-century literature Geoffrey Sill, *The Cure of the Passions and the Origins of the Novel* (Cambridge: Cambridge University Press, 2001).
24. Nutton, 'The Seeds of Disease', p. 15.
25. See the introduction to Jacques Ferrand, *A Treatise on Lovesickness*, eds. Donald Beecher and Massimo Ciavolella (Syracuse: Syracuse University Press, 1990).
26. As explicated in *ibid.*, pp. 32–3.
27. A letter to *The Tatler* of 17 August 1710 from a reader frightened by a masked rider reveals how such precautions could unintentionally misfire. See *The Tatler* ed. *Donald F. Bond*, 3 vols. (Oxford: Clarendon Press, 1987), pp. iii; 118–19.
28. Penelope Aubin, *Charlotta Du Pont* (London, 1739), p. 107.
29. Samuel Richardson, *Sir Charles Grandison*, ed. Jocelyn Harris (Oxford: Oxford University Press, 1986), p. 323 [Vol. 2, Letter XIII].
30. Fuller talks of 'peculiar venemous Particles' that find a fit with the ovula. These consist of 'rigid, infrangible, and unalterable Atoms, so subtle, pointed edged, and perhaps indented, crooked [and] barbed ... as to be ... wholly destructive to the Spirits, Blood and solids of Man' but concedes that 'their real particular, geometrical Figures, measures, and mechanic manner of exerting their Powers' remain 'undiscoverable to us in this our ... State of imperfection' (*Exanthematologia*), pp. 179; 181.
31. Nutton, 'Seeds of Disease', p. 14.
32. Source in Severinus untraced.
33. Gideon Harvey, *A Treatise of the Small-pox and the Measles; describing their Nature, Causes and Signs* (London: 1696), pp. 7–10.

34. Felicity Nussbaum, *Limits of the Human*, pp. 109–32 and Chapter 5 below.
35. For a psychoanalytic approach see Julia Kristeva, *Powers of Horror: An Essay on Abjection* (New York: Columbia University Press, 1982), p. 71ff.
36. Tobias Whitaker, *An Elenchus of Opinions Concerning the Cure of the Small Pox* (Oxford, 1661), p. 8.
37. Elaine Hobby, 'Gender, Science and Midwifery: Jane Sharp, "The Midwives Book" (1671)' in *The Arts of 17th-Century Science*, eds. Claire Jowitt and Diane Watt (Aldershot: Ashgate, 2002), pp. 146–59; 150.
38. *Philosophical Transactions*, vol. 46 (1749), pp. 233–4. Such beliefs persisted at a popular level, but later medical works, such as George Pearson's *Observations on the Effects of Variolus Infection on Pregnant Women* (London, 1794), wholly disregard imprinting.
39. G. S. Rousseau, 'Pineapples, Pregnancy, Pica, and Peregrine Pickle' originally published in *Tobias Smollett: Bicentennial Essays Presented to Lewis M. Knapp*, eds. G. S. Rousseau and P.-G. Boucé (Oxford: Oxford University Press, 1971), pp. 79–109; reprinted in G. S. Rousseau, *Nervous Acts: Essays on Literature, Culture and Sensibility* (Basingstoke: Palgrave Macmillan, 2004).
40. Claude Quillet, *Callipædia. A Poem in Four Books … Written in Latin By Claudius Quillet, Made English By N. Rowe* (London, 1712), p. 18. This popular English translation is elsewhere attributed to William Oldisworth (and others).
41. Rousseau, *Nervous Acts*, pp. 122–3.
42. See also Ambroise Paré, *On Monsters and Marvels*, trans. Janis Pallister (Chicago: University of Chicago Press, 1982); P-G Boucé, 'Imagination, pregnant women, and monsters, in eighteenth-century England and France', in *Sexual Underworlds of the Enlightenment*, eds. G. S. Rousseau and R. Porter (Manchester: Manchester University Press, 1987), pp. 86–100; M.-H Huet, *Monstrous Imagination* (Cambridge MA: Harvard University Press, 1993); Dennis Todd, *Imagining Monsters: Miscreations of the Self in Eighteenth-Century England* (Chicago and London: University of Chicago Press, 1995), (Todd analyses the notorious case of Mary Toft, the 'Rabbit Woman of Godalming' who, in 1726, claimed to have given birth to seventeen rabbits); and Julia Epstein, 'The Pregnant Imagination, Women's Bodies, and Fetal Rights', in *Inventing Maternity: Politics, Science and Literature, 1650–1865*, eds. Susan C. Greenfield and Carol Barash (Lexington, 1999), pp. 111–37.
43. Miller briefly notes the role of the passions in some accounts but 'conceits' find no place in her attempt to impose a pattern upon what she admits is a confusing picture (*Adoption of Inoculation*), p. 248.
44. *A Sermon Preached before his Grace Charles Duke of Marlborough, President, the Vice-Presidents and Governors of the Hospital for the Small-pox and for Inoculation* (London, 1752), p. 18.
45. *Ibid.*, pp. 260–1.
46. 'Uninterested Spectator', *A letter to J. V. Lettsom M. D. occasioned by Baron Dimsdale's remarks* (London, 1779), pp. 22–3.
47. Rosenberg, *Explaining Epidemics*, p. 13.

48. Smith, *Speckled Monster*, p. 98.
49. Robert Houlton, *The Practice of Inoculation Justified* (London, 1767), p. 40.
50. See Raymond Williams, *Marxism and Literature* (Oxford: Oxford University Press, 1977), chapter 8.

CHAPTER 2

1. Henry Bold, *Poems, Lyrique, Macaronique, Heroique* (London, 1664), p. 234.
2. Howard Brody, *Stories of Sickness* (New York, revised second edition 2003), p. 81.
3. Arthur Kleinman, *The Illness Narratives: Suffering, Healing and the Human Condition* (New York, 1988); for reforms see A. W. Frank, *The Wounded Storyteller; Body, Illness and Ethics* (Chicago and London, 1995).
4. Kleinman, *Illness Narratives*, p. xiii.
5. Brody, *Stories of Sickness*, p. 13.
6. Kleinman, *Illness Narratives*, p. 1.
7. Anne Hunsaker Hawkins, *Reconstructing Illness: Studies in Pathography* (West Lafayette Indiana, 1999), p. 229, footnote 1.
8. *Ibid.*, pp. xii; 3; 11–14.
9. Hawkins, *Reconstructing Illness*, ix; and 1. Hawkins finds formal similarities between seventeenth-century spiritual autobiography (conversion narratives) and modern pathographies (pp. 32–4).
10. *Ibid.*, pp. xiv–xv; 49–50.
11. See Ian Watt, *The Rise of the Novel* (London: Chatto and Windus, 1957); Lennard J. Davis, *Factual Fictions: Origins of the English Novel* (New York, 1983) and Michael McKeon, *The Origins of the English Novel* (Baltimore: Johns Hopkins University Press, 1987).
12. G. A. Starr, *Defoe and Spiritual Autobiography* (Princeton: Princeton University Press, 1965).
13. Frances Flood, *The Devonshire Woman; Or, a wonderful narrative of Frances Flood, Shewing how she was taken by the Small-pox in the street of Saltford, near Bath, in the Year 1723* (n.p. 1723–4?), 1. Subsequent references given in brackets.
14. For example, in the churchyard by Strata Florida Abbey, mid-Wales a representational headstone marks the burial site of a cooper's leg amputated after a work accident in the 1770s. The cooper subsequently emigrated to America and never re-united with his leg, at least in this world.
15. For resurrection debates see Roy Porter, *Flesh in the Age of Reason* (London: Allen Lane, 2003), pp. 18; 82.
16. Thompson, who graduated MA from Queen's College in 1739 and held a fellowship before becoming rector of Hampton Poyle in Oxfordshire, thought that the 'date of our English Poetry may with great Justice begin with Spenser' (*Sickness*, 218). Other annotations confirm the influence of Ariosto, Balde, Donne, Cameons, Casimire, Sannazarius and Tasso. Thompson oversaw a 1753 edition of Joseph Hall's *Virgidemiarum* and a posthumous 1772 edition of William Browne's *Works* bears his preface and notes.

17. William Thompson, *Sickness; a Poem in Three Books* (London, 1745), 'Advertisement to the Reader', pp. v–vi.

18. Elizabeth Singer Rowe's 'Hymn of Thanks, On my Recovery from the Small-Pox' appeared posthumously in *The Miscellaneous Works In Prose and Verse of Mrs. Elizabeth Row . . . In Two Volumes* (London, 1739), I, p. 94. The circumstances in which she survived the disease, around 1712, remain obscure. *The Poetical Works of John and Charles Wesley*, 7 vols. (London, 1868), VII, pp. 93–4, [Poems LXXIX and LXXX].

19. *Ibid.*, pp. 94–5.

20. By way of contrast an 'Ode to Health, written on a recovery from the small-pox', first published in *Odes on Various Subjects* (London, 1747), by Thompson's Oxford contemporary, Joseph Warton is an emotionally restrained exercise in literary abstractions shielding the reader from any noisome physical details. See Revd. John Wooll, *Biographical Memoirs of the Late Revd. Joseph Warton* (London, 1806), pp. 13; 131–3.

21. The first edition bears '1745' on the title page, but appeared in early 1746. It was reprinted with some 'alterations' in 'the Divisions' in Thompson's *Poems on Several Occasion to which is added Gondibert and Birtha, a Tragedy* (Oxford, 1757), ('Tome Two' is dated 1751 on the half-title). All subsequent page references, provided in brackets, refer to the final 1757, 'Five Book' version.

22. Frank, *Wounded Storyteller*, as discussed in Brody, *Stories of Sickness*, p. 85.

23. Hawkins, *Reconstructing Illness*, pp. 21; 24, referring to Robert Jay Lifton, *Death in Life, Survivors of Hiroshima* (New York, 1967).

24. *Ibid.*, pp. xiii; 18ff.

25. Frank, *The Wounded Storyteller*, pp. xi–xii; 16–17.

26. Hawkins, *Reconstructing Illness*, p. 4.

27. Thompson's muse 'Ianthe' remains unidentified.

28. Susan Sontag, *Illness as Metaphor* (New York, 1978), p. 3.

29. H. St Maur, *Annals of the Seymours* (London: Kegan Paul, 1902), pp. 250–1; 428–30.

30. Thompson is not mentioned in Hertford's published correspondence, but evidence of their relationship may yet be found amongst her unpublished papers. For literary reciprocations see James Sambrook, *James Thomson, 1700–1748: a Life* (Oxford: Clarendon Press, 1991), p. 264.

31. Alludes to 'The House of Pride' and the figure of 'Despair' in *Faerie Queene* I, iv; I, ix respectively.

32. See *Jusepe de Ribera, lo Spagnoletto, 1591–1652*, eds. Craig Felton and William B. Jordan (Fort Worth: Kimbell Art Museum, 1982) and Alfonso E. Pérez Sánchez and Nicola Spinosa, *Jusepe de Ribera, 1591–1652* (New York: H. Abrams for the Metropolitan Museum of Art, 1992).

33. For the influence of du Bartas on Milton and other English writers see introduction to *The Divine Weeks and Works of Guillame de Saluste Sieur du Bartas translated by Joshua Sylvester*, ed. Susan Snyder, 2 vols. (Oxford: Clarendon Press, 1979). The episode under discussion is in *The Divine Weeks*, 'The III Part of the I Day of the II Week'.

34. For Newtonian terminology as professional rhetoric see Anita Guerrini, ' "A Club of Little Villains": Rhetoric. Professional Identity, and Medical Pamphlet Wars', in *Literature and Medicine during the Eighteenth Century*, eds. Roy Porter and Marie Mulvey Roberts (London, 1993).
35. Hawkins, *Reconstructing Illness*, p. 22.
36. Madeleine Forey, ed. *Ovid's Metamorphoses translated by Arthur Golding* (Harmondsworth: Penguin, 2002), XIV, lines 63–65; 406–407.
37. Samuel Garth, John Dryden, et al., *Metamorphoses*, ed. Garth Tissol (Ware: Wordsworth Editions, 1998), p. 460.
38. *Ibid.*, pp. 74–75 (III, lines 94–5). Thompson must have noted the aptness of the precise wording in the 1717 edition where, in Addison's translation, the teeth-sowing episode (Book III), begins as 'Cadmus beheld him [the serpent] wallow in a flood/Of swimming poison, intermix'd with blood'. Cadmus's wife later witnessed her husband's transformation into a scaly, black serpent.
39. *Ibid.*, pp. 288–9 (IX, lines 161–75) (John Gay's 1717 translation).
40. John Dunton, *A Voyage Round the World*, 2 vols. (London, 1691), II, p. 42. For Dunton see Chapter 7.
41. I read 'Spirits' in the passage just cited as Thompson's poetic shorthand for 'animal spirits', the contemporary term for the purported vehicle by which, as Thomas Willis had recently shown, the nerves carry ideas to the seat of sensation in the brain. For religious enthusiasm and deranged imaginations see Dennis Todd, *Imagining Monsters: Miscreations of the Self in Eighteenth-Century England* (Chicago and London: University of Chicago Press, 1995).
42. Virginia Woolf, 'On Being Ill' in *The Essays of Virginia Woolf*, ed. Andrew McNellie, 4 vols (London, Hogarth, 1994), iv, pp. 317–29.
43. Lucy Bending, *The Representation of Bodily Pain in late Nineteenth-Century English Culture* (Oxford: Clarendon Press Press, 2000), pp. 83–9. Elaine Scarry, *The Body In Pain: the Making and Unmaking of the World* (New York and Oxford: Oxford University Press, 1985).
44. Scarry, *Body in Pain*, p. 5.
45. Woolf, 'On Being Ill', p. 318.
46. Bending, *Representations of Bodily Pain*, pp. 85–6.
47. *Ibid.* p. 184.
48. Edmund Massey, *Sermon Against the Dangerous and Sinful Practice of Inoculation* (London, 1722), p. 6.
49. See Miller, *Adoption of Inoculation*, pp. 103–104.
50. Donne, *Devotions*, as quoted in Hawkins, *Reconstructing Illness*, pp. 52–3; 234.
51. Brody, *Stories of Sickness*, p. 120.
52. Discussing the emergence of the case history, Hawkins describes 'the tendency in modern medical practice to focus primarily not on the needs of the individual who is sick but on the nomothetic condition that we call disease ...' (*Reconstructing Illness.*, p. 6)
53. Thomas Fuller, *Exanthematologia, or an Attempt to Give a Rational Account of eruptive fevers, especially of the measles and smallpox* (London, 1730), p. 263.

54. *The Works of William Cullen, MD*, 2 vols. (Edinburgh and London, 1827), II, pp. 149–516.

55. Walter Lynn M. D., *Essay Towards a More Easie and Safe method of Cure in the Small Pox, Founded on Experiments and a Review of Dr. Sydenham's Works* (London, 1717), p. 4. For another brief autobiographical 'Case' see Thomas Dover MD, *The Ancient Physicians's legacy to his Country being what he has collected himself in Forty-Nine years practice . . . Fourth Edition* (London, 1733), p. 64.

56. *Ibid.*, xvii; Kleinman, *Illness Narratives*, p. 32.

57. Brody, *Stories of Sickness*, p. 115, paraphrasing S. Kay Toombs, *The Meaning of Illness: a Phenomenological Account of the Different Perspectives of Physician and Patient* (Boston: Kluwer, 1992).

58. As cited in *Ibid.*, p. 118.

59. For modern usages see Hawkins, *Reconstructing Illness*, p. 44.

60. John Hoyles, *The Waning of the Renaissance 1640–1740: Studies in the Thought and Poetry of Henry More, John Norris and Isaac Watts* (The Hague: Martinus Nijhoff, 1971), p. 224.

61. Robert Anderson, *The Works of the British Poets with Prefaces Biographical and Critical*, 14 vols. (London and Edinburgh, 1795), X, pp. 353–4.

62. *Ibid.*, p. 353. Alexander Chalmers, 'The Life of William Thompson' in *The Works of the English Poets from Chaucer to Cowper . . . in Twenty-One Volumes* (London, 1810), XV, p. 5.

63. Hawkins, *Reconstructing Illness*, p. 10. Making the same point, Brody cites modern clinical tests in the field of psycho-neuro-immunology proving the efficacy of the so-called 'placebo response' involving 'actual bodily change' in the patient resulting from 'the symbolic or emotional impact of the healing encounter' (*Stories of Sickness*, pp. 12–14).

64. Hawkins, *Reconstructing Illness*, p. 2.

65. Lynn and Dover, as cited in Chapter 2.

CHAPTER 3

1. See Ruth Wallerstein, *Studies in Seventeenth-Century Poetic*, (Wisconsin: University of Wisconsin Press, 1950), p. 132, set against Raymond Anselment, *The Realms of Apollo: Literature and Healing in Seventeenth-Century England* (Newark: University of Delaware Press, 1995), p. 207.

2. For arguments that *Lachrymae Musarum* served as a vehicle for necessarily covert, hence displaced expressions of mourning for Charles I, at a time – a mere six months or so after the regicide – when any open expression of such grief was politically dangerous see John McWilliams, ' "A Storm of Lamentations Writ": Lachrymae Musarum and Royalist Culture After the Civil War' in *Yearbook of English Studies (Modern Language research Association)*, 33 (2003), 273–89; 275.

3. Donald R. Hopkins, *The Greatest Killer: Smallpox in History* (Chicago and London: The University of Chicago Press, 1983), pp. 38–41.

4. Robert Latham and William Matthews, eds. *The Diary of Samuel Pepys*, 11 vols. (London: G. Bell [later Bell & Hyman], 1970–1983), I, p. 244.

5. Thomas Marley, *A Short View of the Lives of the Illustrious Princes, Henry Duke of Glucester, and Mary Princess Deceased* (London, 1661), pp. 54–7.
6. Katherine Philips, 'On the Death of the Duke of Gloucester', *The Collected Works of Katherine Philips*, ed. Patrick Thomas, 2 vols. (Stump Cross: Stump Cross Press 1990), I, p. 76.
7. Martin Lluelyn, *An Elegie On the Death of the Most Illustrious Prince, Henry Duke of Gloucester* (Oxford, 1660), p. 3.
8. *Ibid.*, p. 4.
9. *Ibid.*, pp. 4–5.
10. Tobias Whitaker, *An Elenchus of Opinions Concerning the Cure of the Small Pox Together with Problematicall Questions Concerning the Cure of the French Pest* (London, 1661). The anonymous author of *Hactenus Inaudita: or, Animadversions Upon the new found way of Curing the Small Pox* (London, 1663), cites a 'Mr N. N.' observing that 'Physitians of late have more lost their credit in these diseases then ever: witness the severe judgment of the world in the cases of the Duke of *Gloucester* and the *Princess Royal*' (p. 65).
11. Whitaker, *Elenchus*, [A4, verso-recto].
12. *Ibid.*
13. *Ibid.*, p. 59.
14. *Ibid.*, [A2, verso].
15. See P. M. Rattansi, 'Paracelsus and the Puritan Revolution' and 'The Helmontian-Galenist Controversy in Restoration England' both in *Ambix: The Journal of the Society for the Study of Alchemy*, vol. 2, Issue 1 (February 1963), 24–32; and vol. 12, issue 1 (February 1964), 1–23.
16. Gilbert Burnet, *History of My Own Time* ed. Osmund Airy, 2 vols. (Oxford: Clarendon Press, 1897), I, p. 299.
17. Physicians and others associated the new ferocity of smallpox with modern luxury well into the Hanoverian period. See Miller, *Adoption*, pp. 30–5.
18. *Elegy on the death of Her Highness Mary Princess Dowager of Aurange, daughter to Charles the First* ... (London, 1660), as reprinted in *Poems, Lyrique, Macaronique, Heroique ... by Henry Bold*. (London, 1664), pp. 234–5. Bold (1627–1683) had been dislodged as a probationer fellow of New College Oxford by parliamentary visitors in 1648.
19. Thomas Shipman, *Carolina: or, Loyal Poems* (London, 1683), pp. 78–9.
20. For example, see 'On the Death of her late sacred majesty Mary Queen of England' in Samuel Wesley, *Elegies on the Queen and Archbishop* (London, 1695).
21. The physicians Walter Lynn and Thomas Willis blamed smallpox on upper-class excess. When the latter pronounced *mala stamina vitæ* on a son of James II he was never recalled to court. See Creighton, *History of Epidemics*, pp. 450–2.
22. J. Crouch, *The Muses Tears for the Loss of the Illustrious Prince, Henry Duke of Glocester* (London, 1660), p. 3.
23. Nicholas Amhurst, *Oculus Brittanniae* (London, 1724), p. 8.
24. John Glanville, 'On the Death of the Queen in 1694' (1695), as reprinted in his *Poems* (London, 1725), p. 18; J. S., *A Brief History of ... Princess, Mary Queen of England* (London, 1695), p. 131.

25. Brody, *Stories of Sickness*, p. 90.
26. Whitaker, *Elenchus*, 1; pp. 24–5.
27. Thomas Jordan, *Piety*, [D2 verso].
28. William Strode, *The Poetical Works of William Strode* ed. Bertram Dobell (London, 1907), pp. 86–7.
29. Probably written in 1675, this elegy was published in Oldham's posthumous *Remains* (1684). See *The Poems of John Oldham*, eds. Harold F. Brooks and Raman Selden (Oxford: Clarendon Press, 1987), pp. 291–314. Subsequent references to line numbers are provided in brackets.
30. BL 669, fol. 20 (p. 57), reproduced in John W. Draper, ed. *A Century of Broadside Ballads* (London: Ingpen and Grant, 1928), p. 71. For Nicholas Gray (c. 1590–1660) see *ODNB*.
31. Matthew Stevenson, *Poems: or, A Miscellany of Sonnets, Satyrs, Drollery, Panegyricks, Elegies, &c At the Instance and Request of Several Friends, Times, and Occasions* (London, 1673), pp. 5–6.
32. Anselment, *Realms*, p. 205.
33. *Ibid.*, pp. 205; 173.
34. *Ibid.*, p. 207.
35. Turner, *Body and Society*, p. 198.
36. From *Rabelais and his World*, trans. Helene Iswolsky, as anthologised in *Bakhtinian Thought; An Introductory Reader*, ed. Simon Dentith (London: Routledge, 1995), p. 227. Throughout this study I use the term 'grotesque' in this modern usage. For usage in neo-classical theory see Clark Lawlor, 'The grotesque, reform and sensibility in Dryden, Fielding and Collier' in *British Journal for Eighteenth-Century Studies*, vol. 222 (Autumn 1999), 2, 187–205.
37. Kristeva, *Powers of Horror*, p. 1.
38. *Ibid.*, pp. 53; 3–4. Connor describes the skin as 'the vulnerable, unreliable boundary between inner and outer conditions, and proof of their frightening, fascinating intimate contiguity' (*Book of Skin*), p. 65.
39. Turner, *Body and Society*, pp. 213–14; 222–4.
40. Turner, *Body and Society*, p. 198.
41. Eric Smith, *By Mourning Tongues: Studies in English Elegy* (Ipswich: Boydell with Rowan and Littlefield, 1977), p. 11.
42. As cited in *Ibid.*, p. 90.
43. John W. Draper, *The Funeral Elegy and the Rise of English Romanticism* (New York: New York University Press, 1929), p. 99.
44. *Ibid.*, pp. 101; and 117.
45. Robert Cotesworth to his father, 15 April 1716, quoted in Edward Hughes, *North Country Life in the Eighteenth Century*, (London: Oxford University Press, 1952), I, p. 345.
46. McWilliams, 'A Storm of Lamentations . . .', p. 283.
47. In his brief discussion McWilliams describes an 'urn' ('A Storm of Lamentations . . .', p. 282). My own reading differs significantly.
48. *Ibid.*
49. Anselment, *Realms*, p. 205.

50. For example, Anon, *A Cordial and Epitaph upon the much Lamented Death of the Incomparable Henry Duke of Gloucester* (London, 1660). Anselment discusses the contemporary significance of the Apollonian tradition in his opening (*Realms*11ff.).

51. These read: 'Quãm cuperet, lachrymans augusti Herois in Urnam, / Musa tuum Niobe corpus, et Arge tuum! / Ut flueret Morbi Dolor æmulus; utq(ue) tumebat / Pustula, sic tumeat Lachryma mille oculis / Flete Deæ: Britonum hunc Florem tellure repostu(m) / Expromota in Lachrymas Castalis unda riget'. A literal prose-translation, for which I thank Robert Ireland for his assistance, reads 'How would the Muse, weeping over the noble hero's urn, desire your body, Niobe, and yours, Argus, So that grief might flow, a rival of the sickness, and that, as the pustule swelled, so might the tear swell from a thousand eyes! Weep, goddesses, for this flower of the Britons, buried in the earth: The Castalian stream, poured out in tears, is dry'. This transcript and my interpretation differs from that in McWilliams, 'A Storm . . .', p. 282.

52. Joshua Barnes, 'On the Untimely Death of the Queen' in *Lachrymae Cantabrigiensis in Obitum serenissemæ reginæ Mariæ* (Canterbury, 1695), [V2].

53. Anselment, *Realms*, p. 208; Shipman, *Carolina*, pp. 78–9.

54. Thompson, *Sickness*, Canto II, p. 230.

55. Oldham died of smallpox on 9 December 1683. Other poetic tributes came from, amongst others, Dryden, Waller and Tom Brown.

56. Thompson, *Sickness*, p. 230.

57. Abraham Cowley, *Poems*, ed. A. R. Waller (Cambridge: Cambridge University Press, 1905), p. 441.

58. *Ibid.*

59. This much-discussed poem is compared with his Hastings elegy in Wallerstein, *Studies*, pp. 136–40.

60. Killigrew was not unique in being a gifted young woman whose private literary activities only became public after sudden death from smallpox. When Mary Evelyn succumbed to the disease in the very same 1685 outbreak, her father – the famous diarist – recorded being astonished to find numerous literary papers in her private closet. See *The Diary of John Evelyn*, ed. E. S. de Beer, 6 vols. (Oxford: Oxford University Press 1955), IV, p. 430. When Octavia Walsh died of smallpox in 1706, her unsuspecting family were also surprised to discover her private cache of notebooks containing religious reflections and original poems. See Roger Lonsdale, ed. *Eighteenth-Century Women Poets* (Oxford and New York: Oxford University Press, 1990), pp. 52–3.

61. Further details in my contribution to *Women and Poetry 1660–1750*, eds. Sarah Prescott and David E. Shuttleton, (London: Palgrave Macmillan, 2003), pp. 29–39.

62. See Carol Barash, *English Women's Poetry, 1649–1714* (Oxford: Clarendon Press, 1996).

63. Hammond, ed. *Poems of Dryden*, p. 114.

64. Katherine Philips, *Poems by the most deserved Admired Mrs. Katherine Philips The matchless Orinda* (London, 1667), preface [a1].

65. *Ibid.*

CHAPTER 4

1. See Draper, *The Funeral Elegy*, p. 119, who notes that in 1700, a 55-page volume of elegies to Dryden 'contains hardly any mortuary detail' (p. 188).
2. Johnson, *Lives*, I, pp. 419–20.
3. Draper, *The Funeral Elegy*, p. 126.
4. *Ibid.*, p. 154.
5. Elisabeth Bronfen, *Death, Femininity and the Aesthetic* (Manchester: Manchester University Press, 1992), p. 86.
6. J. G. Barker-Benfield, *The Culture of Sensibility: Sex and Society in Eighteenth-Century Britain* (Chicago: Chicago University Press, 1992).
7. John Thelwall, *Poems Chiefly Written in Retirement*, [1801], facsimile reprint (Oxford: Woodstock Books, 1989), p. 94. The elegy first appeared in Thelwall's *Poems upon Various Subjects* (London, 1787).
8. John Tutchin, *Poems on Several Occasions with a Pastoral; to which is added A Discourse of Life* (London, 1685), pp. 72–3.
9. When Tutchin was tried before Judge Jeffreys at the 'Bloody Assizes', the notorious prosecutor remarked: 'You are a rebel,' said Jeffreys, 'and all your family have been rebels since Adam'. Details in *ODNB*.
10. Isaac Watts, *Horæ Lyricæ: Poems Sacred to Devotion and Piety* [1706; 1711] . . . *with a Memoir of the Author by Robert Southey* (London, 1837), pp. 161–4.
11. From *L'homme devant la mort* (Paris: 1977), as cited in Bronfen, *Over Her Dead Body*, p. 87.
12. *Ibid.*, p. 163.
13. *Ibid.*
14. John Hoyles, *The Waning of the Renaissance 1640–1740: studies in the thought and poetry of Henry More, John Norris and Isaac Watts* (The Hague, 1971), p. 217.
15. Isaac Watts to Revd John Shower, 22 December 1707, in Isaac Watts, *The Works of the Reverend and Learned Isaac Watts, Containing, besides his Sermons, and Essays on Miscellaneous subjects, several additional pieces, Selected from his Manuscripts by the Rev. Dr. Jennings, and the Rev. Dr. Doddridge, in 1753, 6 vols.* (London, 1810), IV, p. 492.
16. See Selma L. Bishop, *Isaac Watt's 'Hymns and Spiritual Songs' 1707, a publishing history* (Ann Arbor, MI: Pierian Press, 1974) and Hoyles, *Waning of the Renaissance*, pp. 143–4.
17. Draper, *The Funeral Elegy*, p. 117.
18. As reproduced in Edwin Paxton Hood, *Isaac Watts; His Life and Writings, His Home and Friends* (London, 1875), p. 342. The entry reads 'Had a Small Pox – 1683'.
19. Watts, *Reliquiæ Juveniles, Miscellaneous Thoughts in prose and verse, on Natural, Moral and Divine Subjects, written chiefly in Younger Years*, p. 121 (first published in 1734, subsequent references are to the seventh, Glasgow edition of 1786).
20. *Ibid.*
21. *Ibid.*, p. 122.
22. Watts, *Works*, IV, 'Elegy LIII'.

23. *Ibid.*

24. Watts, *Works*, IV, 'Prayer LXXIII'.

25. See Samuel Wesley the younger (1691–1739), *Poems on Several Occasions, by Samuel Wesley. The Second Edition, with Additions*, 6 vols. (Cambridge, 1743), VI, p. 411. The victim, Margaret Cavendish (1715–1785), celebrated by Prior as the 'lovely little Peggy', married William Bentinck, second duke of Portland in 1734.

26. In a preface for Rowe's *Devout Exercises of the Heart* (London, 1737) Watts defends her sensationalist religiosity against charges of mysticism and eroticism. See Hoyles, *The Waning of the Renaissance*, pp. 229–32 and Hood, *Isaac Watts*, pp. 182–8.

27. *Correspondence Between Frances, Countess of Hertford (Afterwards Duchess of Somerset) and Henrietta Louisa, Countess of Pomfret, between the years 1738 and 1741*, 3 vols. (London, 1805), I, xii (biographical preface). Two further letters from Hertford discussing her grief are printed in St Maur, *Annals of the Seymours*, note 84, pp. 428–30.

28. Hertford to Hon Mrs Knight, 16 May 1746 in Thomas Hull, ed. *Select Letters Between the late Dutchess [sic] of Somerset, Lady Luxborough and others …* 2 vols. (London, 1778), I, pp. 30–1.

29. Hertford to Lady Luxborough, 20 November, 1748, in *Ibid.*, p. 83.

30. Thompson is not mentioned in any of the many Hertford letters accessible in early printed editions, but archival evidence of their relationship may yet emerge.

31. Robert Gould, *Works of Mr. Robert Gould: In Two Volumes. Consisting of those Poems [and] Satyrs*, (London, 1709), pp. 251–8 (brief discussion in Anselment, *Realms*, pp. 194–5).

32. For rise in seaboard epidemics see Hopkins, *Greatest Killer*, p. 241.

33. For trans-Atlantic context see Watts, *Epidemics and Disease*, pp. 112–14. For Mather and smallpox see *ibid.*, p. 113 and John T. Barrett, 'The Inoculation Controversy in Puritan New England', *Bulletin of the History of Medicine*, XII (1942), pp. 169–90.

34. Hopkins, *Greatest Killer*, p. 246.

35. The mention of Richard Kidder, Bishop of Bath and Wells (1633–1703), places the events of the poem before 1703. Kidder's wife was the deceased Margett's aunt.

36. James Woodhouse, *The Life and Poetical Works of James Woodhouse (1735–1820): Edited by the Rev. R. I. Woodhouse*, 2 vols. (London and New York: The Leadenhall Press, 1896), I, pp. 1–4.

37. *Ibid.*, II, p. 154. All subsequent references to this edition appear in brackets.

38. *Ibid.*, II, p. 154 (Woodhouse's original footnote). Of a further nine babies carried by his wife Hannah, few survived.

39. John Skinner, *Songs and poems, by the Rev. John Skinner. With a sketch of his life, by H. G. Reid* (Peterhead and Edinburgh, 1859), pp. 52–3.

40. Laurence Sterne, *A Sentimental Journey*, introduction by Paul Goring (Harmondsworth: Penguin, 2001), p. 41.

41. The phrase derives from Ian Watt, *The Rise of the Novel: Studies in Defoe, Richardson, and Fielding* (London, 1957).

42. See, for example, the opening of John Cleland, *Memoirs of a Woman of Pleasure*, ed. Peter Sabor (Oxford: Oxford University Press, 1985), where the narrator Fanny Hill explains that she first turned to prostitution after both her parents died of smallpox when she was fourteen, but left 'entirely unmark'd' (p. 2).

43. See sources cited in Chapter 3. The most detailed account is that of the attendant physician Walter Harris, written-up as Observation VII (pp. 178–83) in his *Treatise of the Acute Disease of Infants; to which is added Medical Observations on Several grievous Diseases* (London, 1742).

44. See Janet Todd, *Sensibility, an Introduction* (London: Methuen, 1986); Adela Pinch, *Strange Fits of Emotion; Epistemologies of Emotion, Hume to Austen* (Stanford: Stanford University Press, 1996). For medical background see Sill, *Cure of the Passions*.

45. Henry Brooke, *The Fool of Quality*, 4 vols. (Dublin, 1765), III, Chapter XIV, pp. 48–9. Subsequent quotations all from this one passage.

46. Henry Mackenzie, *The Man of the World* (London, 1773), pp. 30–1. In Vol. II, Chapter XXII surviving smallpox brings about repentance in the victim. The death from smallpox of the child Tommy Clewin while incarcerated with his parents in debtor's prison bears related implications in Tobias Smollett's novel *The Life and Adventures of Sir Launcelot Greaves* (1760–1761) (Chapter XXI). Smollett's pathetic portrayal contributed to a growing debate over prison conditions which was to culminate in a reform bill first introduced to parliament in 1774. In his *The State of the Prisons in England and Wales, with preliminary Observations, and an Account of some Foreign Prisons* (Warrington, 1777), the evangelical philanthropist John Howard reported that smallpox was rife in Britain's Houses of Correction, and City and County gaols.

47. Hopkins notes that in rural areas local authorities came to realise that providing free inoculation of a whole population at risk of epidemic was more cost-effective than mass-burials (*Greatest Killer*, p. 74).

48. *Ibid.*, 58–59. For the debate over *gratis* inoculation of the poor see William Black, *Observations Medical and Political on the Small-Pox, And the Advantages and Disadvantages of General Inoculation, especially in Cities* (London, 1781), pp. 47–67.

49. Miller, *Adoption*, pp. 134–71.

50. When not quoting contemporary sources I use the more accurate 'Lebuu'. He was an adopted son of King Ibedeul. The Pelew Islands recently became the independent pacific Republic of Palau.

51. See 'Introduction' to George Keate, *An Account of the Pelew Islands* eds. Karen L. Nero and Nicholas Thomas (London and New York: Leicester University Press, 2002), p. 31. All references, hereafter in brackets, are to this edition.

52. *Ibid.*, p. 265. This explains why Keate has to rely upon the reports of Wilson's associate, a 'Mr Sharp' who oversaw Lebuu's nursing care.

53. As discussed in Nicholas Thomas's preface to Keate, *Account*, pp. 34–5.

54. James Carmichael Smyth to Keate, 27 December 1784, describing Lebuu's death (and wording on the tombstone) included in Keate, *Account*, pp. 267–8.

55. The excellent editorial matter provided by Karen L. Nero and Nicholas Thomas fully explicates the cultural impact of the 'Lee Boo' story (27ff). A Drury Lane broadsheet advert for 'a Grand Melodramatic Romance, called Prince Lee Boo' dated 1833 is reproduced as Plate 14.

CHAPTER 5

1. For clinical pathology see Fenner et al., *Smallpox and its Eradication*, p. 49. Pock-marks, more common on the face because of a greater frequency of sebaceous glands, are the result of fibrosis of the dermis. Scarring took distinctive forms with only the milder, less fatal strains of the disease being responsible for the classic pitted pock-marks, the scar-tissue left where individual pustules had healed. Number and depth could vary greatly from one or two isolated examples, to widespread pitting across the face, upper-body and arms. Reddish patches, technically termed 'hyper-pigmentation' were characteristic of many survivors with fair skin. Those limited numbers surviving the severe strains were often left with hyper-pigmented sheet scarring over large areas, somewhat like the tissue paper scar left by severe scalding.

2. Lucinda McCray Beier, *Sufferers and Healers; the Experience of Illness in Seventeenth-Century England* (London: Routledge, 1987), p. 78.

3. Phrase borrowed from chapter heading in Grundy, 'Comet of the Enlightenment'.

4. Lady Mary Wortley Montagu, *Essays and Poems and Simplicity, a Comedy*, ed. Robert Halsband and Isobel Grundy (Oxford: Clarendon Press, 1977), p. 203.

5. *The Spectator by Joseph Addison, Richard Steele and others*, 5 vols. ed. Donald F. Bond (Oxford: Clarendon Press, 1965), I, p. 101, footnote.

6. Richard Mead, *Works*, pp. 381–2.

7. Diemerbroeck, *Anatomy*, pp. 21–2.

8. Fuller, *Exanthematalogia*, p. 393.

9. The efficacy of prematurely 'opening' the pustules by such surgical intervention was a frequent matter of dispute amongst medical writers.

10. Diemerbroeck, *Anatomy*, p. 21.

11. Grundy, 'Medical Advance', 15. See also Jill Campbell, 'Lady Mary Wortley Montagu and the "Glass Revers'd" of Female Old Age' in *'Defects': Engendering the Modern Body*, eds. Helen Deutsch and Felicity Nussbaum (Ann Arbor, 2000), pp. 213–51.

12. Nussbaum, *Limits*, p. 117.

13. James Brydges, Duke of Chandos as cited in Robert Halsband, *The Life of Lady Mary Wortley Montagu* (Oxford: Oxford University Press, [1956], 1960), p. 52.

14. Pointon, *Hanging the Head*, p. 143.

15. Ben Jonson, *Discoveries 1641, Conversations with William Drummond of Hawthornden 1619* (Edinburgh: Edinburgh University Press, 1966), p. 15.

16. Quillett, *Callipædia* (London, 1712), pp. 44–6.

17. Lawrence Stone, *The Family, Sex and Marriage in England, 1500–1800* (London and New York: Harper and Row, 1997), pp. 656–7; Robert B. Shoemaker, *Gender in English Society 1650–1850: The Emergence of Separate Spheres* (London and New York: Longman, 1998), pp. 91–113.

18. The diaries of both Pepys and Evelyn are littered with similar speculations the likely disfigurement of court beauties; for example, see Pepys's comments on Lady Richmond for 30 and 31 August 1668.

19. Jonathan Swift, *Journal to Stella* ed. Harold Williams, 2 vols. (Oxford: Clarendon Press, 1963), II, p. 524. Swift took a more sympathetic interest in the fate of 'Biddy Floyd'. See *Ibid.*, II, pp. 223; 262–3; 380; 386. For Pope's gallant concern over Martha Blount when contracting smallpox prevented her from attending the coronation of George I see *The Correspondence of Alexander Pope*, ed. George Sherburn, 5 vols. (Oxford: Clarendon Press 1956), I, pp. 265; 268–9.

20. Mary Pix, *The Different Widows or Intrigue All-a-Mode. a Comedy* (London, 1703), p. 28.

21. Bond, ed. *The Spectator*, pp. 101–102; see also *Complete Letter-Writer*, p. 195.

22. Samuel Johnson, *The Rambler*, [in 3 vols.] *The Yale Edition of the Works of Samuel Johnson, Volume IV*, eds. W. J. Bate and Albrecht B. Strauss (New Haven and London: Yale University Press, 1969), IV, p. 34.

23. Edmund Elys, 'To Mrs K. G. having been lately sick of the small Pox' in *Dia Poemata* (London, 1655), p. 41.

24. As cited in *Ben Jonson, Poems* ed. Ian Donaldson (Oxford, London, New York and Toronto: Oxford University Press, 1975), p. 181.

25. *Ibid.*

26. Thomas Philipot, *Æsop's Fables with his Life* (London, 1687), p. 3.

27. See, for example, William Strode, 'On a Gentlewoman that had had the Small-Poxe' *The Poetical Works of William Strode*, ed. Bertram Dobell (London, 1970), p. 49.

28. Anselment, *Realms*, p. 202, discussing the grotesque example of Owen Feltham's 'Lines On a gentlewoman, whose Nose was Pitted with the Smallpox' (1661).

29. Quillett, *Callipædia* (London 1712), pp. 44–5.

30. For a vicious later example see an 'Elegy to a Friend' (1816), in 'Peter Pindar' (John Wolcot), *The Works of Peter Pindar*, 4 vols. (London, 1816), IV, pp. 364–5.

31. Walter Lynn, *An Essay Towards a More Easie and Safe Method of Cure in the Small Pox* (London, 1714), p. 61.

32. Matthew Hales, *A Letter from Sir Matthew Hale, Kt, sometime Lord Chief Justice of England, To one of his Sons; After his recovery from the Small-Pox* (London. 1684), p. 2.

33. Andrew Tripe, M. D. [William Wagstaffe], *The Small-Pox, a Poem* (London, 1748), pp. 5–7.

34. William Wycherley, *The Country Wife*, Act II, Scene I.

35. John to George Keats, Friday 12 November, 1819, *The Letters of John Keats, 1814–1821*, ed. Hyder Edward Rollins, 2 vols. (Cambridge: Cambridge University Press, 1958), II, p. 230.

36. For earlier associations between wanton women and disease see Healy, *Fictions of Disease*, pp. 136–7.

37. *The London Jilt of Politick Whore* (London, 1683), 'To the Reader', (subsequent references provided in text).

38. Felicity Nussbaum, '*The Brink of all we Hate': English Satires on Women, 1660–1750* (Lexington: Kentucky University Press, 1984). For social attitudes to prostitution see Shoemaker, *Gender in English Society*, pp. 75–9.

39. Robert Bage, *Man as He Is*, 4 vols. (London, 1792), I, p. 251.

40. Samuel Richardson, *Pamela* (London: Everyman, 1978), [vols. III and IV, Letter LXXXI], II, pp. 336–7. Richardson would have known a particularly complex treatment of this male constancy theme, 'The Transformation of Fidelio into a Looking-Glass', in *The Spectator* (No 392, 30 May 1712), discussed in detail in Campbell, 'Lady Mary . . .', pp. 225–6.

41. See Thomas d'Urfey, *The Richmond Heiress: or, A Woman Once in the Right* (London, 1694), [104–105] and Margaret Cavendish, 'The Feminine Description' in *Natures Pictures Drawn by Fancies Pencil to the Life* (London, 1671), pp. 10–12. For genuine cases of male fidelity to disfigured brides see G. C. Moore Smith, ed. *The Letters of Dorothy Osborne to William Temple* (Oxford: Clarendon Press, 1928), pp. 183–4 and Lucy Hutchinson, *Memoirs of the Life of Colonel Hutchinson* (London, 1904), pp. 63–4. A shunned bride has her say in Henry Jones, *Inoculation; or Beauty's Triumph* (Bath, 1768), p. 12.

42. Arthur Friedman, ed. *Collected Works of Oliver Goldsmith*, 5 vols. (Oxford: Clarendon Press, 1966), IV, pp. 237–371.

43. Details in John Dussinger's article in *ODNB*.

44. Samuel Wesley (the younger), 'Memoir of Mrs Charles Wesley' in *Wesleyan Methodist Magazine*, 45 (1822), 509.

45. Campbell, 'Lady Mary . . .', p. 223 and Nussbaum, *Limits*, p. 119.

46. Bond, ed. *The Spectator*, V, pp. 101–104; 101 (subsequent references appear in text).

47. Brody, *Stories of Sickness*, p. 2.

48. Campbell, 'Lady Mary . . .', p. 223 (subsequent references appear in text).

49. Alexander Pope, *The Rape of the Lock and other Poems*, ed. Geoffrey Tillotson (London: Methuen, 1940), p. 195 (1717 version, Canto V, lines 15–22).

50. See E. Pollack, *The Poetics of Sexual Myth: Gender and Ideology in the Verse of Swift and Pope* (Chicago and London, 1985).

51. *The Poems of Ambrose Philips*, ed. M. G. Segar (Oxford: Basil Blackwell, 1937), pp. 126–7.

52. Johnson, *The Rambler*, IV, 326. Subsequent references provided in text.

53. See, for example, *The Complete Letter-Writer containing Familiar Letters on the most common Occasions in Life* (London, 1776), which typically juxtaposes a discussion of ageing with a reassuring letter 'To a lady who had lost her beauty by the smallpox' (p. 195).

54. Nussbaum, *Limits*, p. 116.

55. Shipman, *Carolina*, p. 78.

56. Jonathan Smedley, *Poems on Several Occasions* (London, 1730), pp. 9–10.
57. Campbell observes how the moral essayists 'urge women to imagine them-
    selves as gradually exchanging features of their bodies for spiritual or mental
    attributes over time, as if they could incrementally transfer their existences
    from the realm of the physical to that of the immaterial' ('Lady Mary . . .',
    p. 227).
58. William Pattison, *The Poetical Works of Mr. William Pattison*, 2 vols.
    (London, 1728) II, pp. 217–18. Pattison originated in Rye, so it seems likely
    that Mary Frewen was related to the Rye physician Dr. Thomas Frewen
    (1704–1791), a promoter of inoculation.
59. 'Saturday' was not amongst those 'Town Eclogues' pirated by Curll in his 1716
    volume *Court Poems*. It appeared in Horace Walpole's unauthorised edition of
    Six Town Eclogues with some other Poems (London, 1747). For this complex
    composition and publishing history see Grundy, *Lady Mary*, pp. 103–12.
60. Grundy, 'Lady Mary . . .', p. 98.
61. Halsband, *The Life of Lady Mary Wortley Montagu* , pp. 50–3.
62. Montagu, *Essays and Poems*, pp. 201–204; lines 1–4. Subsequent references to
    line numbers in brackets.
63. Hertford to Pomfret, 17 December 1740, as printed in *Correspondence
    Between Frances, Countess of Hertford (Afterwards Duchess of Somerset) and
    Henrietta Louisa, Countess of Pomfret, between the years 1738 and 1744*, 3 vols.
    (London, 1805), II, p. 233. Montagu was actually twenty-six when she con-
    tracted smallpox.
64. Montagu, *Essays and Poems*, p. 35. This frequently cited statement is from Lady
    Louisa Stuart's 'Biographical Anecdotes of Lady M. W. Montagu', printed to
    preface to the 1837 edition of her grandmother's *Works*. As the only relative
    allowed to read her grandmother's diaries before they were destroyed by Lady
    Mary's daughter Lady Louisa is considered a reliable source.
65. Campbell, 'Lady Mary . . .', p. 236.
66. *Ibid.*
67. *Ibid.*, p. 237.
68. Grundy, *Lady Mary*, p. 102.
69. Campbell, 'Lady Mary . . .' p. 236.
70. Nussbaum, *Limits*, p. 119.
71. The poem is often printed with quotation marks, but the only autograph mss
    (reproduced in *Essays and Poems*, fig. 3), carries none.
72. As quoted in George Sherburn, *The Early Career of Alexander Pope* (Oxford,
    1934), p. 204. See also Grundy, *Lady Mary*, p. 101.
73. First printed with her reassuring lines 'On her attending Miss Charlot
    Clayton, in the Small-Pox' addressed to Jones's 'faultless' patroness Mary
    Lovelace, Lady Beuclerk, in Jones, *Miscellanies in Prose and Verse* (Oxford,
    1750), pp. 79–80. Subsequent references in brackets.
74. See Ros Ballaster, 'Seizing the Means of Seduction: Fiction and Feminine
    Identity in Aphra Behn and Delarivier Manley' in *Women, Writing, History*,
    eds. Isobel Grundy and Susan Wiseman (London: Batsford, 1992), pp. 93–108.

75. Delarivier Manley, *The Adventures of Rivella*, ed. Katherine Zelinsky (Ontario: Broadview, 1999), pp. 43–6; 47. I read this to mean that Rivella no longer puts any value on her scarred face.

76. *Ibid.*, p. 47.

77. Spencer, 'Imagining the Woman Poet', p. 103.

78. Eliza Hayward, *The Wife, the Husband, and The Young Lady*, eds. Alexander Petit and Margo Collins (London: Pickering and Chatto, 2000), p. 275. Hayward adds lines from a 'late poetess' (untraced): 'Nature has been ungentle to my face, / With artless fingers shadow'd every grace / Deep has she left her cruel marks behind, / As if she meant to scar my very mind.' I thank Iona Italia for drawing my attention to this reference.

79. *Ibid.*, p. 276.

80. Nussbaum, *Limits*, p. 120.

81. See Catherine Gallagher, *Nobody's Story: the Vanishing Acts of Women Writers in the Marketplace, 1670–1820* (Oxford: Oxford UniversityPress, 1994) and Sarah Prescott, *Women, Authorship and Literary Culture, 1690–1740* (London: Palgrave Macmillan, 2003).

82. Frances Burney, *Camilla; or a Picture of Youth* eds. Edward A. Bloom and Lillian D. Bloom (London: Oxford University Press, 1972), p. 149. As Nussbaum examines in detail, Burney uses Eugenia to explore the socially anomalous phenomenon of an 'ugly' heiress (*Limits*, pp. 120–32).

83. Discussed in Nussbaum, *Limits*, pp. 118–19. See also the similar case of Harriot Trentham in Scott's Utopian novel *A Description of Millenium Hall* (1762), who rejoices when smallpox saves her from a liaison with a married man and in '. . . a very short time she became perfectly contented with the alteration this cruel distemper had made in her' since her 'love for reading returned'. Sarah Scott, *A Description of Millenium Hall*, ed. Gary Kelly (Ontario: Broadview, 1995; reprinted 1999), p. 241.

84. See Betty Rizzo's introduction to Sarah Scott, *The History of George Ellison* (Lexington: University of Kentucky Press, 1996), pp. ix–xi.

85. Nussbaum, *Limits*, p. 117.

86. Charlotte Smith, *The Old Manor House*, ed. Anne Henry Ehrenpreis (Oxford: Oxford World's Classics, 1989), pp. 507–508. (all quotations from this passage). Ehrenpreis argues convincingly for the target being the dramatist Hannah Cowley (1743–1809).

87. *Ibid.*, pp. 235–6.

88. Jane Spencer, 'Imaging the Woman Poet: Creative Female Bodies' in *Women and Poetry*, eds. Prescott and Shuttleton, pp. 99–120.

CHAPTER 6

1. Gould, *Works*, II, pp. 254–5.

2. *Callipaedia* (1712), p. 45.

3. This homoerotic aspect is addressed in Santesso, 'Lachrymae Musarum', p. 629.

4. Catherine Cockburn, *The Works of Mrs. Catherine Cockburn, Theological, Moral, Dramatic, and Poetical*, 2 vols. (London, 1751), II, p. 557.
5. *Ibid.*, pp. 557–8.
6. *Ibid.*, pp. 558–9.
7. Anselment, *Realms*, p. 209.
8. Brome, *Songs and Poems* (London, 1660), pp. 107–9.
9. Bakhtin adopts this term in *Rabelais and his World* (1965), first English translation 1968.
10. See Dentith, *Bakhtinian Thought*, p. 67; see also pp. 79–84.
11. Bakhtin, *Rabelais*, as cited in *Ibid.*, p. 228.
12. *The Dramatic Works and Poems of James Shirley*, eds. William Gifford and Alexander Dyce, 6 vols. (London: J. Murray, 1833), VI, p. 349.
13. Hales, *A Letter from Sr Matthew Hale, Kt . . . To one of his Sons; After his recovery from the Small-Pox* (London, 1684), p. 2. (page numbers hereafter supplied in brackets).
14. Harris, *Treatise of the Acute Diseases*, p. 183.
15. Connor, *Book of Skin*, p. 76.
16. Montagu to Sarah Chiswell, Adrianople, 1 April 1717 in *Selected Letters*, ed. Halsband, p. 98; Miller, *Adoption*, pp. 62–3.
17. 'George Fox' in *Dictionary of National Biography*, Leslie Stephens and Sidney Lee, eds. 63 vols (London, 1885–1900) (hereafter *DNB*).
18. Dunton was apprenticed to the Presbyterian bookseller Thomas Parkhurst on 7 December 1674. He ran home, but was persuaded to resume and had only just arrived back in London when the disease struck. Temporarily blind, he recognised the voice of a friend sent by his father: 'this gave me such a transport of Joy, that 'twas thought, I shou'd have expired in the excess of it'. See *The Life and Errors of John Dunton* (London, 1705), pp. 39–40.
19. John Dunton, *A Voyage Round the World*, 2 vols. (London, 1691), II, p. 42 (page numbers hereafter supplied in brackets).
20. The same sexual innuendo is at work in the elegy to Hastings when Dryden describes smallpox as the 'very filth'ness of *Pandora's* Box' (line 54).
21. Dunton's source was probably the *Travels* (c. 1366) of Sir John Mandeville who claimed that Prester John married the daughter of 'The Great Cham'.
22. Nussbaum analyses the rhetorical association between the 'defect' of smallpox scarring and 'racial otherness' in *Limits of the Human*, pp. 128–9.
23. Dunton had a successful career as a bookseller, journalist and poet. He travelled widely, including to America, and was twice married.
24. Dunton, *Life and Errors* [ii–iii].
25. See, for example, Henry Fielding, *Joseph Andrews* ed. Douglas Brooks-Davies (Oxford: Oxford University Press, revised 1999), Book II, Chapter xvii, p. 159.
26. Melissa Percival, 'Johann Casper Lavater: Physiognomy and Connoisseurship' in *British Journal of Eighteenth-Century Studies*, vol. 26 (2003), I, pp. 77–90. 'Putting on a Face' in Roy Porter, *Flesh in the Age of Reason* (London, 2003), pp. 244–56 (discusses the culture of physiognomy, but not the role of disfiguring illnesses); and Johann Casper Lavater, *Essays on*

Physiognomy: designed to promote the Knowledge and Love of Mankind, 5 vols. (London: 1789), I, pp. 125–8.

27. *Ibid.*, I, p. 148.

28. See 'Life of Blacklock' by Henry Mackenzie prefacing *Poems by the Late Dr. Thomas Blacklock; together with an Essay on the Education of the Blind* (Edinburgh, 1793) and Robert Chambers, *A Biographical Dictionary of Eminent Scotsmen*, 4 vols. (Glasgow, 1834), I, pp. 218–34; Eunice Smith, entry in *ODNB*.

29. For partisan accounts see Ernest Mossner, 'Hume and the Scottish Pindar' in *The Forgotten Hume; le Bon David* (New York: Columbia University Press, 1953), pp. 13–37 and Austin Wright, *Joseph Spence; a Critical Biography* (Illinois: University of Chicago Press, 1950), pp. 149–57.

30. Joseph Spence *An Account of the Life, Character, and Poems of Mr Blacklock* (London, 1754); 'Blind', *Encyclopaedia Britannica* (Edinburgh, 1783), I, p. 290.

31. See the mocking comments of the dramatist John Home printed in Henry Mackenzie, *An Account of the Life and Writings of John Home Esq.* (Edinburgh and London, 1822), p. 131.

32. James Boswell, *Life of Johnson*, ed. George Birkbeck Hill and revised by L. P. Powell, 6 vols. (Oxford: Clarendon Press, [1934] 1971), V, pp. 46; 394; I, p. 466.

33. In the poem Blacklock mentions not yet having a full beard.

34. Blacklock, *Poems* (London, 1756), p. 191. (references hereafter provided in text).

35. Todd, *Imagining Monsters*, 243; Helen Deutsch, ' "Truest Copies" and "Mean Originals": Pope, Deformity, and the Poetics of Self Exposure', *Eighteenth-Century Studies* 27 (Fall 1993), 1–26.

36. See David T. Mitchell and Sharon L. Snyder, *Narrative Prosthesis: Disability and the Dependencies of Discourse* (Ann Arbor: University of Michigan Press, 2000). Caricatured servants, such as 'Guzzle the butler' in George Colman's *Inkle and Yarico, an Opera* (1787), are frequently portrayed as pitted with smallpox. The comic actor James Spiller (1692–1729) successfully exploited the fact that losing an eye to smallpox meant he had to abandon serious heroic roles, going on to specialise in low-life characters, most successfully, Matt-o'the-Mint in *The Beggar's Opera*. See George Akenby, *The Life of Mr James Spiller, the late famous comedian* (London, 1729), pp. 7; 28. In James Grainger's influential classificatory system for fashionable collectors of engraved historical 'heads', 'deformed Persons' are included in the twelfth and very last category alongside 'the lowest order of People'. See James Grainger, *Biographical History* (1769) as discussed in Pointon, *Hanging the Head*, p. 56.

37. See Hume to Spence, 15 October 1754, on quizzing Blacklock over what associations he attached to the word 'love', in John Burton Hill, *The Life and Correspondence of David Hume*, 2 vols. (Edinburgh, 1846), I, p. 392. Blacklock married Sarah Johnston, a surgeon's daughter, in 1762.

38. My illustration reproduces that by William Bonnar (1800–1853), (Scottish Portrait Gallery, B19). A related version, engraved by W. F. Holl (1815–1884), was published in John Wilson, *The Land of Burns; a Series of Landscapes and Portraits Illustrative of the Life and Writings of the Scottish Poet* (Glasgow: 1846).

The Scottish Portrait Gallery recently acquired another watercolour sketch, probably made direct from life, which may have been the basis for both (PG 3264).

39. Blacklock and Saunderson were often discussed in tandem, for example, in James Wilson *Biography of the Blind: including all who have distinguished themselves as poets, Philosophers, Artists etc.* (Birmingham, 1833). Wilson lost his own sight to smallpox aged six. For traditional iconography see Jacques Derrida, *Memoirs of the Blind; the Self-Portrait and other Ruins*, trans. Pascale-Anne Brault and Michael Naas (Chicago and London: University of Chicago Press, 1993).

40. Nicholas Saunderson, *The Elements of Algebra in Ten Books, to which is Prefix'd, An Account of the Author's Life and Character* (Cambridge, 1749), ii. An oil portrait of Saunderson by J. Vanderbanck, painted for Martin Folkes in 1718 (bequeathed to Cambridge University in 1823), was originally engraved by G. Vandergucht to form the frontispiece to Saunderson's *Elements*.

41. Joseph Spence, *Observations, Anecdotes, and Characters of Books and Men, collected from conversation*, ed. James M. Osborn (Oxford: Clarendon Press, 1966), pp. 429–30.

42. *Ibid.*, p. xiii.

43. *Ibid.*, p. x.

44. Overview in Carolyn Williams, *Pope, Homer and Manliness; Some Aspects of Eighteenth-Century Learning* (London and New York: Routledge, 1993), Part I. William Hay, *Deformity; an Essay* (1754), as discussed in my Appendix.

45. Quoted in Anselment, *Realms*, p. 199.

46. In the context of a middle-class call for the reformation of manners symptomatic disfigurements such as pock-marks and eroded noses served as ready indicators of syphilitic libertinism, as in Hogarth's narrative paintings, but the evidence I am about to present indicates that smallpox scars on men could be accorded positive aesthetic value.

47. Discussed in Anselment, *Realms*, p. 209.

48. Thompson, *Sickness*, p. 286.

49. For this tradition see Pope's 'Verses Occasioned by Mr. Addison's Treatise on Medals', as quoted in Pointon, *Hanging the Head*, p. 66 (and Illustration 72).

50. Connor, *Book of Skin*, p. 55.

51. Thomas Dale, *Nine Commentaries Upon Fevers, and Two Epistles Concerning the Small-Pox addressed to Dr. Mead* (London, 1730), Case I, p. 103.

52. Tobias Smollett, *The Adventures of Peregrine Pickle*, ed. James L. Cliffold, revised by Paul-Gabriel Boucé (Oxford and New York: Oxford University Press, 1983), I, chapter 30, p. 148. In the same novel however (Bk I, chapter 88, p. 449) smallpox scars contribute to the 'ludicrous figure' of Viscount Vane.

53. Frances Brooke, *The Adventures of Emily Montague* [1769], ed. Mary Jones Edwards (Carleton: Carleton University Press, 1985), [vol. I, Letter xxxvii], pp. 86–7.

54. The only example I have found of smallpox being said to enhance a woman's beauty is in the anonymous novel *Virtue Rewarded; or, the Irish Princess* (London, 1693), p. 12.

CHAPTER 7

1. The standard study remains Miller, *Adoption*; see also Smith, *Speckled Monster* (pp. 30–9) for inoculation in England up to 1752.
2. The title of Genevieve Miller's essay 'Putting Lady Mary in her Place: a Discussion of Historical Causation', *Bulletin of the History of Medicine* 55 (1981), 2–16, based upon her presidential address to the American Association for the History of Medicine in 1980 just after global eradication, speaks for itself. Miller's pro-institutional approach is countered by Isobel Grundy in 'Medical Advance and Female Fame: Inoculation and its After-Effects', *Lumen XIII* (1994), 13–42.
3. Grundy, 'Medical Advance', 14 and Nussbaum *Limits*, pp. 113–15.
4. For folk-practice amongst slaves see Miller, *Adoption*, pp. 53–4.
5. Richard Blackmore, 'A Dissertation Upon the Modern Practice of Inoculation' in *A Treatise Upon the Smallpox* (London, 1723), Part II, pp. 81ff.
6. *Philosophical Transactions*, 29, no. 339, pp. 72–82; Miller, *Adoption*, pp. 48–69 (and Appendix B).
7. Samuel Whyte, *The Shamrock; or, Hibernian Cresses* (Dublin, 1772), p. 185.
8. Alexander Hamilton, *A Treatise on the Management of Female Complaints, and of Children in Early Infancy* (Edinburgh, 1792), p. 483.
9. Jones, *Inoculation*, p. 5.
10. Amhurst, *Oculus Britanniae* (London, 1724), p. 9.
11. Prose references, provided in brackets, are to *The Plain Dealer being Select Essays on Several Curious Subjects ... Now First collected in two Volumes* (London, 1734), vol. I.
12. I quote these verses as reprinted in *The Works of the Late Aaron Hill*, 4 vols. (London, 1753), pp. 53–5. For attribution see Christine Gerard, *Aaron Hill: The Muse's Projector, 1685–1750* (Oxford, 2003).
13. Grundy, 'Medical Advance', p. 30.
14. Jurin used the bills of mortality to set about calculating the death rate from smallpox over the previous half-century. Between 1721 and 1727 he compiled and published the accumulating annual statistics on the number and success rate of inoculations from which he argued on rational, evidential grounds in favour of inoculation as a safe way of reducing smallpox. See Creighton, *History of Epidemics*, p. 481 and Miller, *Adoption*, pp. 111–18. Grundy argues that even Jurin's apparently objective statistical reports reveal an element of 'Enlightenment exclusion' in downplaying local British traditions of 'buying the smallpox' and related West African folk practices in order to claim inoculation for a 'male professional establishment' ('Medical Advance', 25–6).
15. Hill, *Works*, pp. 54–5.
16. Lipscomb's choice of a medical theme reflected inherited family concerns: his father was a surgeon at Winchester where smallpox had 'raged furiously' back in 1742 when nearly 2,000 people were reportedly inoculated. The poet's cousin George Lipscomb M.D. (1773–1844), was also a staunch promoter of inoculation, publishing several pamphlets denouncing Jennerian vaccination.

17. William Lipscomb, *The Beneficial Effects of Inoculation* (London, 1772), p. 2 (all references to first edition).
18. First published in three parts between 1774 and 1776. All references are to *Infancy, or the Management of Children: a Didactic Poem in Six Books, The sixth edition* ... (Exeter and London, 1803). Citations, provided in brackets, use book and line numbering in this edition.
19. Details in Grundy, *Lady Mary*, p. 162.
20. Wendy Frith, 'Sex, smallpox and seraglios: a monument to Lady Mary Wortley Montagu' in *Femininity and Masculinity in Eighteenth-Century Art and Culture*, eds. Gill Perry and Michael Rossington (Manchester: Manchester University Press, 1994), p. 113.
21. *Infancy* ends with a rebuke to Europe and America for not erecting a single statue in honour of Montagu. The only known near-contemporary monument erected to commemorate Montagu as medical pioneer – a semi-public obelisk erected in the gardens of Wentworth Castle, Yorkshire – is discussed in Frith, 'Sex, smallpox and seraglios', pp. 99–122.
22. Downman includes a tribute to Blacklock in his *The Land of the Muses* (London, 1768) and in *Infancy* compliments him as he who 'Forbid the external sight of things' is 'within / Illumed by goodness' (III: lines 623–8).
23. In his 'Introductory Lectures on Nosology' Cullen suggest that 'the specific nature of contagions, and the dependence of the variety of the disease upon the nature of the body, are presumptions in favour of the inoculation of all specific contagions'. *The Works of William Cullen, M.D. Professor of the Practice of Physic in the University of Edinburgh, Containing his Physiology, Nosology, and First Lines of the Practice of Physic*, ed. John Thomson, 2 vols. (Edinburgh and London, 1827), I, pp. 451–2. See also 'First Lines of The Practice of Physic' [1784] (Bk III: Exanthemata or Eruptive Fevers: [DLXXXVII–DCXXX] Chapter I, 'Of the Smallpox'), as reprinted in *ibid.*, II, pp. 149–160 (quotation at p. 149).
24. See Francis M. Lobo, 'John Haygarth, Smallpox and Religious Dissent in Eighteenth-Century England'. *The Medical Enlightenment of the Eighteenth Century*, ed. Andrew Cunningham and Roger French (Cambridge: Cambridge University Press, 1990), pp. 220–2; 231–3; 240. (*Infancy* commends Haygarth's associate Hewson). Downman also commends Thomas Glass M.D. (1709–1786). (*Infancy* VI: lines 109–15). Glass, who became Downman's colleague at the Devon and Exeter Hospital, was considered one of the greatest English authorities on inoculation.
25. For a later satire on the neglectful mother who condones her daughter foregoing inoculation see Lady Emmeline Stuart-Wortley's poem 'A Visit to a County House' in *Lays of Leisure Hours* (London, 1838).
26. In 1722, at Montagu's prompting, Queen Caroline arranged for the inoculation of orphans and later the royal children. Grundy, *Lady Mary* ..., p. 214.
27. Dover, *Ancient Physician's Legacy*, pp. 48–9.
28. *Correspondence Between Frances, Countess of Hertford ... and Henrietta Louisa, Countess of Pomfret*, III, p. 190.

29. Montagu to Lady Mar, July 1723, in *Selected Letters of Lady Mary Wortley Montagu*, ed. Robert Halsband (London: Longman, 1960), p. 128. Montagu's attack on the vested interest of male doctors and their macho approach to inoculation in her anonymous article 'A Plain Account of the Inoculating of the Small pox by a Turkey Merchant', first published in *The Flying Post* in September 1722, was toned-down by editors. See Grundy, *Lady Mary*, p. 217.

30. Elizabeth Griffith, *The Delicate Distress*, ed. Cynthia Booth Ricciardi and Susan Staves (Lexington: University of Kentucky Press, 1997). Subsequent references to this edition provided in brackets.

31. For a romantic treatment see 'Invocation to Oberon; Written on the Recovery of My Daughter from Inoculation' in Mary Robinson, *The Poetical Works* (London, 1806), pp. 311–17.

32. Clarence Tracy, ed. *The Poetical Works of Richard Savage* (Cambridge: Cambridge University Press, 1962), pp. 77–9. This poem first appeared in Savage's *Miscellaneous Poems* (1726) alongside 'A POEM on the Recovery of her Grace the Dutchess [sic] of RUTLAND from the Small-Pox'.

33. *Ibid.*, headnote, p. 77.

34. *Ibid.*, p. 69. Savage does not mention Montagu's role as inoculator, but both poems appeared in his *Miscellaneous Poems and Translations* (London, 1726), dedicated to her.

35. Bowden, *Poems*, pp. 49–53 (references hereafter provided in text).

36. Dr. Bowden (c.1732–1761) was probably a younger brother of the dissenting minister John Bowden who preached Rowe's funeral sermon in 1737.

37. According to Roger Lonsdale in *Eighteenth Century Women Poets: an Oxford Anthology* (Oxford, 1989), Lewis was the only child of the Revd John Lewis of Holt, Wiltshire, 1714–1761. Within a year of her father's death she married Robert Clark of Tetbury, Gloucestershire, moving to his estate in Tetbury (now Highgrove). He supported the posthumous publication of *Poems Moral and Entertaining, written long since by Miss Lewis, then of Holt . . .* (Bath, 1799), for the benefit of local charities.

38. By 1749, her poems had appeared in the *Bath Journal* and in various London periodicals under the pseudonym 'Sylvia'.

39. In Bowden's poem 'The Young Lady's Tryal', he jokingly hauls 'Sylvia' before a heavenly court of poets for hiding her literary gifts under a bushel. See also his 'On a Young Lady at Holt (a Place Famous For Mineral Waters) on her late Ingenious POEMS' (dated March 1749), with her 'Answer' in his *Poems* (1754), pp. 98–102 (these and further verse-exchanges are reprinted in her 1799 *Poems*).

40. See Bowden to Lewis, dated June, 1749 in Bowden, *Poems*, pp. 291–2.

41. *Ibid.*, pp. 296–7.

42. Bowden's poem implies that Lewis's inoculation produced a severe case of symptomatic smallpox. I have been unable to establish a precise date for the operation, probably prompted by the epidemic of 1752.

43. Lewis, *Poems*, p. 98.

44. 'A Hymn of Thanks, On my Recovery from the Small-Pox' Elizabeth Rowe (1674–1737), *The Miscellaneous Works In Prose and Verse of Mrs. Elizabeth Rowe . . . in Two Volumes* (London, 1739), I, p. 95.
45. *Ibid.*, p. 96.
46. *Ibid.*, p. 97.
47. Anna Seward, *The Poetical Works of Anna Seward; With Extracts from her Literary Correspondence*, 3 vols. (Edinburgh and London, 1810), I, p. 186.
48. Henry Jones, *Inoculation; or Beauty's Triumph* (London, 1768), p. 11.
49. Nussbaum's confusing attribution of this poem to 'Henry Jones Bath' [sic] is compounded by her claim that it celebrates 'Sir Robert Sutton' (*Limits*, pp. 117; 320) (the surgeon remained a commoner).
50. Smith, *Speckled Monster*, chapter 4. Smith considers the epidemic of 1752 as marking the start of what he terms 'The Age of Inoculation'.
51. For example, John Galt's *Annals of the Parish* (Edinburgh, 1821), for the 'Year 1774', reflects the situation in rural Ayrshire: '. . . the inoculation was not in practice yet among us, saving only in the genteel families that went into Edinburgh for the education of their children, where it was performed by the faculty there'.
52. As quoted in Smith, *Speckled Monster*, p. 68.
53. Elizabeth (née Seymour) Duchess of Northumberland, had become heiress to the barony of Percy upon the death from smallpox of her brother Lord Beauchamp in 1744. Jones also calls on her to bring to its fulfilment 'Gracious MONTAGUE's serene Millenium / That Peaceful Paradise, which booming reigns / Within her sainted and seraphic Soul / As calm and pure, as Eden's blissful Grove' (p. 9). This must allude to Lady Barbara Montagu's vision of an ideal community of virtuous women, including several seeking retreat after being scarred by smallpox, as portrayed in the Utopian novel *Millenium Hall* (1762). Though Montagu had died in 1765 and *Millenium Hall* is now attributed wholly to Montagu's companion Sarah Scott, at this time the novel was invariably thought of as co-authored.

CHAPTER 8

1. Tim Fulford and Debbie Lee 'The Jenneration of Disease: Vaccination Romanticism and Revolution' in *Studies in Romanticism*, Spring 2000, vol. 39, 1, 139–63; 140. (hereafter 'Jenneration'). Subsequent references are provided in brackets.
2. John Baron, *The Life of Dr. Jenner*, 2 vols. (London, 1838), II, p. 119.
3. Thomas Frognall Dibdin, *Reminiscences of a Literary Life*, 2 vols. (London: 1836), I, pp. 343–4.
4. Benjamin Moseley, *Medical Tracts* (London, 1800), p. 1. Subsequent references are to this second edition.
5. Moseley, *Medical Tracts*, pp. 179–81. Moseley began his medical career as a surgeon, in which capacity he made a quick fortune in Jamaica before returning home to purchase an MD from St Andrews and publish on tropical diseases.

He spent thirty years as a London society physician attached to the Royal Medical Hospital, Chelsea.

6. William Rowley, *Cow-Pox Inoculation no Security Against Small-Pox Infection, to which is added the Modes of Treating the Beastly New Diseases Produced from Cow-Pox* (London, 1805), p. vii (hereafter referenced in brackets).

7. Baron, *Life*, II, p. 111.

8. Anon., *Physic and Physicians, a Medical Sketch Book*, 2 vols. (London, 1839), II, p. 80.

9. Richard B. Fisher, *Edward Jenner, 1749–1823* (London: André Deutsch, 1991), p. 120 (hereafter 'Jenner').

10. *Ibid.*, pp. 97–9.

11. Diedre Le Faye, ed. *Jane Austen's Letters* (London: Folio Society, 2003), p. 62.

12. Fulford and Lee, 'Jenneration', pp. 140–2.

13. Dibdin, *Reminiscences*, I, p. 199.

14. Discussed in Ludmilla Jordanova, *Defining Features: Scientific and Medical Portraits 1660–2000* (London: Reaktion, 2000), pp. 87–99.

15. *Ibid.* Fig. 55 reproduces James Northcote's 1802 oil portrait, owned by Plymouth Medical Society. Jenner exchanged pastoral paintings with the anatomist John Hunter. See Fisher, *Jenner*, p. 34.

16. John Coakley Lettsom, *Observations on the Cow-Pock* (London, 1801), pp. 2–4; 15.

17. Wellcome Library MS3016 and MS3017. A volume of Jenner's verse was printed at the expense of Thomas Pruen. At least one appeared in Dibdin's journal *The Museum* (I, 255–256). See Fisher, *Jenner*, p. 26.

18. Fisher, *Jenner*, pp. 31–3.

19. *Biographia Literaria, or Biographical Sketches of My Literary Life and Opinions*, eds. James Engell and W. Jackson Bate, 2 vols. (London: Routledge and Kegan Paul, 1983), II, p. 85.

20. Coleridge to Jenner, September, 1811, in *Collected Letters*, VI, pp. 1025–1026.

21. *Ibid.*, p. 1026. Fulford and Lee, 'Jenneration', pp. 153–5.

22. Fisher, *Jenner*, p. 156.

23. For example, John Walker's 'Jenneric Opera', serialised in the *Medical Observer* (1808), found a response in *The Vaccine Scourge* (1815) from the surgeon-poet John Ring who also translated Christopher Anstey's Latin 'Ode to Jenner'. In *Il Trionfo della Vaccinia* (Parma: 1810), by the Neapolitan admirer Gioachino Ponta, a vast machinery of gods, goddesses, spirits and fates are brought into play to tell the epic story of the discovery of vaccination. See Baron *Life*, II, pp. 169–73; 41–2.

24. *Ibid.*, p. 179.

25. James Sheridan Knowles, *A Collection of Poems on Various Subjects* (Waterford, 1810), pp. 29–48; 32.

26. First published as a review in 1804, expanded as a two-part essay in Nathan Drake, *Literary Hours, or Sketches, Critical, Narrative and Poetical*, 3 vols. (London, 1820), II, pp. 304; 308–309. Lofft's notes to the third edition of *The Farmer's Boy* make liberal use of Drake's glowing comments.

27. *Ibid.*, p. 309.
28. See *Selections from the Correspondence of Robert Bloomfield, the Suffolk Poet*, ed. W. H. Hart, F. S. A. (London, [1870] facsimile reprint Walton-on-Thames: for Robert F. Ashby, 1968), p. 20. Hereafter cited as 'Bloomfield, *Correspondence*'. Drake originally practised medicine in Bloomfield's native Suffolk but had since settled at Hadleigh, Surrey. See *The Farmer's Boy* (third edition), p. xxv.
29. Bloomfield, *Correspondence*, p. 20.
30. Dibdin, *Reminiscences*, I, p. 200.
31. *Ibid.*, p. 201.
32. All quotations in this paragraph, Jenner to Dibdin, 10 October 1803 printed in Dibdin, *Reminiscences*, I, p. 201.
33. Bloomfield, *Correspondence*, pp. 28–9.
34. *Ibid.*, p. 29.
35. *Ibid.*, p. 25. On 29 February 1803, Bloomfield reports that 'Dr. Jenner is in town, and has written to me'.
36. Letter to George Bloomfield, *Ibid.*, pp. 33–4.
37. Nathaniel Bloomfield, *An Essay on War in Blank Verse; Honington Green, a Ballad; The Culprit, an Elegy and other Poems, on Various Subjects* (London, 1803), pp. x–xi.
38. Jonathan Lawson, *Robert Bloomfield* (Boston: Twayne Publishers, 1980), pp. 33–34 (quoting BL Add. MSS. 28, 268, 113).
39. *Ibid.*, p. 34. Bloomfield's youngest child was vaccinated in 1802 (BL Add. MS 28, 268, 69).
40. Preface to N. Bloomfield, *Essay on War*, pp. xxiii–xxiv (dated 'Troston Hall, 2 Jan: 1803').
41. All quotations this paragraph from *Ibid.*, p. vii.
42. See *The Farmer's Boy*, third edition, pp. viii; ix–x (footnotes).
43. Bloomfield, *Correspondence*, p. 9 (hereafter referenced in brackets).
44. *Ibid.*, pp. 8–9; 17. Bloomfield couched his objections in terms of protecting his own reputation for modesty.
45. *Ibid.*, p. 17.
46. Sales of the first edition were relatively poor. Bloomfield complained that the booksellers did not advertise it because they did not own it. But *Good Tidings* reached a wider readership when it was 'improved' and included in the 1806 volume *Wildflowers; or, Pastoral and Local Poetry*. See Lawson, *Robert Bloomfield*, p. 25.
47. Robert Bloomfield, *Good Tidings, or News From the Farm, a Poem* (London, 1804), 'Advertisement'. Subsequent page references given in brackets.
48. *Extract from a Poem, entitled 'Good Tidings, or News From the Farm' by Robert Bloomfield. Recited at the Anniversary Meeting of the Royal Jennerian Society, Thursday 17th May, 1804* (London, 1804).
49. Wickett and Duvall, *The Farmer's Boy*, p. 35.
50. Fulford and Lee, 'Jenneration', p. 150.

51. There appears to be no evidence of Bloomfield reading Thomas Blacklock's poetry, but this picture of a blind boy who has been denied access to the visual wonders of the natural world resembles the blind poet's autobiographical musings.

52. *Ibid.*

53. Arthur Aiken, ed. *The Annual Review and History of Literature for 1804* (London, 1805), III, p. 574, which then reprints the passage I have just discussed.

54. *Ibid.*, pp. 32–3.

55. 'Song Sung by Mr. Bloomfield at the Anniversary of Doctor Jenner's Birthday, 1803', printed posthumously in *The Remains of Robert Bloomfield* (London, 1824), p. 50.

56. Bloomfield, *Correspondence*, pp. 33–2.

57. Dibdin, *Reminiscences*, I, p. 202; *Physic and Physicians*, II, p. 79. The use of this metaphor probably derives from Sydenham.

58. William Hazlitt, *The Round Table: a Collection of Essays on Literature, Men and Manners*, 3 vols. (Edinburgh, 1817), [No XXVIII], II, p. 12.

59. Lofft to Robert Bloomfield, 10 July 1803, *Correspondence*, p. 31.

60. John Goodridge and John Lucas, eds. *Robert Bloomfield, Selected Poems* (Nottingham Trent University: Trent Editions, 1998), p. 7.

61. Drake, *Literary Hours*, p. 316.

62. Woodville was physician to St Pancras smallpox hospital from March 1791. He abandoned a proposed second volume of his *History* after confirming Jenner's findings in his *Reports of a Series of Inoculations for the Variolæ Vaccinæ or Cow-pox* (London, 1799). Dibdin also consulted Woodville's *History* at Jenner's prompting.

63. Examining Rowley's 'Ox-faced, cow-poxed boy' Moseley remarked that 'he has frequently seen distortions from that terrible distemper, the yaws, in the African race, where there has been the resemblance of various animals'. Rowley, *Cow-Pox*, p. vii.

64. For the 1806 'vaccine expedition' of the Spanish Surgeon-Royal, Dr. Francis Xavier see Baron, *Life*, II, pp. 79–80.

65. Jenner to Baron, 23 December 1804, in Baron, *Life*, II, p. 24. For 'Inkle and Yarico' see Moira Fergusson, *Subject to Others: British Women writers and Colonial Slavery, 1670–1834* (London: Routledge, 1992), pp. 73ff.

66. The pathetic response of 'Abba Thulle' to the news of his son's death is recorded in a 'Supplement' to Keate's *Account*.

67. As Keate's recent editor observes, with this aim the East India Company sent a return expedition of 1790, led by Captain John McCluer, who delivered a copy of Keate's *Account* to the tribal father.

68. See Keate, *Account*, p. 268.

69. Baron, *Life*, II, pp. 101–104.

70. *Annual Review* (1805), III, p. 574 and Lawson, *Robert Bloomfield*, pp. 31–3.

71. Robert Southey, *A Tale of Paraguay* (London, 1825), p. 19. Southey arranged for his own children to be vaccinated.

72. *Ibid.*, p. 240.

73. *Ibid.*, pp. 159–60.

EPILOGUE

1. Gilman, *Disease and Representation*, pp. 6–7.
2. See also Cotterell's use of such a tropes in his preface to Philips's *Poems* as discussed at end of Chapter 3.
3. Thomas Philipot, *Æsop's Fables with his Life* (London, 1687), p. 3.
4. Brome, *Songs*, pp. 106–8.
5. Connor, *Book of Skin*, p. 73.
6. *Ibid.*, p. 53.
7. *Ibid.*, pp. 14–15.
8. Temple Luttrell, in *The Edinburgh Magazine, or Literary Amusement* (1774), pp. 306–9.
9. Lavater, *Essays*, I, p. 125.
10. See Michael S. Gurney, 'Disease as Device; the Role of Smallpox in Bleak House' in *Literature and Medicine* 9 (1990), 80–92.
11. The fate of the beautiful Frances, Lady Aubrey in Mary Robinson's novel *Walsingham; or the Pupil of Nature* (1797), for whom 'the mirror which reflected her deformity looked like the fiat of total annihilation' exemplifies many such novelistic episodes (vol. I, chapter 2).
12. Smith, *Speckled Monster*, p. 21.
13. Jonathan B. Tucker, *Scourge: The Once and Future Threat of Smallpox* (New York: Atlantic Monthly Press, 2001) and Richard Preston, *The Demon in the Freezer: the Terrifying Truth about the Threat of Bioterrorism* (London, 2003). Calls for the destruction of viral stocks were debated throughout the 1980s, but the current global political climate makes this increasingly unlikely.

APPENDIX

1. She was canonized as such in a 1779 painting of contemporary women writers and artists by Richard Samuel (details in *ODNB*).
2. William Wycherely, *The Country Wife*, Act III, Scene 2. For the culture of portraiture see Pointon, *Hanging the Head*, pp. 43 and 80 and Jordanova, *Defining Features, passim*. Pointon observes how Rowlandson and caricaturists exploited the idea of the portrait painter's studio as a site of 'grotesque flattery' (p. 48).
3. See Katherine Gibson, 'John Bushnell', *ODNB*.
4. Pointon, *Hanging*, p. 113.
5. See Sarah Cooper, 'John Pinkerton', *ODNB*. The same applies to portraits of the radical philosopher William Godwin.
6. Cited in *ODNB*.
7. Pointon, *Hanging*, p. 5.
8. Alexander Pope 'Peri Bathous; or Martinus Scriblerus his Treatise of the Art of Sinking in Poetry' [1725] in *Miscellanies in Prose and Verse by Pope, Swift and Gay*, ed. Alexander Petit, 4 vols. (London, 2002), III, p. 25.
9. From Dibdin's *Bibliomania* (1811) as cited by Peter Hayworth in 'Humphrey Wanley' *ODNB* (includes this portrait).

10. Robin Reilly, *Josiah Wedgwood 1730–1795* (London, 1992), p. 4. The most famous portrait of Wedgwood, that painted from the life by Joshua Reynolds in 1780 shortly after the potter had undergone the amputation of his leg, does portray premature ageing, but as Reilly notes (p. 219), it does not obviously indicate scars. Some high-colouring on Wedgwood's face could be read as Reynolds's way of suggesting sheet scarring. Similarly, Reynold's portrait of Joseph Warton, later engraved by A. Cardon to provide the frontispiece to Revd. John Wooll, *Biographical Memoirs of the Late Revd. Joseph Warton* (London, 1806), may also subtly suggest scarring on the subject's left cheek and jaw line.

11. Campbell, 'The Glass Revers'd', p. 224.

12. William Hazlitt, 'On the Pleasures of Painting', *Table Talk, or Original Essays on Men and Manners*, 2 vols. (London, 1821–1822), I, p. 20.

13. Tom Paulin, *The Day-Star of Liberty; William Hazlitt's Radical Style* (London: Faber and Faber, 1998), p. 5. Portrait reproduced as plate 2.

14. British Museum Print Collection (Inventory no. 1889-4-9-145; under portraits Class IV, Sub 2. Period 4).

15. Brief discussions in Todd, *Imagining Monsters*, pp. 234–7 and *'Defects'*, eds. Deutsch and Nussbaum, pp. 2–3; 115–16.

16. *The Works of William Hay Esq.*, 2 vols. (London, 1794), I, Preface, p. iv; Mead, 'De Variolis et Morbillis' or *Discourse on the Small-pox and Measles* (1747).

17. Hay, *Deformity*, p. 4.

18. *Ibid.*, p. 37. Hay's action contrasts with that of Pope who ensured that his curvature of the spine was 'written-out' of his many commissioned portraits. Only one or two pencil sketches quickly executed 'from the life', presumably made without Pope's knowledge, escaped this effort to police his public image.

Select bibliography

This list excludes modern scholarly editions of the novels, essays, poems, collected correspondence and diaries of canonical writers, but full references for these, and all works consulted are provided in the footnotes. Unless otherwise stated, place of publication is London.

Anon. *A Cordial and Epitaph upon the much Lamented Death of the Incomparable Henry Duke of Gloucester*. 1660.

Anon. *Hactenus Inaudita: or, Animadversions Upon the new found way of Curing the Small Pox*. 1663.

Anon. *The London Jilt or Politick Whore*. 1683.

Anon. *A Short Treatise of the Smallpox, showing the means how for to govern and cure those which are infected therewith*. 1652.

Anon. *A Letter to J. C. Lettsom, M.D. F.R.S. S.A.S. & c. occasioned by Baron Dimsdale's Remarks on Dr. Lettsom's letter to Sir Robert Barker . . . upon general inoculation. By an uninterested spectator*. 1779.

Anon [J. S.]. *A Brief History of . . . Princess Mary Queen of England*. 1695.

Aiken, Arthur, ed. *The Annual Review and History of Literature for 1804*. 1805.

Anderson, Robert. *The Works of the British Poets with Prefaces Biographical and Critical*. 14 vols. London and Edinburgh: 1794–1795.

Anselment, Raymond. *The Realms of Apollo: Literature and Healing in Seventeenth-Century England*. Newark: University of Delaware Press, 1995.

Aubin, Penelope. *Charlotta Du Pont*. 1739.

Bakhtin, Michel. *Rabelais and his World*, trans. H. Iswolsky. Cambridge, MA: MIT Press, 1968.

Ballaster, Ros. 'Seizing the means of seduction: fiction and feminine identity in Aphra Behn and Delarivier Manley'. *Women, Writing, History, eds*. Isobel Grundy and Susan Wiseman. Batsford, 1992, pp. 93–108.

Barash, Carol. *English Women's Poetry, 1649–1714*. Oxford: Clarendon Press, 1996.

Barker-Benfield, J. G. *The Culture of Sensibility: Sex and Society in Eighteenth-Century Britain*. Chicago: Chicago University Press, 1992.

Baron, John. *The Life of Dr. Jenner, 2 vols*. 1838.

Beier, Lucinda McCray. *Sufferers and Healers; the Experience of Illness in Seventeenth-Century England*. Routledge, 1987.

Black, William. *Observations Medical and Political on the Small-Pox, and the Advantages and Disadvantages of General Inoculation, especially in Cities.* 1781.

Bending, Lucy. *The Representation of Bodily Pain in late Nineteenth-Century English Culture.* Oxford: Clarendon Press, 2000.

Blacklock, Thomas. *Poems by the Late Dr. Thomas Blacklock; together with an Essay on the Education of the Blind.* Edinburgh: 1793.

Blackmore, Richard. *A Treatise Upon the Smallpox.* 1723.

Bloomfield, Nathaniel. *An Essay on War in Blank Verse; Honington Green, a Ballad; The Culprit, an Elegy and other Poems, on Various Subjects.* 1803.

Bloomfield, Robert. *Extract from a Poem, entitled 'Good Tidings, or News From the Farm' by Robert Bloomfield. Recited at the Anniversary Meeting of the Royal Jennerian Society, Thursday 17th May, 1804.* 1804.

Good Tidings, or News From the Farm, a Poem. 1804.

Selections from the Correspondence of Robert Bloomfield, the Suffolk Poet, ed. W. H. Hart, FSA. London: Spottiswoode and Co., 1870 [facsimile reprint Walton-on-Thames for Robert F. Ashby, 1968].

Bold, Henry. *Poems, Lyrique, Macaronique, Heroique.* 1664.

Boucé, P-G. 'Imagination, pregnant women, and monsters, in eighteenth-century England and France'. *Sexual Underworlds of the Enlightenment,* eds. G. S. Rousseau and R. Porter. Manchester: Manchester University Press, 1987, pp. 86–100.

Bowden, Samuel. *Poetical Essays on Several Occasions,* 2 vols. 1733; 1735.

Poems on Various Subjects; with some Essays in Prose. Bath: 1754.

Brieger, Gert H. 'The Historiography of Medicine'. *Companion Encyclopaedia of the History of Medicine,* eds. W. F. Bynum and Roy Porter. Routledge, 1993.

Brody, Howard. *Stories of Sickness.* Oxford and New York: Oxford University Press, [1987] revised second edition, 2003.

Brody, Saul Nathaniel. *The Disease of the Soul: Leprosy in Medieval Literature.* Ithaca: Cornell University Press, 1974.

Brome, Alexander. *Songs and other Poems.* 1661.

Brome, Richard, ed. *Lachrymae Cantabrigiensis in Obitum serenissemæ reginæ Mariæ.* Canterbury: 1695.

Bronfen, Elisabeth. *Death, Femininity and the Aesthetic.* Manchester: Manchester University Press, 1992.

Brooke, Henry. *The Fool of Quality,* 4 vols. Dublin: 1765.

Campbell, Jill. 'Lady Mary Wortley Montagu and the "glass revers'd" of female old age'. *"Defects": Engendering the Modern Body,* eds. Helen Deutsch and Felicity Nussbaum. Ann Arbor: University of Michigan Press, 2000, pp. 213–51.

Chalmers, Alexander. *The Works of the English Poets from Chaucer to Cowper . . . in Twenty-One Volumes.* 1810.

Chambers, Robert. *A Biographical Dictionary of Eminent Scotsmen,* 4 vols. Glasgow: 1834.

Cockburn, Catherine. *The Works of Mrs. Catherine Cockburn, Theological, Moral, Dramatic, and Poetical,* 2 vols. 1751.

Connor, Steven. *The Book of Skin.* Reaktion Books, 2004.

Conrad, Lawrence I. and Michael Neve, *et al.* eds. *The Western Medical Tradition, 880 BC to AD 1800*. Cambridge: Cambridge University Press, 1995.

Cowley, Abraham. *Poems*, ed. A. R. Waller. Cambridge: Cambridge University Press, 1905.

Creighton, Charles. *A History of Epidemics in Britain*, 2 Vols., [1891, 1894]. Frank Cass and Co., reprinted 1963.

Crookshank, M. *History and Pathology of Vaccination*. Philadelphia: 1889.

Crouch, J. *The Muses Tears for the Loss of the Illustrious Prince, Henry Duke of Glocester*. 1660.

Cullen, William. *The Works of William Cullen, M.D. Professor of the Practice of Physic in the University of Edinburgh, Containing his Physiology, Nosology, and First Lines of the Practice of Physic*, ed. John Thomson. 2 vols. Edinburgh and London: 1827.

Davis, Lennard J. *Factual Fictions: Origins of the English Novel*. New York: Columbia University Press 1983.

Dentith, Simon, ed. *Bakhtinian Thought; An Introductory Reader*. Routledge, 1995.

Deutsch, Helen. 'Truest copies' and 'mean originals': Pope, deformity, and the poetics of self exposure'. *Eighteenth-Century Studies* 27, Fall 1993, 1–26.

Dibdin, Thomas Frognall. *Reminiscences of a Literary Life*, 2 vols. 1836.

Diemerbroeck, Ysbrand van. *The Anatomy of Human Bodies . . . To which is added a particular treatise of the small-pox and measles . . . Translated [from original Latin] by William Salmon*. 1694.

Dixon, C. W. *Smallpox*. J. and A. Churchill, 1962.

Dover, Thomas. *The Ancient Physicians's legacy to his Country being what he has collected himself in Forty-Nine years practice . . . Fourth Edition*. 1733.

Downman, Hugh. *Infancy, or the Management of Children: a Didactic Poem in Six Books, The sixth edition, to which are added poems not before published*. Exeter and London: 1803.

Drake, Nathan. *Literary Hours, or Sketches, Critical, Narrative and Poetical*, 3 vols. 1820.

Draper, John W. *The Funeral Elegy and the Rise of English Romanticism*. New York: New York University Press, 1929.

Drewitt, F. D. *The Life of Edward Jenner*. Longmans, 1931.

Dunton, John. *A Voyage Round the World*. 1691.

The Life and Errors of John Dunton. 1705.

Athenianism; or, the new projects of Mr. Dunton. 1710.

Edwardes, Edward J. *A Concise History of Small-pox and Vaccination in Europe*. 1902.

Elys, Edmund. *Dia Poemata: Poetick Feet standing upon Holy Ground; or, Verses on certain Texts of Scripture*. 1655.

Encyclopaedia Britannica, or a Dictionary of Arts and Sciences, 10 vols. Edinburgh: J. Balfour *et al.*, 1778–1783.

Felltham, Owen. *Resolves; Divine, Moral, Political. The Eighth Impression. With New . . . Additions Both in Prose and Verse*. 1661.

Fenner, F. *et al. Smallpox and its Eradication*. Geneva: World Health Organisation, 1988.

Fergusson, Moira. *Subject to Others: British Women writers and Colonial Slavery, 1670–1834*. Routledge, 1992.

Fisher, Richard B. *Edward Jenner, 1749–1823*. André Deutsch, 1991.

Flood, Frances. *The Devonshire Woman; Or, a wonderful narrative of Frances Flood*. NP, 1723.

Forey, Madeleine. *Ovid's Metamorphoses translated by Arthur Golding*. Harmondsworth: Penguin, 2002.

Frank, A. W. *The Wounded Storyteller: Body, Illness, and Ethics*. Chicago: Chicago University Press, 1995.

Frith, Wendy. 'Sex, smallpox and seraglios: a monument to Lady Mary Wortley Montagu'. *Femininity and Masculinity in Eighteenth-Century Art and Culture*, eds. Gill Perry and Michael Rossington. Manchester: Manchester University Press, 1994, 99–122.

Fulford, Tim and Debbie Lee. 'The Jenneration of disease: vaccination romanticism and revolution'. *Studies in Romanticism*. Boston: Spring 2000, vol. 39, I, 139–63.

Fuller, Thomas. *Exanthematologia, or an Attempt to Give a Rational Account of eruptive fevers, especially of the measles and smallpox*. London: 1730.

Gallagher, Catherine. *Nobody's Story: the Vanishing Acts of Women Writers in the Marketplace, 1670–1820*. Oxford: Clarendon Press, 1994.

Gearin-Tosh, Michael. 'Marvell's "upon the death of Lord Hastings"', *Essays and Studies*, 34, 1981, 105–22.

George Keate. *An Account of the Pelew Islands*, eds. Karen L. Nero and Nicholas Thomas. London and New York: Leicester University Press, 2002.

Gilman, Sander L. *Disease and Representation: Images of Illness from Madness to AIDS*. Ithaca and London: Cornell University Press, 1988.

Glanville, John. *Poems*. 1725.

Goodridge, John and John Lucas, eds. *Robert Bloomfield, Selected Poems*. Nottingham Trent University: Trent Editions, 1998.

Gould, Robert. *Works of Mr. Robert Gould: In Two Volumes. Consisting of those Poems [and] Satyrs*. 1709.

Griffith, Elizabeth. *The Delicate Distress*, eds. Cynthia Booth Ricciardi and Susan Staves. Lexington: University of Kentucky Press, 1997.

Grundy, Isobel. *Lady Mary Wortley Montagu: Comet of the Enlightenment*. Oxford: Oxford University Press, 1999.

'Medical advance and female fame: inoculation and its after-effects'. *Lumen* XIII (1994), 13–42.

Gurney, Michael S. 'Disease as device; the role of smallpox in Bleak House'. *Literature and Medicine* 9 (1990), 80–92.

Hales, Matthew. *A Letter from Sir Matthew Hale, Kt, sometime Lord Chief Justice of England, To one of his Sons; After his recovery from the Small-Pox*. London: 1684.

Halsband, Robert, ed. *Selected Letters of Lady Mary Wortley Montagu*. Longman, 1960. *The Life of Lady Mary Wortley Montagu*. Oxford: Oxford University Press, [1956] Galaxy Edition, 1960.

Hamilton, Alexander. *A Treatise on the Management of Female Complaints and of Children in Early Infancy*. Edinburgh: 1792.

Harvey, Gideon. *A Treatise of the Small-pox and the Measles; describing their Nature, Causes and Signs.* 1696.

Harris, Walter. *Treatise of the Acute Disease of Infants; to which is added Medical Observations on Several grievous Diseases.* 1742.

Hatfield, Elaine, John Cacioppo and Richard Rapson, eds. *Emotional Contagion.* Cambridge: Cambridge University Press, 1994.

Hay, William. *The Works of William Hay Esq.* 2 vols. 1794.

Hayward, Eliza. *The Wife, the Husband, and The Young Lady*, eds. Alexander Petit and Margo Collins. Pickering and Chatto, 2000.

Hazlitt, William. *Table Talk, or Original Essays on Men and Manners*, 2 vols. 1821–1822.

Healy, Margaret. *Fictions of Disease in early Modern England: Bodies, Plagues and Politics.* Basingstoke: Palgrave, 2001.

[Hertford] *Correspondence Between Frances, Countess of Hertford Afterwards Duchess of Somerset and Henrietta Louisa, Countess of Pomfret, between the years 1738 and 1741*, 3 vols. 1805.

Hill, Aaron. *The Plain Dealer being Select Essays on Several Curious Subjects ... Now First collected in two Volumes.* 1734.

The Works of the Late A[aron] H[ill], 4 vols. 1753.

Hill, John Burton. *The Life and Correspondence of David Hume*, 2 vols. Edinburgh: 1846.

Hobby, Elaine. 'Gender, science and midwifery: Jane Sharp, *"The Midwives Book", 1671' The Arts of 17th-Century Science*, eds. Claire Jowitt and Diane Watt. Aldershot: Ashgate, 2002.

Holmes, Richard. *Coleridge; Early Visions.* London, Sydney, Auckland and Toronto: Hodder and Stoughton, 1989.

Hood, Edwin Paxton. *Isaac Watts; His Life and Writings, His Home and Friends.* London: 1875.

Hopkins, Donald R. *The Greatest Killer: Smallpox in History.* Chicago and London: University of Chicago Press, 2002.

Howard, John. *The State of the Prisons in England and Wales, with preliminary Observations, and an Account of some Foreign Prisons.* Warrington: 1777.

Hoyles, John. *The Waning of the Renaissance 1640–1740: studies in the thought and poetry of Henry More, John Norris and Isaac Watts.* The Hague: Martinus Nijhoff, 1971.

Huet, M.-H. *Monstrous Imagination.* Cambridge, MA: Harvard University Press, 1993.

Hughes, Edward. *North Country Life in the Eighteenth Century.* 2 vols. London: Oxford University Press, 1952.

Hull, Thomas, ed. *Select Letters Between the late Dutchess [sic] of Somerset, Lady Luxborough and others*, 2 vols. 1778.

Jarcho, Saul. *The Concept of Contagion in Medicine, Literature, and Religion.* Malabar, Florida: Krieger Publishing Company, 2000.

Jones, Henry. *Inoculation; or Beauty's Triumph: a Poem in Two Cantos.* London and Bath: 1768.

Jones, Mary. *Miscellanies in Prose and Verse.* Oxford: 1750.

Jonson, Ben. *Discoveries 1641, Conversations with William Drummond of Hawthornden 1619.* Edinburgh: Edinburgh University Press, 1966.

Jordan, Thomas. *Piety and Poesy, Contracted.* 1643.

Jordanova, Ludmilla. *Defining Features: Scientific and Medical Portraits 1660–2000.* Reaktion, 2000.

Jurin, James. *A Letter to the Learned Caleb Cotesworth, M.D. ... Containing, a comparison between the mortality of the natural small pox, and that given by inoculation.* 1723.

Kleinman, Arthur. *The Illness Narratives: Suffering, Healing and the Human Condition.* New York: Basic Books, 1988.

Knowles, James Sheridan. *A Collection of Poems on Various Subjects.* Waterford: 1810.

Kristeva, Julia. *Powers of Horror: An Essay on Abjection.* New York: Columbia University Press, 1982.

Lamport, John. *Direct Method of Ordering and Curing People of that loathsome Disease the Small Pox.* 1685.

Latham, Robert and William Matthews, eds. *The Diary of Samuel Pepys.* 11 vols. London: G. Bell [later Bell & Hyman], 1970–1983.

Lavater, Johann Casper. *Essays on Physiognomy: designed to promote the Knowledge and Love of Mankind,* 5 vols. 1789.

Lawson, Jonathan. *Robert Bloomfield.* Boston: Twayne Publishers, 1980.

Lefebure, Molly. *Bondage of Love; a Life of Mrs Samuel Taylor Coleridge.* Victor Gollancz, 1986.

Lettsom, John Coakley. *Observations on the Cow-Pock.* 1801.

Lewis, Esther. *Poems Moral and Entertaining, written long since by Miss Lewis, then of Holt, Now, and for almost Thirty years past, the Wife of Mr. Robert Clark, of Tetbury with a few others addressed to her.* Bath: 1799.

Lipscomb, William. *The Beneficial Effects of Inoculation.* 1772.

Lleulyn, Martin. *An Elegie On the Death of the Most Illustrious Prince, Henry Duke of Gloucester.* Oxford, 1660.

Lobo, Francis M. 'John Haygarth, smallpox and religious dissent in eighteenth-century England'. *The Medical Enlightenment of the Eighteenth Century,* eds. Andrew Cunningham and Roger French. Cambridge: Cambridge University Press, 1990, 217–53.

Luyendijk-Elshout, Antoine. 'Of masks and mills: the enlightenment doctor and his frightened patient'. *The Languages of Psyche: Mind and Body in Enlightenment Thought,* ed. G. S. Rousseau. Berkeley and Oxford: University of California Press, 1990.

Lynn, Walter. *An Essay Towards a More Easie and Safe Method of Cure in the Small Pox.* 1714.

Mackenzie, Henry. *An Account of the Life and Writings of John Home Esq.* Edinburgh and London: 1822.

Manley, Delarivier. *The Adventures of Rivella,* ed. Katherine Zelinsky. Ontario: Broadview, 1999.

Marley, Thomas. *A Short View of the Lives of the Illustrious Princes, Henry Duke of Gloucester, and Mary Princess Deceased, late brother and sister of His Majesty, the King.* 1661.

Massey, Edmund. *Sermon Against the Dangerous and Sinful Practice of Inoculation.* 1722.

McWilliams, John. 'A storm of lamentations writ: lachrymae musarum and royalist culture after the civil war'. *Yearbook of English Studies Modern Language research Association* 33, 2003, 273–89.

Miller, Genevieve. *Adoption of Inoculation for Smallpox in England and France.* Philadelphia: University of Pennsylvania Press, 1957.

Miller, Genevieve. 'Putting Lady Mary in her place: a discussion of historical causation'. *Bulletin of the History of Medicine* 55, 1981, 2–16.

Mitchell, David T. and Sharon L. Snyder. *Narrative Prosthesis: Disability and the Dependencies of Discourse.* Ann Arbor: University of Michigan Press, 2000.

Montagu, Lady Mary Wortley. *Essays and Poems and Simplicity, a Comedy,* eds. Robert Halsband and Isobel Grundy. Oxford: Clarendon Press, 1977.

Moore, James. *The History of the Smallpox.* 1815.

Moseley, Benjamin. *Medical Tracts.* 1800.

Treatise on Sugar, with Miscellaneous Medical Observations. 1799.

Mossner, Ernest. *The Forgotten Hume; le Bon David.* New York: Columbia University Press, 1953.

Murdoch, Brian. *Adam's Grace: Fall and Redemption in Medieval Literature* (London: D. S. Brewer, 2000).

Nussbaum, Felicity A. *'The Brink of all we Hate': English Satires on Women, 1660–1750.* Lexington: Kentucky University Press, 1984.

The Limits of the Human; Fictions of Anomaly, Race and Gender in the Long Eighteenth Century. Cambridge: Cambridge University Press, 2003.

Nutton, Vivian. 'The seeds of disease; an explanation of contagion and infection from the Greeks to the Renaissance'. *Medical History* vol. 27, 1983, 1–34.

'Did the Greeks have a word for it'. *Contagion: Perspectives from Pre-Modern Societies,* eds. Lawrence Conrad and Dominik Wujastyk. Aldershot: Ashgate, 2000, 137–62.

Paré, Ambroise. *On Monsters and Marvels,* trans. Janis Pallister. Chicago: University of Chicago Press, 1982.

Pattison, William. *The Poetical Works of Mr. William Pattison,* 2 vols. 1728.

Paulin, Tom. *The Day-Star of Liberty; William Hazlitt's Radical Style.* Faber and Faber, 1998.

Percival, Melissa. 'Johann Casper Lavater: physiognomy and connoisseurship'. *British Journal of Eighteenth-Century Studies,* 26(1), 2003, 77–90.

Petit, Alexander, ed. *Miscellanies in Prose and Verse by Pope, Swift and Gay,* 4 vols. Pickering and Chatto, 2002.

Philipot, Thomas. *Æsop's Fables with his Life: In English, French and Latin. Newly translated.* 1687.

Philips, Ambrose. *The Poems of Ambrose Philips,* ed. M. G. Segar. Oxford: Basil Blackwell, 1937.

Philips, Katherine. *Poems by the most deserved Admired Mrs. Katherine Philips, the Matchless Orinda.* 1667.

[Philosophical Transactions of the Royal Society]. *The Philosophical Transactions and Collections, to the end of the year MDCC, abridged [etc].* 46, 1749, 233–4.

Pix, Mary. *The Different Widows or Intrigue All-a-Mode; a Comedy.* 1703.

Pointon, Marcia. *Hanging the Head: Portraiture and Social Formation.* New Haven and London: Yale University Press, 1988.

Pope, Alexander. *The Rape of the Lock and other Poems,* ed. Geoffrey Tillotson. Methuen, 1940.

Porter, Roy and G. S. Rousseau. *Gout, The Patrician Malady.* New Haven and London: Yale University Press, 1998.

Porter, Roy. 'The eighteenth century' in Lawrence I. Conrad, Michael Neve, Vivian Nutton, Roy Porter and Andrew Wear, *Western Medical Tradition 800BC to AD 1800.* Cambridge: Cambridge University Press, 1995.

  Bodies Politic; Disease, Death and Doctors in Britain, 1650–1900 Reaktion, 2001.

  Flesh in the Age of Reason. Allen Lane, 2003.

Prescott, Sarah and David E. Shuttleton, eds. *Women and Poetry 1660–1750.* Basingstoke: Palgrave Macmillan, 2003.

Prescott, Sarah. *Women, Authorship and Literary Culture, 1690–1740.* Basingstoke: Palgrave Macmillan, 2003.

Quillet, Claude. *Callipædia: A Poem in Four Books . . . Written in Latin by Claudius Quillet, made English by N. Rowe, Esq.* 1712.

Rattansi, P. M. 'Paracelsus and the Puritan Revolution' in *Ambix: The Journal of the Society for the Study of Alchemy,* vol. II, issue 1, February 1963, 24–32.

  'The Helmontian-Galenist controversy in Restoration England' in *Ambix: The Journal of the Society for the Study of Alchemy,* vol. XII, issue 1, February 1964, 1–23.

Reilly, Robin. *Josiah Wedgwood 1730–1795.* Macmillan, 1992.

Roberts, Marie Mulvey and Roy Porter, eds. *Literature and Medicine During the Eighteenth Century.* Routledge, 1993.

Rosenberg, Charles E. and Janet Golden, eds. *Framing Disease: Studies in Cultural History.* New Brunswick: Rutgers University Press, 1992.

Rosenberg, Charles E. *Explaining Epidemics and other Studies in the History of Medicine.* Cambridge: Cambridge University Press, 1992.

Rousseau, G. S. 'Pineapples, pregnancy, pica, and peregrine pickle'. *Tobias Smollett: Bicentennial Essays Presented to Lewis M. Knapp,* eds. G. S. Rousseau and P.-G. Boucé. Oxford: Oxford University Press, 1971, 79–109.

Rousseau, G. S., Miranda Gill, David Haycock and Malte Herwig, eds. *Framing and Imagining Disease in Cultural History.* Basingstoke: Palgrave Macmillan, 2003.

Rowe, Elizabeth Singer. *The Miscellaneous Works In Prose and Verse of Mrs. Elizabeth Row. To Which are Added, Poems on Several Occasions . . . In Two Volumes.* 1739.

Rowley, William. *Cow-Pox Inoculation no Security Against Small-Pox Infection, to which is added the Modes of Treating the Beastly New Diseases Produced from Cow-Pox.* 1805.

Sánchez, Alfonso E. Pérez and Nicola Spinosa. *Jusepe de Ribera, 1591–1652*. New York: H. Abrams for the Metropolitan Museum of Art, 1992.

Santesso, Aaron. 'Lachrymae musarum and the metaphysical Dryden'. *The Review of English Studies*. New Series vol. 54, no. 217 (November 2003), 615–38.

Savage, Richard. *The Poetical Works of Richard Savage*, ed. Clarence Tracy. Cambridge: Cambridge University Press, 1962.

Scarry, Elaine. *The Body In Prose and Verse by Pain: the Making and Unmaking of the World*. New York and Oxford: Oxford University Press, 1985.

Seward, Anna. *The Poetical Works of Anna Seward; With Extracts from her Literary Correspondence*, ed. Walter Scott, 3 vols. Edinburgh and London: 1810.

Shipman, Thomas. *Carolina: or, Loyal Poems*. 1683.

Shoemaker, Robert B. *Gender in English Society 1650–1850: The Emergence of Separate Spheres*. London and New York: Longman, 1998.

Shuttleton, David E. 'A culture of disfigurement: imagining smallpox in the long eighteenth century'. *Imagining and Framing Disease in Cultural History*, eds. G. S. Rousseau *et al*. Basingstoke: Palgrave Macmillan, 2003, 68–91.
   'Contagion by conceit: menstruosity and the rhetoric of smallpox into the age of inoculation'. *Imagining Contagion in Early Modern Europe*, ed. Claire L. Carlin. Basingstoke: Palgrave Macmillan, 2005, 228–42.

Skinner, John. *Songs and poems, by the Rev. John Skinner. With a sketch of his life*, by H. G. Reid. Peterhead and Edinburgh: 1859.

Smedley, Jonathan. *Poems on Several Occasions*. 1730.

Smith, Eric. *By Mourning Tongues: Studies in English Elegy*. Ipswich: Boydell with Rowan and Littlefield, 1977.

Smith, J. R. *The Speckled Monster: Smallpox in England, 1670–1970, with particular reference to Essex*. Chelmsford: Essex Record Office, 1987.

Sontag, Susan. *Illness as Metaphor / AIDS and its Metaphors*. Harmondsworth: Penguin, 1983.

Southey, Robert. *A Tale of Paraguay*. 1825.

Spence, Joseph. *An Account of the Life, Character, and Poems of Mr Blacklock*. 1754. *Observations, Anecdotes, and Characters of Books and Men, collected from conversation*, ed. James M. Osborn. Oxford: Clarendon Press, 1966.

St Maur, H. *Annals of the Seymours*. Kegan Paul, 1902.

Stevenson, Matthew. *Poems: or, A Miscellany of Sonnets, Satyrs, Drollery, Panegyricks, Elegies, &c.* 1673.

Strode, William. *The Poetical Works of William Strode*. ed. Bertram Dobell. Dobell, 1907.

Swedenberg Jr., H. T. 'More tears for Lord Hastings'. *Huntingdon Library Quarterly*, November 1952, XVI, 43–51.

Thelwall, John. *Poems Chiefly Written in Retirement [1801]*. Oxford: Woodstock Books, 1989.

Thomas, Patrick. *The Collected Works of Katherine Philips*, 2 vols. Stump Cross: Stump Cross Press, 1990.

Thompson, William. *Sickness; a Poem in Three Books*. 1745.

Poems on Several Occasion to which is added Gondibert and Birtha, a Tragedy. Oxford: 1757.

Tissol, Garth, ed. *Metamorphoses.* Ware: Wordsworth Editions, 1998.

Todd, Dennis. *Imagining Monsters: Miscreations of the Self in Eighteenth-Century England.* Chicago and London: University of Chicago Press, 1995.

Toombs, S. Kay. *The Meaning of Illness: a Phenomenological Account of the Different Perspectives of Physician and Patient.* Boston: Kluwer, 1992.

Tucker, Jonathan B. *Scourge: The Once and Future Threat of Smallpox.* New York: Atlantic Monthly Press, 2001.

Tutchin, John. *Poems on Several Occasions with a Pastoral; to which is added A Discourse of Life.* 1685.

[Wagstaffe, William]. *The Small-Pox, a Poem by Andrew Tripe, M. D.* 1748.

Wallerstein, Ruth. *Studies in Seventeenth-Century Poetic.* Wisconsin: University of Wisconsin Press, 1950.

Watts, Isaac. *Reliquiæ Juveniles, Miscellaneous Thoughts in prose and verse, on Natural, Moral and Divine Subjects, written chiefly in Younger Years.* London: 1734.

    The Works of the Reverend and Learned Isaac Watts, Containing, besides his Sermons, and Essays on Miscellaneous subjects, several additional pieces, Selected from his Manuscripts by the Rev. Dr. Jennings, and the Rev. Dr. Doddridge, in 1753, 6 vols. 1810.

    Horæ Lyricæ: Poems Sacred to Devotion and Piety [1706; 1711] . . . with a Memoir of the Author by Robert Southey. 1837.

Watts, Sheldon. *Epidemics and History: Disease, Power and Imperialism.* New Haven and London: Yale University Press, 1997.

Wesley, Samuel. *Elegies on the Queen and Archbishop.* 1695.

Wesley, Samuel. *Poems on Several Occasions, by Samuel Wesley. The Second Edition, with Additions,* 6 vols. Cambridge: 1743.

[Wesley]. *The Poetical Works of John and Charles Wesley,* 7 vols. The Wesleyan-Methodist Conference Office, 1868.

Wesley, Samuel [the younger]. 'Memoir of Mrs Charles Wesley' in *Wesleyan Methodist Magazine* 45, 1822.

Whitaker, Tobias. *An Elenchus of Opinions Concerning the Cure of the Small Pox Together with Problematicall Questions Concerning the Cure of the French Pest.* 1661.

Williams, Caroline. *Pope, Homer and Manliness; Some Aspects of Eighteenth-Century Learning.* London and New York: Routledge, 1993.

Williams, Raymond. *Marxism and Literature.* Oxford: Oxford University Press, 1977.

Woodhouse, James. *The Life and Poetical Works of James Woodhouse 1735–1820: Edited by the Rev. R. I. Woodhouse,* 2 vols. London and New York: The Leadenhall Press, 1896.

Woodward, John. *The State of Physick and of Diseases; with an inquiry into the causes of the late increase of them, but more particularly of the small-pox.* 1718.

Woolf, Virginia. 'On being ill' in *The Essays of Virginia Woolf,* ed. Andrew McNellie, 4 vols. Hogarth, 1994.

Index

Printed in the United States
By Bookmasters